An Introduction to Infectious Disease Modelling

Emilia Vynnycky and Richard G. White

with an introduction by
Professor Paul E.M. Fine

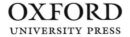

OXFORD
UNIVERSITY PRESS

OXFORD

UNIVERSITY PRESS

Great Clarendon Street, Oxford ox2 6dp

Oxford University Press is a department of the University of Oxford.
It furthers the University's objective of excellence in research, scholarship,
and education by publishing worldwide in

Oxford New York

Auckland Cape Town Dar es Salaam Hong Kong Karachi
Kuala Lumpur Madrid Melbourne Mexico City Nairobi
New Delhi Shanghai Taipei Toronto

With offices in

Argentina Austria Brazil Chile Czech Republic France Greece
Guatemala Hungary Italy Japan Poland Portugal Singapore
South Korea Switzerland Thailand Turkey Ukraine Vietnam

Oxford is a registered trade mark of Oxford University Press
in the UK and in certain other countries

Published in the United States
by Oxford University Press Inc., New York
© Oxford University Press, 2010

British Library Cataloguing in Publication Data

Data available

Library of Congress Cataloging in Publication Data

Data available

Typeset in Minion by Cepha Imaging Private Ltd., Bangalore, India
Printed in Great Britain
on acid-free paper by
CPI Anthony Rowe, Chippenham, Wiltshire

ISBN 978–0–19–856–576–5

10 9 8 7 6 5 4 3 2

Oxford University Press makes no representation, express or implied, that the drug dosages in this book
are correct. Readers must therefore always check the product information and clinical procedures with
the most up-to-date published product information and data sheets provided by the manufacturers and
the most recent codes of conduct and safety regulations. The authors and the publishers do not accept
responsibility or legal liability for any errors in the text or for the misuse or misapplication of material in
this work. Except where otherwise stated, drug dosages and recommendations are for the non-pregnant
adult who is not breastfeeding.

From Emilia
For my mother, brother, and in memory of my father
Дякую за все!!!

From Richard
This book is dedicated, with love, to four very special people.
Janifer, who gave me the best upbringing a child could ever want.
Catherine, who showed me such strength of character over
the years, beyond anything I could ever muster myself. Martin, who
showed me, first to find something I love to do, and then to find
someone to pay me to do it. And finally Sally, who showed me
that there is so much more to life than work, much to this
book's benefit! I could not have done it without you all.

Contents

Preface *xv*

Acknowledgements *xix*

Abbreviations and glossary *xxi*

Symbols and notation *xxvii*

1 Introduction. The basics: infections, transmission
and models *1*

   1.1 Overview and objectives *1*

   1.2 Infections *1*

   1.3 Transmission *5*

   1.4 Models *8*

   1.5 Summary *10*

2 How are models set up? I. An introduction to
difference equations *13*

   2.1 Overview and objectives *13*

   2.2 How are models set up? *13*

   2.3 Identify relevant facts about the infection in question *14*

   2.4 Choose the model structure *15*

       2.4.1 Consideration 1: the natural history of
the infection *15*

       2.4.2 Consideration 2: the accuracy and the time period
covered by model predictions *16*

       2.4.3 Consideration 3: the research question *17*

   2.5 Choose the type of modelling method *18*

   2.6 Setting up deterministic models *19*

       2.6.1 Equation for the number of susceptible
individuals at time $t+1$: *21*

       2.6.2 Equation for the number of pre-infectious
individuals at time $t+1$ *21*

       2.6.3 Equations for the number of infectious individuals
at time $t+1$ *22*

       2.6.4 Equations for the number of immune
('recovered') individuals at time $t+1$ *23*

2.7 Specify the model's input parameters *23*

    2.7.1 Calculating the risk (or force) of infection, λ_t *26*

    2.7.2 Estimating the rate of onset of infectiousness, the recovery rate etc *33*

    2.7.3 Time step size *34*

2.8 Setting up the model *35*

2.9 Final stages in model development: model validation, optimization and prediction *35*

2.10 Summary *37*

2.11 Exercises *37*

3 How are models set up? II. An introduction to differential equations *41*

3.1 Overview and objectives *41*

3.2 How reliable are difference equations? *41*

    3.2.1 The effect of the size of the time step on model predictions *43*

3.3 What are differential equations and how are they written? *44*

3.4 How do we write down differential equations? *49*

    3.4.1 Differential equations for the rate of change in the number of susceptible individuals *50*

    3.4.2 Differential equations for the rate of change in the number of pre-infectious individuals *50*

    3.4.3 Differential equations for the rate of change in the number of infectious and immune individuals *51*

    3.4.4 Methods for checking differential equations *51*

3.5 How do we use differential equations to make predictions? *54*

    3.5.1 A simple differential equation model: exponential decline or growth *55*

3.6 Final word *58*

3.7 Summary *59*

3.8 Exercises *59*

4 What do models tell us about the dynamics of infections? *63*

4.1 Overview and objectives *63*

4.2 The short-term dynamics of infections *63*

    4.2.1 The theory of epidemics *63*

    4.2.2 Factors influencing trends in incidence *65*

    4.2.3 What can we learn from the early stages of an epidemic? *69*

    4.2.4 What is likely to be the size of an epidemic? *77*

    4.2.5 Estimating R_0 or other unknown parameters by fitting models to data *79*

4.3 The long-term dynamics of acute infections *82*

   4.3.1 Why does the incidence of immunizing infections cycle over time? *82*

   4.3.2 Factors influencing the cycles in incidence of immunizing infections *89*

4.4 The dynamics of acute non-immunizing infections *97*

4.5 Summary *99*

4.6 Exercises *100*

5 Age patterns *105*

   5.1 Overview and objectives *105*

   5.2 Age patterns—analysing cross-sectional data *105*

      5.2.1 The acute immunizing infections *105*

      5.2.2 Estimating the average force of infection *106*

      5.2.3 Applying estimates of the average force of infection *111*

      5.2.4 Age patterns for non-immunizing infections *125*

      5.2.5 Practical considerations when analysing data *125*

   5.3 The effect of vaccination on the dynamics of infections *126*

      5.3.1 The indirect effects of vaccination *126*

      5.3.2 The effect of vaccination on the age-specific proportion of individuals that are susceptible *128*

      5.3.3 The effect of vaccination on the age-specific numbers of new infections per unit time *137*

      5.3.4 The importance of including the effects of herd immunity in models *141*

      5.3.5 Extending the logic to other pathogens *143*

   5.4 Summary *143*

   5.5 Exercises *143*

6 An introduction to stochastic modelling *149*

   6.1 Overview and objectives *149*

   6.2 A simple problem *149*

   6.3 Individual-based models (method 1) *150*

      6.3.1 The principles of method 1 *150*

      6.3.2 Calculating the risk of infection in each time step—the Reed–Frost equation *151*

      6.3.3 Example: an illustration of the individual-based approach—method 1 *154*

      6.3.4 Interpreting findings from stochastic models *157*

6.4 Discrete-time stochastic compartmental models (method 2)—
allow chance to determine the number of secondary cases
resulting from each generation of cases *160*

  6.4.1 Overview of method 2 *160*

  6.4.2 Calculating the distribution of the number of susceptible
individuals infected during a given time step *161*

  6.4.3 An illustration of method 2 *163*

6.5 Extensions to methods 1 and 2 *166*

6.6 Continuous time ('time to next event') compartmental
models (method 3) *167*

6.7 Which approach is best? *169*

6.8 Insights and applications of stochastic models *169*

  6.8.1 Inferring reproduction numbers from distributions
of outbreak sizes *169*

  6.8.2 Modelling transmission in small populations and the
persistence of infection *172*

  6.8.3 Individual-based microsimulation models *173*

6.9 Summary *174*

7 How do models deal with contact patterns? *177*

7.1 Overview and objectives *177*

7.2 Why might mixing patterns be important? *177*

7.3 What is the evidence for age-dependent contact for infections
transmitted via the respiratory route? *178*

  7.3.1 Age dependencies in presumed
transmission-linked cases *178*

  7.3.2 Time trends in morbidity following the
(re)introduction of a pathogen *179*

  7.3.3 Age-dependencies in the force of infection *180*

  7.3.4 Social contact surveys *180*

7.4 How do we incorporate age-dependent mixing into models? *181*

  7.4.1 Expressions for the force of infection *181*

  7.4.2 How do we calculate the β parameters? *184*

  7.4.3 Which WAIFW matrix structure(s) should we use? *198*

7.5 How do we calculate R_0 if mixing is assumed to
be non-random? *203*

  7.5.1 Writing down the Next Generation Matrix *203*

  7.5.2 Calculating R_0 *206*

  7.5.3 The mechanics of calculating R_0 when we assume that
individuals do not mix randomly *211*

  7.5.4 Methods for calculating the net reproduction number *215*

7.6   Summary *218*

7.7   Exercises *219*

8 Sexually transmitted infections *223*

8.1   Overview and objectives *223*

8.2   Characteristics of sexually transmitted infections *223*

8.3   What prevalence of gonorrhoea infection might we expect?
       Insights from the Hethcote–Yorke model *226*

8.4   The importance of heterogeneity in sexual activity for STI
       transmission dynamics *231*

    8.4.1   Incorporating risk heterogeneity in the Hethcote
             and Yorke model—key assumptions *232*

    8.4.2   Calculating R_0 in a population with heterogeneity
             in sexual activity *234*

    8.4.3   Proportion of infections due to the
             high-activity group *239*

8.5   Mixing by sexual activity *241*

    8.5.1   Mixing patterns and mixing matrices *242*

    8.5.2   A summary measure of mixing—Q *243*

    8.5.3   Data on mixing by sexual activity *244*

    8.5.4   Modelling mixing by sexual activity *244*

    8.5.5   Effects of mixing on R_0, rate of STI spread and
             equilibrium STI prevalence *247*

    8.5.6   Effects of mixing on rate of STI spread
             and equilibrium STI prevalence
             (for a given R_0 value) *249*

    8.5.7   Effects of mixing on equilibrium STI prevalence
             (for a given STI natural history and partner
             change rates) *252*

    8.5.8   Implications of heterogeneity in sexual
             activity on STI control *254*

8.6   Mixing on gender (heterosexual mixing model) *255*

    8.6.1   Calculating R_0 for a heterosexually mixing
             population (host-vector) *256*

8.7   Summary of predictions using simple curable STI models *259*

8.8   Simple transmission models of human
       immunodeficiency virus/AIDS *259*

    8.8.1   Simple transmission model of HIV/AIDS *260*

8.9   Concurrency *265*

8.10   Network modelling *268*

8.11   Summary *275*

9 Special topics in infectious disease modelling *283*

9.1 Overview and objectives *283*

9.2 The effect of vaccination on the dynamics of infections *283*

  9.2.1 Varicella vaccination and boosting *283*

  9.2.2 Serotype replacement *285*

9.3 Diseases with long incubation periods: tuberculosis *285*

  9.3.1 The long-term dynamics *285*

  9.3.2 Predicting the impact of control for tuberculosis *293*

9.4 Models of HIV/STI coinfection *296*

  9.4.1 Predictions for the impact of cofactor STIs on the HIV epidemic *297*

  9.4.2 The changing role of curable STI treatment for HIV prevention *303*

9.5 Case study: how models of the control of sexually transmitted HIV in sub-Saharan Africa have evolved with the epidemic *306*

9.6 Summary *308*

Further reading *317*

Appendix

A.1 Differential equations *319*

A.2 The dynamics of infections *321*

A.3 Age patterns *328*

A.4 Stochastic modelling *334*

A.5 Age-dependent contact patterns *335*

A.6 Sexually transmitted infections *337*

Basic maths *339*

B.1 Overview *339*

B.2 The equation of a straight line *339*

B.3 The constant '*e*' *340*

B.4 Logarithms *341*

B.5 Differentiation *342*

B.6 Integration *345*

B.7 Matrices *348*

Summary of the key equations used in the text *357*

Index *365*

List of panels

Panel 2.1 The classification of models   20
Panel 2.2 Technical issues relating to models   24
Panel 2.3 Notation—Greek or the Latin alphabet, lower case
          versus upper case?   25
Panel 2.4 The definition of an effective contact and factors affecting β 27
Panel 2.5 Expressions for the risk of infection: scaling parameters,
          density and frequency dependence   30
Panel 2.6 Other notation for difference equations   35
Panel 3.1 Avoiding problems with the size of the time step for a model
          set up using difference equations 45
Panel 3.2 A comparison between difference and differential equations   48
Panel 3.3 Derivation of the discrete-time equivalent of $N(t) = N(0)e^{-mt}$ 56
Panel 3.4 The relationship between risks and rates   57
Panel 3.5 Age-structured models and partial differential equations   58
Panel 4.1 The relationship between the growth rate and the doubling time   74
Panel 4.2 Fitting models and sensitivity analyses   81
Panel 4.3 Incorporating births and deaths into a model describing
          the transmission dynamics of an immunizing infection   84
Panel 4.4 The Hamer model—the model whose predictions never
          damp out   90
Panel 4.5 Evidence for seasonal transmission of infections   91
Panel 5.1 What is a catalytic model?   109
Panel 5.2 Determining whether the force of infection is age-dependent   121
Panel 5.3 Why might the force of infection differ between children and
          adults and between settings?   123
Panel 5.4 Methods for incorporating age-structure into models   131
Panel 5.5 Modelling the impact of meningococcal vaccination in the UK   135
Panel 5.6 The impact of vaccinating individuals at different ages   140
Panel 6.1 Extensions to the Reed–Frost equation   153
Panel 6.2 Interpreting findings from stochastic models   158
Panel 6.3 How many runs from a stochastic model do we need?   160
Panel 6.4 Sampling random numbers from a distribution   162
Panel 6.5 Derivation of the general equation for the probability that
          exactly k_i out of S_t individuals will be infected in the next
          time step   164
Panel 7.1 Derivation of the equations $\lambda_{yy}(t) = \beta_{yy} I_y(t)$ and $\lambda_{yo}(t) = \beta_{yo} I_o(t)$ 184
Panel 7.2 Notation for $\beta_{yy}, \beta_{yo}, \beta_{oy}, \beta_{oo}$ 185
Panel 7.3 Expressions for the force of infection when contact is assumed
          to differ between more than two subgroups in the population   186

Panel 7.4   Methods for calculating the numbers of susceptible and
            infectious individuals in specific age groups   188
Panel 7.5   Extending the logic to deal with different kinds of
            non-random mixing   193
Panel 7.6   Estimating β parameters using contact and
            serological data   194
Panel 7.7   Analyses of the impact of varicella vaccination in
            Canada—an example of the sensitivity of model
            predictions to the assumed mixing patterns   200
Panel 7.8   Worked calculation of the number of infectious individuals
            predicted in each generation following the introduction
            of infectious persons into a totally susceptible population
            using a given Next Generation Matrix   207
Panel 7.9   What is a typical infectious person in the definition of R_0?   212
Panel 7.10 Extending the methods for calculating R_0 to populations
            stratified into more than two subgroups   214
Panel 8.1   Per-act and per-partnership transmission probabilities   228
Panel 8.2   Derivation of R_0 for simple gonorrhoea model   230
Panel 8.3   Maintaining overall partner change rate   233
Panel 8.4   The probability that a partner will be a member of the high
            or low-activity group assuming proportionate mixing   234
Panel 8.5   Calculating R_0 in a population with heterogeneity in sexual
            activity and proportionate mixing   236
Panel 8.6   Immunity and 'pre-emptive saturation'   240
Panel 8.7   Modelling purely with-unlike mixing by both activity groups   248
Panel 8.8   Calculating R_0 in a population with heterogeneity in sexual
            activity and any mixing pattern   250
Panel 8.9   Model equations for simple HIV/AIDS model   261
Panel 8.10 Derivation of HIV epidemic doubling time   266
Panel 8.11 Pair-wise approximation models   271
Panel 8.12 Network modelling terminology   274
Panel 9.1   Estimates of the risk of developing tuberculosis disease soon
            after recent initial infection, reinfection and through reactivation 289
Panel 9.2   Predicting the effect of antiretrovirals for HIV on the incidence
            of tuberculosis   295
Panel 9.3   Calculation of the per-partnership STI cofactor effects on HIV
            transmission   297
Panel 9.4   Equations for model of HIV/STI coinfection   300

Preface

Mathematical models are increasingly being used to examine questions in infectious disease control. Applications include predicting the impact of vaccination strategies against common infections and determining optimal control strategies against HIV and pandemic influenza. However, relatively few public health and infectious disease researchers have had any formal training in mathematical modelling.

Several texts on the mathematical modelling of infectious diseases have been published to date, most notably, *Infectious diseases of humans. Dynamics and control* by Anderson and May in 1992, and, recently *Modeling infectious diseases in humans and animals* by M. J. Keeling and P. Rohani. However, to get the most out of these texts, individuals typically need to have had a fairly advanced training in mathematics.

This book is intended to bring the modelling world closer to people working in infectious diseases or public health. By reading this book and completing the accompanying exercises, we hope that readers will understand the basic methods for setting up mathematical models and how and where models can be applied. We hope that they will also gain a better understanding of the factors which influence the patterns and trends in infectious diseases.

The layout of the book

It is impossible to write a book on mathematical modelling without including some mathematical equations and derivations. With our target audience in mind, we have kept the mathematical level of the book as simple as possible, which, we hope, will make it accessible to someone who has not studied mathematics to university level. We have included only the proofs which we have considered important in the main text. Other proofs or derivations which are interesting, but which some readers may want to skip on initial reading of the text, are provided either in panels or in the Appendices. We have provided references to proofs which have been too detailed to reproduce in the text. We have also included a brief chapter entitled "Basic maths" at the end of the book, which is intended to refresh reader's memories of concepts that they may have covered in previous studies, and which are relevant for the text. A glossary, a table summarizing the notation and the key equations are also provided.

Each chapter includes panels of text, which are intended to discuss some aspect of the infectious disease area or a given method in more depth. Exercises, which can be answered using pen and paper are included in the text; the solutions to the exercises, model files which require Excel or the computer package Berkeley Madonna, and a link to Berkeley Madonna are provided online at : www. anintroductiontoinfectiousdiseasemodelling.com. The exercises are designed to improve understanding. However, whilst we encourage readers to attempt them, it is not essential to work through all of them.

This book consists of nine chapters which are intended to follow a logical sequence.

It begins with an introduction to the epidemiology of infections and models, which is written by Paul E. M. Fine, Professor of Infectious Disease Epidemiology at the London School of Hygiene and Tropical Medicine. In this chapter, readers are introduced to the key features of infections and the occurrence of epidemics. In addition, it discusses the key concepts in infectious disease epidemiology and factors influencing control, namely the basic and net reproduction numbers and the herd immunity threshold. This is followed by a discussion of what we mean by a mathematical model.

The next two chapters focus on how models can be set up and the data that they may require. Readers are led through the key stages of model development from identifying the question to data collection, developing the model structure and equations, key assumptions, prediction, and validation. The key types of models are discussed and the chapters introduce readers to the two specific types of equations which are used to build the majority of (deterministic) models, namely difference and differential equations, with a discussion of the relative merits of the two approaches. Any readers who are already familiar with these methods may wish to skim through these early chapters.

The fourth chapter discusses the insights that models provide into the dynamics of acute infections and the impact of control. It begins by considering the short-term dynamics, discussing why epidemics occur, how data from the early stages of an epidemic can be analysed to infer the basic reproduction number and the future number of cases, and the level of control required to control an infection. It then focuses on the long-term dynamics of infections in the absence of control, discussing why cycles in immunizing infections occur, and contrasts these against the patterns seen for non-immunizing infections. Examples of diseases that are discussed in this chapter include influenza, measles, rubella, syphilis, and pertussis.

Chapter five discusses the age patterns of infections in humans. It begins by illustrating how age-stratified data on the proportion of individuals who have been infected and other data can be analysed to obtain estimates of the rate at which individuals are infected. It then illustrates how these estimates are used to obtain key model input parameters and other insights into the epidemiology of an infection. In addition, it illustrates how the basic reproduction number determines the age patterns in the proportion of individuals that are susceptible and the infection incidence. The chapter then goes on to describe how control may influence the dynamics of infections and the age distribution of individuals who are susceptible to infection, which, can have both beneficial and unexpected outcomes.

The sixth chapter discusses how chance influences the dynamics of infections and the methods for developing stochastic models, which incorporate the effects of chance. The interpretation of output from such models is discussed, together with the insights that these models provide into how outbreak data can be interpreted and analysed. In addition, we discuss the use of microsimulation models, such as those which have been developed during the early 2000s to explore the impact of control against pandemic influenza.

Contact patterns in the population greatly influence the transmission of infections, and many interventions, such as vaccination or school closures during an influenza pandemic, are targeted at children. To make accurate predictions of the impact of such interventions, models need to make accurate assumptions about age-dependent contact patterns. Chapter 7 begins with a review of the evidence for age-dependent mixing, illustrating how contact patterns influence the impact of control and how the impact can be predicted using simple reproduction number measures.

Chapter 8 continues with the theme of contact patterns, this time with how they influence the transmission and control of sexually transmitted infections (STIs). Specifically, it describes how models predict that, without the presence of a risk heterogeneity, short-duration STIs would be unlikely to persist in populations. This has important implications for STI control, suggesting that control can best be achieved by targeting core groups. It goes on to describe simple HIV models and the use of network models in STI epidemiology

The final chapter provides examples of several 'special' topics in infectious disease modelling. Specifically, it discusses varicella and the impact of vaccination on zoster, serotype replacement for pneumoccal disease following vaccination, the dynamics of tuberculosis and the effect of HIV, and the role of coinfections for STIs. The chapter concludes with a discussion of how models have evolved with the HIV epidemic.

What this book does not cover

When we first started writing this book, we aimed to include everything that fascinated us about modelling infectious diseases, and to bring the modelling world closer to those who are interested in modelling but do not have time to become modellers themselves. However, more fascinated us than we had time to include. Specifically, whilst making occasional reference to vector-borne infections and malaria, the key focus is on directly transmitted infections. We have also focused entirely on human infections; readers interested in models of infections in animals may want to read the text by Keeling and Rohani. There have been some exciting recent developments in the field of fitting models to data. To sustain the interest of our target audience, we have simply referred to these developments or provided a brief description intended to provide a conceptual understanding of the principles.

Acknowledgements

The material in this book stems from the lecture notes and computer practicals that we wrote for an MSc module called 'Modelling and the dynamics of infectious diseases', and an intensive summer short course, 'An introduction to infectious disease modelling and its applications', that we set up whilst working at the London School of Hygiene and Tropical Medicine (RW, EV) and at the Health Protection Agency (EV). We therefore wish to thank both our institutions for providing the opportunity to develop these courses.

Over the years, we have been privileged to work with numerous talented colleagues and students who have influenced our ideas and ways of thinking and writing.

We are particularly indebted to Professor Paul Fine who, many years ago, was the PhD supervisor for one of us (EV). In addition to generously giving up time to share some of his immense knowledge about the epidemiology of infectious diseases and modelling, he has taught us how to think critically and how to be sensitive to the needs of a non-mathematical audience. We are also immeasurably grateful to him for writing the first chapter of this book on the basics of infections and models.

Particular thanks are also due to the colleagues who, over the years, have helped to shape our ideas, specifically Paddy Farrington, Nigel Gay, Ben Cooper, Eduardo Massad, Marie-Claude Boily, Richard Hayes and Hans Heesterbeek.

We are also indebted to Professor Laura Rodrigues who provided much-needed encouragement when we first discussed developing a modelling course and writing a book.

Each year that we have taught the courses, we have been fortunate to have had very keen and enthusiastic students, who have never failed to ask interesting and perceptive questions. In the pages that follow, former students will undoubtedly recognize some of the answers to the questions that they asked in class, and some of the answers to the questions that we were unable to answer at the time!

We are extremely grateful to the colleagues or previous students who willingly gave up their time to read drafts or commented on this manuscript, specifically Paul Fine, Ben Cooper, John Edmunds, Paddy Farrington, Punam Mangtani, Charlotte Jackson, Kimberley Nucifura, Sara Thomas, Nigel Gay, Laura Rodrigues, Richard Hayes, Leigh-Anne Shafer, Marie-Claude Boily, Ken Eames, Katie O'Brien, Geoff Garnett, Michael White, Roel Bakker, and Wim Delva. We also wish to thank Hans Heesterbeek and Hiroshi Nishiura for providing historical material relating to R_0 and to Erol Yusuf (Health Protection Agency) for providing access to notification data. We also thank Fiona Marquet for providing administrative assistance and LSHTM for providing financial assistance. We are also grateful to Janifer White and Sally Oldfield for proof-reading.

We also wish to thank Oxford University Press and its editors (Georgia Pinteau, Nic Wilson, Angela Butterworth and Jen Wright) for their patience at each stage in the production of this book.

Finally, ultimate thanks are due to our families and friends for their endless support and patience throughout the years. Special thanks are due to Emilia's brother who willingly read and commented on drafts and provided a summer retreat with his cat for a short period whilst this book was being written, and to Emilia's mother for her amazing tolerance of the entire book-writing process.

Abbreviations and glossary

The following summarizes the definitions of some of the key terms used in the book, compiled from various sources.[1-4]

Assortative (mixing patterns) See **With-like (mixing patterns)**. See Section 7.4.2.1 and 8.5.1.

Asymptomatic (individual) An infected person who does not have any recognized signs of the infection.

Basic reproduction number (R_0) Average number of secondary infectious persons resulting from one infectious person following their introduction into a totally susceptible population. It is sometimes referred to using different names, e.g. the basic reproductive number, the basic reproductive rate, the basic reproduction ratio, etc. It is a number, rather than a rate, since there are no units of time in the definition. See Section 1.3.

Beta (β) The rate at which two specific individuals come into effective contact per unit time. Technically it is the *per capita* rate at which two specific individuals come into effective contact per unit time. It is also sometimes referred to using other names, such as the transmission coefficient, transmission rate, contact parameter, etc. See Section 2.7.1.

Carrier An individual who sheds an infectious agent but does not have any clinical symptoms.

Case An individual who has clinical symptoms of an infection (e.g. cough, fever etc.). Note that not all 'cases' are infectious. See Section 1.2.

Catalytic model A model that is typically used to describe data on the prevalence of previous infection at age a ($z(a)$), where λ is the force of infection. The equation for a simple catalytic model is $z(a) = 1-e^{-\lambda a}$. See Section 5.2.2.

Closed population model A model in which it is assumed that there is no migration into or out of the population, and in which there are no births or deaths.

Compartmental model A model in which individuals in the population are subdivided into broad subgroups (compartments) and the model tracks individuals collectively. See Section 2.6.

Concurrency (of sexual partnerships) Temporal overlap of sexual partnerships or simultaneity of partnerships. See Section 8.9.

Core group Group of individuals with particularly high contact rates.

CRS Congenital Rubella Syndrome.

Damp out Typically refers to the progressive reduction in the size of the peaks in incidence of immunizing infections, usually predicted using deterministic models which do not include seasonal contact patterns. See Section 4.3.1.

Density dependence assumption The assumption that the risk of infection increases as the population size increases. This might occur if the boundary in which the population is confined remains unchanged with increasing population size, and therefore crowding increases. It is sometimes referred to as the 'pseudo mass action' assumption. See Panel 2.5.

Deterministic model A model which describes what happens on average in a population and does not incorporate the effects of chance. See Section 2.6.

Disassortative (mixing patterns) See **With-unlike (mixing patterns)**. See Section 7.4.2.1 and 8.5.1.

Doubling time (of an epidemic) The time taken for the number of infected individuals to double. See Panel 4.1 and Chapter 8.

Dynamic model A model which describes changes in given quantities over time. The term is frequently used to describe models which describe contact between individuals and therefore for which changes in the prevalence of infectious persons are fed back into changes in the force of infection. See Panel 2.1.

Effective contact A contact that is sufficient to lead to transmission if it occurs between an infectious and a susceptible person. See Panel 2.4.

Effective reproduction number See **Net reproduction number**.

Efficacy (vaccine) The direct protection provided by vaccination against infection or other outcome of interest. It excludes any indirect (herd) effect.

Effectiveness (vaccine) The reduction in incidence of the infection (or other outcome) in a population resulting from the combined direct and indirect (herd immunity) effect of vaccination.

Eigenvalue(s) Values which are an intrinsic property of a matrix, so that when a matrix is multiplied by some vector, the result is some factor (the eigenvalue) multiplied by that vector. Eigenvalues are also known as the 'characteristic values'. See Basic maths (section B.7) for a discussion of matrices and vectors.

Elimination Reduction in the incidence of an infection to very low (close to zero) levels. The precise criteria are disease-specific (e.g. the WHO declared the criterion for leprosy to be a prevalence of registered cases below 1 per 10,000).

Endemic infection An infection that is present in a population at a similar level over a prolonged period.

Epidemic The increase and subsequent decrease in incidence following the (re)introduction of an infection in a population. Also refers to the occurrence of cases in a given locality at a frequency which greatly exceeds that expected.

Epidemic threshold Minimum proportion of the population that needs to be susceptible for the infection incidence to increase, calculated as $1/R_0$. See Sections 1.3 and 4.3.1.

Epidemiology This term is used to refer to the study of patterns of diseases (including those which are non-communicable) or infections in a population.

Equilibrium A situation whereby all acting influences are cancelled by others, resulting in a stable, balanced, or unchanging state. For example, the equilibrium prevalence of infection predicted in the long-term by simple SEIR models (see Section 4.3.1) is the result of the balance between the infection, birth, death, and recovery rates.

Eradication Reduction in the incidence of an infection to zero.

Force of infection The rate at which susceptible individuals become infected per unit time. It is also known as the incidence rate or the hazard rate. See Section 2.7.1 and 5.2.2.

Freqency dependence assumption The assumption that the risk of infection remains unchanged as the population size increases. This might occur if the boundary in which the population is confined increases with increasing population size, and therefore crowding remains unchanged, or if the behaviour of individuals does not change as the population size increases. It is sometimes referred to as the 'true mass action' assumption. See Panel 2.5.

Generation time See definition for the serial interval. See Section 1.2.

Growth rate of an epidemic Rate at which the prevalence of infectious persons increases, typically calculated during the early stages of an epidemic. See Section 4.2.3.1.

Herd immunity This is also commonly used to refer to the indirect protection experienced by unvaccinated individuals resulting from the presence of immune individuals in a population. See Section 1.3. In infectious disease epidemiology, it also sometimes refers to the proportion of a population that is immune.

Herd immunity threshold (H) The proportion of the population which needs to be immune in the population for the infection incidence to be stable, calculated as $1-1/R_0$. See Sections 1.3 and 4.2.2.1. Also referred to as the critical immunization threshold. To eradicate an infection, the proportion of the population that is immunized must exceed this threshold value.

Heterogeneous mixing Non-random mixing, whereby the rate at which individuals come into effective contact depends on their age, sex, or some other characteristic. See Section 2.7.1.

HIV Human immunodeficiency virus.

Homogeneous mixing See **Random mixing**. See Section 2.7.1.

HSV-2 Herpes simplex virus Type 2.

Immune (individual) A person who has complete protection to an infection, which results from either vaccination or previous infection. Individuals are said to be 'partially immune' if they are not fully protected. See Section 1.2.

Immunization Successful vaccination, i.e. with the vaccinated person becoming completely immune to the infection.

Immunizing infection An infection which induces near-perfect immunity. Examples of such infections include measles, mumps, rubella (German measles).

Incidence (rate) The number of new events, such as infections or cases in the population at risk (usually susceptibles), per unit person per unit time. Note that the number of new events per person in the general population per unit time is also frequently referred to as the "incidence" in epidemiological and medical literature and surveillance reports. For rare events, this measure is identical to the incidence defined using the strict epidemiological definition. See ref[1] for further details.

Incubation period The time period between infection and onset of clinical symptoms. Note that for many infections, including measles, individuals can be infectious before they show any clinical symptoms. See Section 1.2.

Infectious period The time period during which individuals are infectious. See Section 1.2.

Integer A whole number, i.e. 1, 2, 3, 4 etc.

Latent period See **Pre-infectious period**. See Section 1.2.

Lattice network models Models which are created by placing individuals on a regular grid in space and linking neighbouring individuals. See Panel 8.12.

Microsimulation model A model which tracks every individual in the population separately. See Panel 2.1 and Section 6.2. This is also called an individual or agent-based model.

Mixing matrices See **WAIFW**.

MMR Measles, mumps, rubella.

Network model A model that explicitly tracks the network of contacts between individuals. Infection can only occur between infected individuals and the subset of the total population with which they are in contact. See Section 8.10 for the types of network models.

Net reproduction number (R_n or R) average number of secondary infectious persons resulting from one infectious person in a given population in which some individuals may already be immune because of infection or vaccination. In the modelling literature, this quantity is also often referred to as the 'effective reproduction number'. It is often denoted by the letter R or R_n. See Section 1.3.

Next Generation Matrix Matrix of the number of secondary infectious persons generated by an infectious person in each subgroup in the model. See Section 7.5.1.

Pair-wise approximation models These are created by using the compartmental modelling approach and adding compartments for pairs or triplets of individuals in contact with each other. See Panel 8.11.

Pandemic An epidemic that occurs worldwide.

Pre-infectious period Time period between infection and onset of infectiousness. Sometimes referred to as the 'latent' period. See Section 1.2.

Prevalence The proportion of individuals in a population that have the outcome of interest at a given time. If an infection is endemic, then prevalence ≈ incidence × duration of the condition.

Prophylaxis Medication typically provided to someone either before or after they have been exposed to an infectious person, which is intended to prevent them from developing disease. Prophylaxis is sometimes also referred to as post-exposure or pre-exposure prophylaxis.

Proportionate mixing Contact pattern whereby the rate at which groups of individuals (characterized by age, gender or some other criterion etc.) come into contact with others depends on the proportion of the total contacts generated by each group. See Section 8.5.1.

Q. A summary measure of mixing between individuals. See Section 8.5.2.

Random mixing Contact pattern whereby individuals are equally likely to contact all individuals, irrespective of their age or other characteristic. See Section 2.7.1 and 8.5.1.

Random network models Network models that are created by connecting individuals irrespective of their spatial or social position. See Figure 8.25.

(Pre-emptive) saturation A process which limits the rise in prevalence of STIs, whereby infectious individuals contact individuals who are already infected.

Scale-free networks Networks which can be created by connecting individuals with a probability that is directly proportional to their current number of contacts. See Figure 8.25.

Serial interval Time interval between successive infections in a chain of transmission. Also referred to as the generation time. See Section 1.2.

SEIRS Susceptible–pre-infectious–infectious–recovered–susceptible model structure. See Section 2.4.1.

SI Susceptible–infectious model structure. See Section 2.4.1.

SIR Susceptible–infectious–recovered model structure. See Section 2.4.1.

SIS Susceptible–infectious–susceptible model structure. See Section 2.4.1.

Small world networks Network models that can be created by adding a small number of long-range partnerships to a lattice model. See Panel 8.12.

Solution to an equation The unknown quantities in an equation. For example, the solution to the equation $x^3 - 8 = 0$ is $x = 2$.

Solve an equation To obtain the unknown quantities in the equation. For example, the equation $x^3 - 8 = 0$ can be solved to obtain $x = 2$.

Spatial network model A network model that is created by placing individuals in geographic space and connecting them with a probability that depends on the distance between them. See Panel 8.12.

Stable population model A model in which it is assumed that the population size does not change.

Static model A model which does not describe changes in given quantities in the model over time. The term is also often used to refer to models which do not explicitly describe contact (and therefore transmission) between individuals and so the risk or force of infection takes a fixed value. These models cannot adequately assess the effect of interventions that reduce the prevalence of the infection on the incidence.They are sometimes used for the modelling of non-communicable diseases where there is no feedback from the prevalence of disease to the incidence. See Section 5.3.4.

STI Sexually transmitted infection. See Chapter 8.

Stochastic (model) A model which incorporates the effects of chance, for example, in determining the number of individuals that are infected, become infectious per unit time, recover etc per unit time. See Panel 2.1 and Chapter 6.

Susceptible An individual who has not yet been infected and is at risk of infection.

TB Tuberculosis.

Transmission dynamics Changes in the transmission of an infection over time.

Typical infectious person The theoretical average of all infectious persons in a population, averaging over, for example, infectious individuals in different contact groups. See Panel 7.9.

WAIFW matrix Matrix describing 'Who Acquires Infection from Whom'. See Section 7.4.1.

With-like (mixing patterns) Also referred to as 'assortative' mixing. Refers to contact patterns whereby individuals with a given characteristic are more likely to contact other individuals sharing those characteristics than individuals who do not have those characteristics. e.g. if children are more likely to contact other children than they are to contact adults. See Section 7.4.2.1 and 8.5.1.

With-unlike (mixing patterns) Also referred to as 'disassortative' mixing. Refers to contact patterns whereby individuals with a given characteristic are less likely to contact other individuals sharing those characteristics than individuals who do not have those characteristics, e.g. if children are less likely to contact other children than they are to contact adults. See Section 7.4.2.1 and 8.5.1.

References

1 Hennekens CH, Buring JE. *Epidemiology in medicine.* Boston, MA: and Toronto: Little, Brown and Company; 1987.

2 Heymann DL. *Control of communicable diseases manual,* 18th edn. Washington, DC: American Public Health Association; 2004.

3 Giesecke J. *Modern infectious disease epidemiology,* 2nd edn. London: Arnold; 2002.

4 Halloran ME. Concepts on infectious disease epidemiology. In Rothman KJ, Greeenland S, eds, Philadelphia, PA: Lippincott Williams & Williams; 1998.

Symbols and notation

Table 1 Summary of the commonly used mathematical symbols

Symbol	Definition
$\approx$	Approximately equal to
e	The mathematical constant 2.71828 (see Basic maths section B.3)
$ln(x)$	The natural log of x i.e. $\log_e(x)$ (see Basic maths section B.4)
π	Pi, the mathematical constant 3.14159…
$\geq$	Greater than or equal to
$\leq$	Less than or equal to
!	Factorial. n! equals $n \times (n-1) \times (n-2) \times (n-2) \times \ldots \times 2 \times 1$
$\neq$	Not equal to
Σ	Sum
$\sqrt{}$	Square root
∞	Infinity

Table 2 Summary of the commonly used symbols. The subscript 't' is used when the model is set up using difference equations; the 't' is enclosed in parentheses when the model is set up using differential equations.

Symbol	Definition
A	(a) Average age at infection (all chapters except 8 and 9) (b) Number of individuals with AIDS (Chapter 8)
b	*Per capita* birth rate
β	Rate at which two specific individuals come into effective contact per unit time (equivalent to the *per capita* rate at which two specific individuals come into contact). This notation is used when we assume that individuals mix randomly
β_{yo}	If 'y' and 'o' reflect 'young' and 'old' people respectively, this reflects the rate at which a specific (susceptible) young person comes into effective contact with a specific (infectious) old person. Note that the first part of the subscript reflects the category of the susceptible person (the recipient of the infection) and the second part of the subscript reflects the category of the infectious person. The notation which is used to reflect the rate at which a specific old (susceptible) person and an (infectious) young person come into effective contact is analogous, i.e. β_{oy}

Table 2 Summary of the commonly used symbols. The subscript '*t*' is used when the model is set up using difference equations; the '*t*' is enclosed in parentheses when the model is set up using differential equations. *(continued)*

Symbol	Definition
β_p or β_a	The probability of transmission of a sexually transmitted infection during a sexual partnership (β_p) or sexual act (β_a) between one infectious and one susceptible partner. See Panel 8.1.
β_{WM} or β_{MW}	Per partnership transmission probability from men to women (β_{WM}) or women to men (β_{MW}) (Section 8.6)
B_t, $B(t)$	Number of births at time *t*.
c_e	Number of individuals effectively contacted by each person per unit time; related to β and the population size through the expression $\beta = c_e/N$
c	Average sexual partner change rate (see Section 8.3)
D'	Pre-infectious period, also known as the latent period (defined as the time interval between infection and onset of infectiousness)
D	Duration of infectiousness
E_t, $E(t)$	Number of individuals who are infected but not yet infectious ('pre-infectious') at time *t*.
f	Rate of onset of infectiousness.
g_H, g_L	Probabilities that a sexual partner, selected according to proportionate mixing, will be a member of the high (g_H) or low (g_L) activity group (see Section 8.4.1 and Panel 8.4)
g_{jk}	Probability that someone in the group *k* forms a sexual partnership with someone in group *j* (see section 8.5.1)
I_t, $I(t)$	Number of individuals who are infectious at time *t*.
λ_t or $\lambda(t)$	Force of infection at time *t* (rate at which susceptible individuals are infected per unit time).
$\lambda_{yo}(t)$	Force of infection among young individuals which is attributable to contact with old individuals at time *t*. The notation which is used to reflect the force of infection among old individuals attributable to contact with young individuals is analogous, i.e. $\lambda_{oy}(t)$
$\overline{\lambda_y}(t)$	The overall force of infection among young individuals experienced among individuals at time *t*. In Chapter 7, this is given by the sum of the force of infection among young individuals which is attributable to contact with other children and that attributable to contact with adults, i.e. $\overline{\lambda_y}(t) = \lambda_{yy}(t) + \lambda_{yo}(t)$

The notation which is used to reflect the overall force of infection among old individuals is analogous, i.e. $\overline{\lambda_o}(t) = \lambda_{oy}(t) + \lambda_{yo}(t)$ |
| λ_j^{cSTI-} or λ_j^{cSTI+} | Force of HIV infection on cofactor STI uninfected individuals (λ_j^{cSTI-}) or cofactor STI infected (λ_j^{cSTI+}) in sexual activity group *j* (Panel 9.4) |

Table 2 Summary of the commonly used symbols. The subscript 't' is used when the model is set up using difference equations; the 't' is enclosed in parentheses when the model is set up using differential equations. *(continued)*

Symbol	Definition
Λ	Growth rate in the prevalence of infectious individuals
γ	Progression rate to AIDS per year (e.g. see Section 8.8.1.2 and Panel 8.9 and Panel 9.4)
L	Average life expectancy
m	*Per capita* mortality rate
N_t, $N(t)$	Total population size at time t.
n	Number of sex acts per partnership (see Panel 8.1)
Q	Summary measure of mixing (see Section 8.5.2)
τ	Average partnership duration
r	Rate at which individuals recover from being infectious
R_t, $R(t)$	Number of individuals who are immune ('recovered') at time t
R_0	Basic reproduction number (average number of secondary infectious persons resulting from the introduction of an infectious person into a totally susceptible population)
R_n	Net reproduction number (average number of secondary infectious persons resulting from one infectious person in a given population, i.e. in which some individuals may be immune)
R_{yo}	Number of infectious young persons resulting from each infectious old person in a totally susceptible population. As is the case for β_{yo}, the first part of the subscript reflects the category of the susceptible person (the recipient of the infection) and the second part of the subscript reflects the category of the infectious person
R_H or R_L	Number of secondary infections generated in a totally susceptible population by an infected high (R_H) or low (R_L) activity group member (see Section 8.4.2)
R_{WM}	Number of secondary infections generated in a totally susceptible population in women due to an infected man. Similar definition for R_{MW} (see Section 8.6.1)
R_{LH}	Number of secondary infections in low-activity members generated by an infected high-activity member. Similar definitions for R_{LH}, R_{HH} and R_{LL} (see Panels 8.5 and 8.8)
S_t, $S(t)$	Number of susceptible individuals at time t
S_j^{cSTI-} or S_j^{cSTI+}	Number of individuals HIV-uninfected and cofactor-STI-uninfected (S_j^{cSTI-}) or cofactor-STI-infected (S_j^{cSTI+}) in activity group j (Chapter 9, Panel 9.4)
[SI]	Example of terminology used in pair-wise approximation models. Number of pairs of individuals in a population in which one individual is infected and one individual is susceptible. See Panel 8.12

Table 2 Summary of the commonly used symbols. The subscript 't' is used when the model is set up using difference equations; the 't' is enclosed in parentheses when the model is set up using differential equations. *(continued)*

Symbol	Definition
s, s_0, s_f	Proportion of individuals who are susceptible. The subscript 0 or f is used to denote the proportion who are susceptible at the start or end of a given time period
T_d	Doubling time—typically used as the time required for the number of infectious individuals to double (e.g. see Section 8.8.1.2 and Panel 8.10)
T_s	Serial interval or generation interval (time interval between successive cases in a chain of transmission)
U	The number of sexually active individuals
y_j	Screening rate of group j (see Section 8.5.8)
z	Proportion of individuals who have experienced infection in the past. Infection in the past may or may not reflect immunity
Φ_j	Force of cofactor STI infection on individuals in activity group j. See Panel 9.4
μ	(1) Rate at which newborns lose their maternal immunity (Chapter 5) (2) Death rate due to AIDS (Chapters 8 and 9)

Chapter 1

Introduction

The basics: infections, transmission and models

1.1 Overview and objectives

This chapter provides an introduction to infections and key concepts in infectious disease epidemiology. By the end of this chapter you should:

♦ Be aware of the different kinds of infectious agents;

♦ Be able to define the pre-infectious, infectious and incubation periods and the serial interval for an infection;

♦ Be able to define the basic and net reproduction numbers and the herd immunity threshold for an infection;

♦ Know what models are.

1.2 Infections

Infection may be defined as the invasion of one organism by a smaller (infecting) organism. It is a ubiquitous phenomenon in nature. In fact, all species of plants, animals and even microbes carry infections of many sorts. Many of these infections are harmless, and some are even beneficial (for example, we all carry bacteria in our intestines which assist in digestion of food). But some, the pathogenic infectious agents, or pathogens, harm their hosts and cause disease. Though this book is primarily about these pathogenic infections, it is useful to recognize the ubiquity of the phenomenon.

Infectious agents come in a bewildering array of shapes and sizes, as shown in Table 1.1. Microparasites are small, invisible to the naked eye and found in very large (effectively uncountable) numbers in their hosts, whereas the macroparasites are much larger, visible to the naked eye and are generally found in countable numbers in or on their hosts.

This book will concentrate mainly upon the microparasite infections of humans.

Though some infectious agents which affect humans live in the environment, from which they may be transmitted to human hosts (examples are the bacteria which cause tetanus), the large majority live only in humans, or in other vertebrate animals and humans. Transmission between human or animal hosts occurs in a variety of ways, the most important being by direct contact (scabies, leprosy), the respiratory route

Table 1.1 Summary of the different kinds of infectious agents

Type of agent	Characteristics	Examples
Microparasites		
Virus	Small, simple, obligatory parasites of larger cells	Measles, mumps, rubella, smallpox, severe acute respiratory syndrome (SARS), influenza
Bacteria	Larger and more complex than viruses—many are able to grow independently but some require a cell host	*Bordetella pertussis* (whooping cough), *Mycobacterium tuberculosis* (tuberculosis) *Salmonella typhi* (typhoid fever)
Protozoa	Larger single-celled organisms, more complex than bacteria—many are able to grow independently but some require a cell host	*Plasmodium falciparum* (malaria); *Entamoeba histolytica* (dysentery)
Macroparasites		
Helminths (worms)	Large (1mm to 10m) multicellular organisms	*Schistosoma mansoni* (schistosomiasis)
Arthropods	Insects, lice, ticks and their relatives	*Ixodes* spp (ticks)

(influenza, whooping cough, tuberculosis) the faecal–oral route (typhoid, dysentery, many helminths), through sexual contact (HIV, gonorrhoea) or through insect vectors (malaria, dengue). The relationship between individuals allowing transmission of infection is typically called *contact.*

Once inside a (human) host, the infectious agent typically must replicate for a period of time before being able to be transmitted on to a subsequent individual, or before causing disease. The details of these events are extremely important in understanding disease, but will not be described here.[1] Suffice it to say that different infectious agents typically travel (for example, in the respiratory tract or bloodstream) to favoured sites within the host's body, where they multiply.

For the purposes of understanding infectious disease dynamics, it is important to distinguish three important time periods involved in these processes: the *pre-infectious* (sometimes called *latent*) *period,* defined as the time from infection to when a host is able to transmit the agent on to another host; the *incubation period,* defined as the time from infection to the onset of clinical disease; and the *infectious period,* defined as the period from the end of the pre-infectious period until the time when a host is no longer able to transmit the infection to others.

These periods are illustrated in Figure 1.1, showing the events in two successive hosts in a chain of transmission. Importantly, the time from onset of such a primary to a secondary case is known as the *serial interval.* It is evident that this is determined largely by the duration of the pre-infectious and infectious periods (which determine when infection leaves the source or primary case) as well as the incubation period (which determines when the recipient or secondary case has clinical onset). It is generally

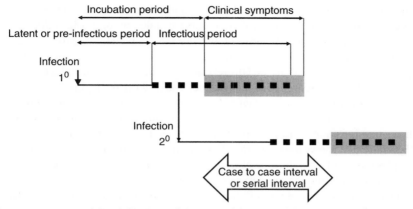

Fig. 1.1 Summary of the definitions of the pre-infectious, incubation and infectious periods for an infection. Note that the relationship between, and the relative durations of, these periods differ between different infections. The dotted lines refer to the infectious period and the shaded blocks refer to clinical disease. Adapted from Fine, 2003.[2]

clinical onsets of disease which are reported and are thus the basis of infectious disease statistics. Sometimes, early in an outbreak or in a small epidemic, the relationship between successive cases, or groups of cases may be evident (Figure 1.2a), but more often the details of the person to person chains of transmission are lost in the larger number of cases and clinical onsets over time.

The outcome of infections has crucially important features. Some infections may be mild, causing little or no illness in their host—and thus may never be recorded. The proportion of such inapparent infections may be quite high (e.g. more than 99 per cent in polio) or quite low (less than 5 per cent in measles). At the other extreme infections may be fatal, the proportion varying between populations (e.g. measles is rarely fatal now in wealthy countries but may be fatal in up to 10 per cent of cases in young children in poor populations). The duration of infectiousness or of disease are typically determined by the ability of the infected host to mount an immune response. The nature of immunity developed to different infections is itself a complicated issue, well beyond the scope of this book, but for our purposes we need to recognize three broad sorts of immune outcomes.

First, infected individuals may become solidly immune, such that they can never again be infected (this sort of immunity is found in some virus infections like measles, rubella and mumps). Secondly, individuals may rid themselves of the infections but remain susceptible to greater or lesser degree to a subsequent infection (this occurs with whooping cough, and with malaria). Thirdly, individuals may develop little or no immunity and so remain infected and infectious effectively for life (as happens with HIV). There are many variations on these themes—for example, in tuberculosis an individual may remain infected for many years, but only become infectious late in life, or may be *superinfected* by another exposure, thus ending up infected simultaneously with two or more strains of tubercle bacilli. It is important to appreciate the details of these immune responses and courses of events when describing any infection.

Figure 1.2a–d shows four patterns of infections in populations. Figure 1.2a shows a measles epidemic in a school, revealing successive 'crops' or 'generations' of cases. Figure 1.2b shows measles in the UK, revealing that prior to the introduction of vaccination in 1968, there were major epidemics every two years. Figure 1.2c shows the trend of tuberculosis in the UK. Figure 1.2d shows the rise and fall in the notifications of influenza during the 1957 influenza pandemic, following the typical pattern seen when a new infection is introduced into a totally susceptible population.

Figure 1.3a–d shows four patterns of infections by age, namely measles, influenza, toxoplasmosis and HIV, showing how the prevalence of infection depends on both age and time. We will find that models help us to understand such patterns.

One further comment about infections is essential before considering the modelling approach: heterogeneity. Every reader of this book is aware from personal experience that there are tremendous differences between people in their biological constitution, behaviour and disease history. These differences are undeniably important in determining patterns of disease in populations, but we will see that much can be learned about patterns of infections by assuming away heterogeneity, and considering that populations were made up of large numbers of similar individuals mixing at random

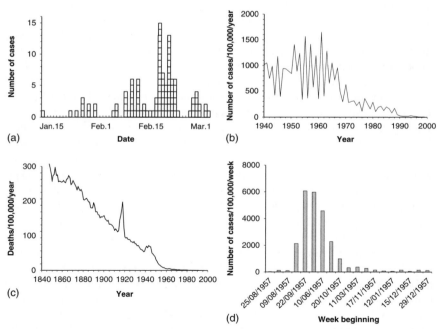

Fig. 1.2 (a) Measles epidemic in a boarding school in the north-eastern United States in 1934;[3] (b) Notification rates of measles in England and Wales;[4] (c) Mortality rates from tuberculosis in England and Wales since 1850;[5] (d) Notification rates of influenza in a general practice in Wales during the 1957 ('Asian') influenza pandemic.[6]

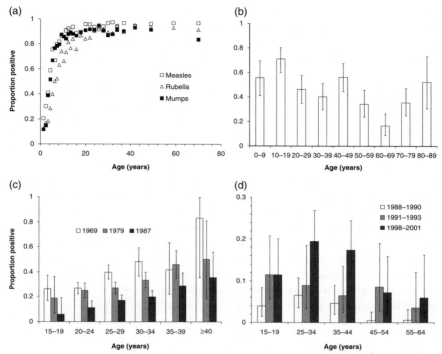

Fig. 1.3 (a) Proportions of individuals in different age groups who were found to be seropositive for measles, mumps and rubella antibodies in England and Wales in 1988;[7] (b) Proportions of individuals who had antibodies to the 1957 (Asian) influenza strain in Sheffield (UK) in 1957;[8] (c) Proportions of individuals found to be positive to *Toxoplasma gondii* in Norway in 1969, 1979 and 1987;[9] (d) Proportions of women found to be HIV positive in the community during the periods 1988–1990, 1991–1993 and 1998–2001 in Karonga district, Malawi.[10]

together. We will move in later parts of this book to consider more realistic heterogeneous populations, in which individuals belong to various groups which interact in various ways.

1.3 **Transmission**

The frequency of infections, as of diseases in general, in populations is generally described in terms of incidence and prevalence: prevalence being defined as the number or proportion of affected individuals in a population at any point in time and incidence being defined in terms of the risk or rate of new cases per unit time per 100 (or 1000) susceptible (at risk) individuals. These statistics, typically broken down by age, sex and other groups (e.g. by area or occupation) are reported routinely for many infectious diseases. They are invaluable—but they do not tell us how transmissible an infection may be. For this we need different measures.

The best known measure of transmissibility is the *secondary attack rate*, defined as the proportion infected among those susceptibles in (e.g. household or other) contact with a primary case.[11] Such statistics are available for many infections. They range from low risks of transmission (e.g. below 5 per cent for monkeypox) to high levels (80 per cent or greater for measles in some contexts).

Another measure of transmissibility is the *reproduction number*, defined as the (average) number of successful transmissions per infectious person. This number should be maximum when an infectious person is introduced into a totally susceptible population, in which circumstance it is defined as the *basic reproduction number* or R_0[12, 13]. Clearly, the value of R_0 must exceed unity if an infection is to persist in a population. R_0 values differ greatly for different infections, and under different circumstances. They range from very low levels for infections which cannot persist in populations up to numbers as high as 100 for malaria in parts of central Africa.

The basic reproduction number is defined in the context of a totally susceptible population, as may occur with the introduction of a new infection. It may be formally defined as the average number of secondary infectious persons resulting from a typical infectious person following their introduction to a totally susceptible population.

If the newly-introduced infection induces immunity in infected individuals, the proportion immune will increase with time, resulting in fewer transmissions from each infectious person—as some of their potential transmissions will fall on immune individuals. In such circumstances, the number of actual transmissions will be some number less than R_0, and is defined as the *net* or *effective* reproduction number, often (and in this text) given the symbol R_n. In simplest terms,

$$R_n = R_0 \times s \qquad 1.1$$

Here, s is defined as the proportion of the population that is susceptible. This relationship and its implications is illustrated in Figure 1.4, which shows three generations of transmission of an infectious agent whose R_0 is equivalent to 4.

This equation shows a fundamental relationship, that when the proportion susceptible, s, is equal to $1/R_0$, then each infectious person should lead to just a single transmission, i.e. $R_n = 1$. If the proportion susceptible is less than this proportion, incidence will decrease; if it is greater than this proportion then incidence will increase. This critical threshold of susceptibles is typically described in terms of its converse, or the proportion immune (*Proportion immune = 1 − s*). The critical threshold immune, defined as the *herd immunity threshold* (*HIT*), is then given by the following equation:

$$HIT = 1 - \frac{1}{R_0} = \frac{R_0 - 1}{R_0} \qquad 1.2$$

In theory, this herd immunity threshold provides a target for immunization programmes—as if this proportion of immunes is exceeded, then incidence of an infection should decrease.

Table 1.2 gives examples of serial intervals, R_0 values and crude herd immunity thresholds for several common infections. These are included to give a general idea of

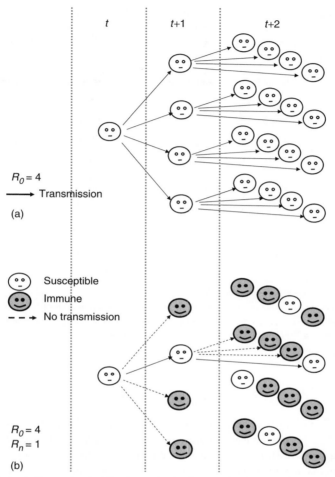

Fig. 1.4 Cartoon illustrating implications of a basic reproduction number $R_0 = 4$. In each successive time (serial) interval, each individual has contact which is sufficient to transmit infection to four other individuals. If the population is entirely susceptible (a), incidence increases exponentially, fourfold each generation (until the accumulation of immunes slows the process). If 75 per cent of the population is immune (b), then only 25 per cent of the contacts lead to successful transmissions, and the net reproduction number is $R_n = R_0 \times s = R_0 \times 0.25 = 1$. Adapted from Fine, 1993.[14]

the magnitude of these parameters, but should not be taken as gospel. Several of the infections, in particular malaria, pertussis, polio, and tuberculosis do not induce solid lifelong immunity to infection, which raises complex issues in defining realistic herd immunity thresholds.

Changes in the size of the susceptible population explain why we see epidemics of infections similar to those shown in Figure 1.2a, b and d. For example, when an infection

Table 1.2 Approximate serial intervals, basic reproduction numbers and implied crude herd immunity thresholds (calculated as $1-1/R_0$) for common potentially vaccine-preventable diseases. Estimates drawn from [16, 12, 17, 18, 19, 20]. Adapted from Fine, 1993.[14]

Infection	Serial interval (range)	R_0	Herd immunity threshold (%)
Diphtheria	2–30 days	6–7	85
Influenza	2–4 days	2–4	50–75
Malaria	20 days	5–100	80–99
Measles	7–16 days	12–18	83–94
Mumps	8–32 days	4–7	75–86
Pertussis	5–35 days	12–17	92–94
Polio	2–45 days	2–4,* 8–14†	‡
Rubella	7–28 days	6–7	83–85
Smallpox	9–45 days	5–7	80–85
Tuberculosis§	Months–years	–	–

* populations with good hygiene; † populations with poor hygiene.[20]

‡ The herd immunity threshold for polio is controversial because immunity to infection is not solid.

§ R_0 and herd immunity threshold for tuberculosis are not well defined because of changes in contact over time and the long serial interval, as well as controversial issues over immunity and the extent of reinfection.

for which $R_0 >1$ is introduced into a totally susceptible population, the incidence rises as each infectious person leads to more than one other infectious person. The incidence decreases once the susceptible population has been depleted so much so that the proportion that is susceptible is less than $1/R_0$ and the net reproduction number is less than one.

Though real life is typically rather more complicated than described by these thresholds (which assume a randomly mixing population), the relationship is nonetheless an important one.[15] We will meet it repeatedly in the pages which follow.

1.4 Models

A model is just a simplified representation of a complex phenomenon. We are all familiar with the use of models in various contexts—by architects, economists and many branches of biomedicine—for example, the use of laboratory animals as models when carrying out research on drugs or toxic materials. The more complex a phenomenon is, or the more difficult and expensive it is to study, or the greater the ethical implications of carrying out research, then the greater is the motive to explore models. By such logic, infectious diseases in humans are obvious subjects for modelling—they are complex, research in human populations is difficult and expensive, and such research raises many ethical issues. Thus it is no surprise that there is a long history of modelling relevant to human infectious diseases.

Three sorts of models have been used. *Animal models*—populations of mice into which infections were introduced—were popular in the first half of the twentieth century,[21] but were very expensive and this approach is now rarely used. *Mechanical models* were developed first at Johns Hopkins University to explore the implications of chance for infection transmission in populations.[22] The original mechanical models consisted of coloured beads arranged in trays and were very clumsy—but this approach has been continued with the use of computers and computer simulation, and is now an important method of analysis of infectious disease phenomena. Finally, there are *mathematical models*—in which the population parameters are described by symbols and linked by algebraic formulae, and nowadays, analysed using computers. These models are the most abstract, but they allow analysis and logical proofs in a way which other approaches do not permit. There is a long tradition of such models. This book emphasizes the mathematical models.

Models begin with a (simple) description of the subject under study, and move on to describe the essential elements which determine real life behaviour. These simplification and logical analysis steps are crucial, and determine the utility of the outcome. The opportunity which models provide to analyse a complex subject is itself one of the important benefits of a modelling approach—the model becomes, in effect, a logical structure which mimics the real world. If this process is wisely considered, and the most important features of the phenomenon are recognized, then the model may provide a realistic representation of the real world. If the model ends up not behaving like the real world, then this is evidence that its basic assumptions were either wrong or insufficient in some important way—a recognition which should encourage revision and redescription of the problem.

Let us consider a very simple infectious disease circumstance: an infection is introduced into a group of (susceptible) individuals (for example, people in a village, or children in a school). Infected children become infectious a short time after infection, and subsequently recover to become immune. We will consider what happens in successive serial intervals of this event, using the notation S_t and I_t to reflect the numbers of susceptible and infectious individuals at time t.

Suppose we know the circumstance at time t—is there any way to predict what the circumstance will be in time $t+1$? This requires some assumptions, effectively a model. The simplest assumption would be that the risk of infection among the susceptibles (i.e. the proportion of susceptibles who become infected) in any time period is a simple function of the number of infectious persons present during that time period. Assuming that individuals are infectious for only one time period, then we would express this as:

$$I_{t+1} = kS_t I_t \qquad\qquad 1.3$$

In this description, the 'k' is a sort of proportionality coefficient, sometimes called a 'contact rate'. It is, in effect, the proportion of all possible contacts between infectious persons and susceptibles (this total is given by the product $S_t \times I_t$) which lead to the susceptible person becoming infectious.

Following on with this logic, we would predict that the number of susceptibles remaining in the next period is as follows:

$$S_{t+1} = S_t - I_{t+1} \qquad\qquad 1.4$$

We will see that this very simple description of infection transmission, whereby incidence is a function of the product of the number of infectious individuals and the numbers of susceptibles turns out to be very widely used in infectious disease modelling, although the letter k is usually replaced with the letter (see Chapter 2).

The formulation described in Equation 1.3 will appear frequently in the pages that follow. It is called the *mass action principle* as applied to epidemiology, taking that name from the physical–chemical principle that the rate of a reaction is a function of the product of the concentrations of the reagents. Indeed, the use of this simple chemical principle in epidemiology, with its implication that people are like molecules of an ideal gas, nicely illustrates the simplification philosophy of modelling.

1.5 **Summary**

Infection may be defined as the invasion of one organism by a smaller (infecting) organism. There are many types of infectious agents and many ways in which transmission can occur. For understanding the dynamics of infectious diseases, it is important to distinguish three important time periods: the *pre-infectious* (sometimes called *latent*) *period*, defined as the time from infection to when a host is able to transmit the agent on to another host; the *incubation period*, defined as the time from infection to the onset of clinical disease; and the *infectious period*, defined as the period from the end of the pre-infectious period until the time when a host is no longer able to transmit the infection to others.

There are three broad sorts of immune outcomes of infection:

1) Solid immunity (individuals can no longer become infected);

2) Individuals may rid themselves of infection but can remain susceptible to some extent to further infection;

3) Individuals develop little or no immunity and can be infected and infectious for life.

The best known measure of transmissibility is the secondary attack rate, defined as the proportion infected among those susceptibles in contact with a primary case. Two other measures of transmissibility are frequently used: the basic reproduction number (R_0) and the net or effective reproduction number (R_n). R_0 describes the transmission potential of an infection under ideal conditions and is defined formally as 'the average number of secondary infectious persons resulting from the introduction of a typical infectious person into a totally susceptible population'. The net reproduction number is defined as the average number of secondary infectious persons resulting from each infectious person in a given population, e.g. in which some individuals may be immune because of previous infection.

R_0 is used to define the herd immunity threshold ($HIT = 1-1/R_0$), which provides a theoretical target threshold for an immunization programme—if the proportion of immunes in a population exceeds this threshold, then the incidence of the infection should decrease.

References

1 Mims CA, Nash A, Stephen J. *Mims' pathogenesis of infectious disease, 5th edn.* London: Academic Press; 2001.

2 Fine PE. The interval between successive cases of an infectious disease. *Am J Epidemiol* 2003; 158(11):1039–1047.

3 Aycock WL. Immunity to poliomyelitis. Heterologous strains and discrepant neutralization tests. *Am J Med Sci* 1942; 204(3):455–467.

4 Office for Population Censuses and Surveys. *Communicable disease statistics. A review of communicable disease statistics for 1980.* Series MB2 no. 7. 1980. London, Her Majesty's Stationery Office.

5 Registrar General. *Annual report of the Registrar General of births, deaths and marriages in England and Wales.* 1939. London, England, Her Majesty's Stationery Office.

6 Ministry of Health. *The influenza pandemic in England and Wales 1957–58.* 100. 1960. London, Her Majesty's Stationery Office. Reports on Public Health and Medical Subjects.

7 Farrington CP. Modelling forces of infection for measles, mumps and rubella. *Stat Med* 1990; 9(8):953–967.

8 Clarke SK, Heath RB, Sutton RN, Stuart-Harris CH. Serological studies with Asian strain of influenza A. *Lancet* 1958; 1(7025):814–818.

9 Forsgren M, Gille E, Ljungstrom I, Nokes DJ. *Toxoplasma gondii* antibodies in pregnant women in Stockholm in 1969, 1979, and 1987. *Lancet* 1991; 337(8754):1413–1414.

10 White RG, Vynnycky E, Glynn JR et al. HIV epidemic trend and antiretroviral treatment need in Karonga District, Malawi. *Epidemiol Infect* 2007; 135(6):922–932.

11 Frost W. The familial aggregation of infectious disease. *Am J Public Health* 1938; 28:7–13.

12 Anderson RM, May RM. *Infectious diseases of humans. Dynamics and control.* Oxford: Oxford University Press; 1992.

13 Diekmann O, Heesterbeek JA, Metz JA. On the definition and the computation of the basic reproduction ratio R_0 in models for infectious diseases in heterogeneous populations. *J Math Biol* 1990; 28(4):365–382.

14 Fine PE. Herd immunity: history, theory, practice. *Epidemiol Rev* 1993; 15(2):265–302.

15 Fine P, Mulholland K. Community immunity. In Plotkin SA, Orenstein WA, Offit PA, eds, *Vaccines.* Philadelphia, PA: Saunders Elsevier; 2008, pp. 1573–1592.

16 Heymann DL. *Control of Communicable Diseases Manual, 18th edn.* Washington DC, USA: American Public Health Association; 2004.

17 Ferguson NM, Cummings DA, Cauchemez S et al. Strategies for containing an emerging influenza pandemic in Southeast Asia. *Nature* 2005; 437(7056):209–214.

18 Mills CE, Robins JM, Lipsitch M. Transmissibility of 1918 pandemic influenza. *Nature* 2004; 432(7019):904–906.

19 Grassly NC, Fraser C, Wenger J et al. New strategies for the elimination of polio from India. *Science* 2006; 314(5802):1150–1153.

20 Fine PE, Carneiro IA. Transmissibility and persistence of oral polio vaccine viruses: implications for the global poliomyelitis eradication initiative. *Am J Epidemiol* 1999; 150(10):1001–1021.

21 Greenwood M, Hill AB, Topley WWC, Wilson J. *Experimental epidemiology*. 209. 1936. London, HMSO. MRC Special Report Series.

22 Fine PE. A commentary on the mechanical analogue to the Reed–Frost epidemic model. *Am J Epidemiol* 1977; 106(2):87–100.

How are models set up?
I. An introduction to difference equations

2.1 Overview and objectives

This chapter is designed to introduce the key steps for setting up models, the main types of models and the key input parameters. We will use a model describing the transmission of pandemic influenza as an example.

By the end of this chapter you should:

♦ Know the key steps which are used to set up models;

♦ Be aware of the different types of models;

♦ Be able to write down the difference equations for simple models of the transmission of an infection;

♦ Be able to define the main input parameters for such models.

2.2 How are models set up?

Figure 2.1 shows a list of steps which might be involved in developing a model. It is based on one compiled by a group in Rotterdam[3] following its experience of setting up detailed models of the transmission and control of onchocerciasis and schistosomiasis, for use by policy makers and programme managers. Each step in this list may need to be revisited many times before the model is completed and (as was the case for the modelling group in Rotterdam) the development of large models may take many years.

To illustrate this process, we consider how we might approach setting up a model to answer the following research questions:

An influenza problem

(a) If one infectious person infected with a new strain of influenza enters a town of 100,000 susceptible individuals, how will the average number of people who are susceptible, infectious and immune to this strain change during the subsequent few weeks?

(b) What proportion of individuals is likely to have been infected by the end?

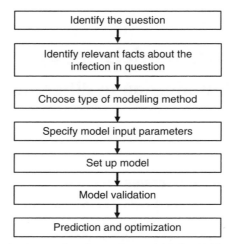

Fig. 2.1 Steps in the development and use of a model (after Habbema *et al.* 1996).[3]

2.3 **Identify relevant facts about the infection in question**

When developing a model, it is important to start by identifying key features of the epidemiology of the infection, such as:

- ◆ What is the pre-infectious period (the time period between infection and onset of infectiousness, often called the 'latent' period) (See section 1.2)?
- ◆ For how long are individuals normally infectious?
- ◆ What is the basic reproduction number?
- ◆ Are all age groups (or other social groups) affected equally by the infection?

Influenza example

For our influenza problem, as we are considering the introduction of a new strain into a population, no data are available. At best, we can base our model on data from previous influenza pandemics or inter-pandemic ('seasonal') influenza, as follows:

- ◆ The pre-infectious period is 1–2 days, as implied by the time interval between infection and viral shedding in experimental studies and challenge studies among individuals in the placebo arm of controlled studies.[4]
- ◆ The duration of infectiousness is variable; the duration of viral shedding based on a meta-analysis of challenge studies is about five days, with the amount of virus shed typically peaking on the second day after infection.[4] The duration of shedding may also be longer for children than for adults.[5]
- ◆ The basic reproduction number in previous pandemics was 1.5–3.[6–10]

◆ The age groups most affected by influenza have differed substantially during previous pandemics. Young adults had the highest mortality rates during the 1918 (Spanish) influenza pandemic, children had the highest clinical attack rates during the 1957 (Asian) influenza pandemic, whereas all age groups seemed equally affected during the 1968 (Hong Kong) influenza pandemic.[11]

A model provides a convenient framework in which we can put all the above information together to make predictions of changes in the number of susceptible, infectious and immune individuals and the likely number of cases. To develop the model, we need to write down equations relating the number of susceptible, infectious and immune individuals at some later time (e.g. tomorrow) to the number today, and evaluate these equations for each time (today, tomorrow, the next day…). To do this, we first need to decide on the structure of the model.

2.4 **Choose the model structure**

There are three main considerations when considering the model structure:

1) The natural history of the infection.

2) The accuracy and time period over which model predictions are required.

3) The research question.

2.4.1 **Consideration 1: the natural history of the infection**

The model structure should reflect the natural history of the infection and therefore important disease categories and transitions need to be described as well as important categories in the population itself. Figure 2.2 shows some of the most common and simplest model structures. For simplicity, these do not account for births into and deaths out of the population; we shall return to this complication later.

The Susceptible–Infectious (SI) model structure is the simplest way to describe the natural history of HIV, since, once infected, HIV-positive individuals remain infected and infectious for life. The Susceptible–Infectious–Susceptible (SIS) model structure is often used for curable sexually transmitted infections, such as gonorrhoea, for which infected individuals are infectious until they are treated or recover.[12]

For the so-called 'immunizing infections' (i.e. those for which individuals are immune to further infection after they have been infected), the Susceptible–Pre-infectious–Infectious–Recovered (SEIR) or Susceptible–Infectious–Recovered (SIR) model structures would be appropriate, where the pre-infectious category reflects the individuals who have been infected but who are not yet infectious. In the modelling literature, these individuals are referred to as those in the 'infected' or 'exposed' class; however, this terminology is not ideal, since infectious individuals are also, by definition, infected and everyone can be considered to be exposed. However, to retain some consistency with the conventional notation, we shall use the letter 'E' when referring to these individuals in abbreviations.

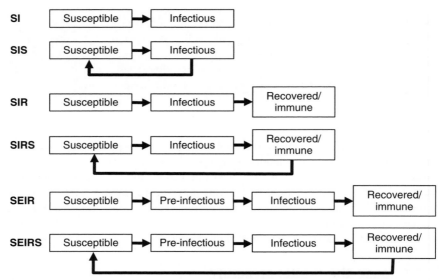

Fig. 2.2 Common structures for models used to describe the transmission of infections.

The Susceptible–Pre-infectious–Infectious–Recovered–Susceptible (SEIRS) or Susceptible–Infectious–Recovered–Susceptible (SIRS) model structures have been used for pertussis and seasonal influenza, to explore the changes in the immunity of individuals to the infection. Such changes might occur because of changes in the strains circulating in the population or waning immunity.[13–16]

The recovered class in the SIR or SEIR models is also sometimes referred to as the 'removed' class, since those who are immune no longer contribute to the infection process.

Any dependency on age or other social group may also need to be accounted for, depending on the research question. For example, to explore the impact of age-related interventions (e.g. vaccinating schoolchildren or the elderly) each of the categories in the model should be stratified by age. For sexually transmitted infections, on the other hand, it is important to distinguish between individuals in the so-called 'core group', who contact many individuals and are therefore at high risk of infection, and those who are less active. Methods for incorporating these stratifications are discussed in Chapters 5, 7 and 8.

2.4.2 Consideration 2: the accuracy and the time period covered by model predictions

The structure also depends on how accurate the model predictions need to be. For example, estimates of the daily numbers of influenza cases based on an SIR model are likely to be less reliable than those from an SEIR model, since the SIR model does not account for the time lag between infection and onset of infectiousness. Therefore, keeping everything else the same, we would expect our model to predict that influenza would spread more rapidly if we used an SIR model structure rather than a SEIR model structure. On the other hand, since (in theory!) every infected individual eventually becomes immune, SEIR and SIR models should produce identical estimates of the *total* number of cases which are likely to be seen by the end of an epidemic.

In addition, to describe the *long-term* transmission of an infection, a model may need to incorporate key aspects of the demography of the population being modelled (births, deaths, and migration) and possibly seasonal variation in contact patterns (e.g. resulting from changes in school attendance because of school terms and holidays). For example, the number of susceptible individuals changes substantially in a population during a year because of births and deaths, but changes little during one month. Consequently, we may find that to make predictions of the spread of influenza over a short period (e.g. a few months) we can safely ignore births and deaths, but that predictions spanning a period of several years are very sensitive to assumptions about births and deaths.

A further consideration for influenza is that strains change through antigenic drift and so the population's immunity to the circulating strains also changes over time. An SEIR or SIR model might therefore be appropriate for describing transmission following the introduction of a new strain of influenza into a population over a 2–3-year period; a SEIRS model would be needed to make predictions over a period spanning 10 or more years.

2.4.3 Consideration 3: the research question

The research question strongly determines the structure of the model, as illustrated in Figure 2.3. This shows a model of the transmission dynamics of *M. tuberculosis*, which is based on the model of Dye *et al.*[17] after removing one key feature (see below). This is a complex variant of the SEIRS model structure in Figure 2.2, which we shall discuss in Chapter 9.

In the model represented in Figure 2.3, individuals develop infectious disease either soon after initial infection with *M. tuberculosis* or many years later. The model is structured so that it can explore the impact of treating cases, for example, having a compartment for "treatment failures" and allowing those treated successfully to return to the so-called "latent" compartment. Infectious individuals can also cure naturally without treatment.

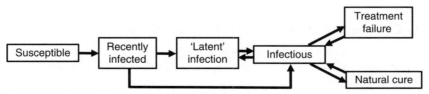

Fig. 2.3 A simplified version of the model of the transmission dynamics of *M. tuberculosis* of Dye *et al.*[17] Note that for tuberculosis, the term 'latent' is used in a different way from the way it is used for acute immunizing infections, since individuals who have 'latent' infection can go on to develop either infectious or non-infectious disease. Adapted from Dye *et al*, 1998.[17]

However, in reality, not all tuberculosis cases are infectious[18] and thus the feature that is missing from this model diagram (and which was present in the original model) is a compartment representing the non-infectious cases. Thus, the model described in Figure 2.3 can be used to explore the impact of treatment on the burden of *infectious disease*; however, to examine the impact of treatment on the burden of *both infectious and non-infectious* disease, we would need to add a compartment for non-infectious cases to the model (see [17]).

This leads on to the question of how complex models should be. The quote, often attributed to Einstein, that '*models should be as simple as possible and no simpler*' should be borne in mind when trying to design a model. A model is a simplification of reality that allows us to explore patterns in data and, hopefully, discover fundamental insights that explain these patterns. The greater the complexity of the model, the more difficult this is to achieve.[19]

Advances in computing power are allowing the development of some very detailed models. The ONCHOSIM model, which was developed during the 1980s to explore control options for onchocerciasis, for example, tracks the life history of every worm present in diseased individuals in given villages.[20] Some models of influenza transmission developed during the early 2000s attempt to capture detailed movements of individuals to schools, cinemas, etc. in populations comprising millions of individuals.[7, 21–23]

Such models can be difficult and time-consuming to set up, requiring many input parameters and data (much of which may not be readily available). On the other hand, an attraction of these models is that they are relatively easy to understand, being close to reality and, once the model is set up, many different scenarios can be explored.

Influenza example

For now, we will keep the objective of our influenza modelling exercise simple—to make predictions over a short time period (a few weeks) in a population without stratifying the predictions by age. We will assume random mixing, no seasonal variation and no age dependencies in the parameters.

Because we are making predictions over the short term, we will ignore demography (births/deaths/migration) and, to avoid inaccuracies which might result from using an SIR model, we will use an SEIR model structure.

2.5 **Choose the type of modelling method**

Models may be deterministic or stochastic.

Deterministic models describe what happens 'on average' in a population. In these models, the input parameters (e.g. the rate of disease onset or the rate at which people recover) are fixed, and therefore the model's predictions, such as the number of cases which will be seen over time, are 'predetermined'.

Stochastic models, on the other hand, allow the number of individuals who move between compartments to vary through chance, for example, the rate at which people are infected or infectious individuals recover from disease may vary randomly.

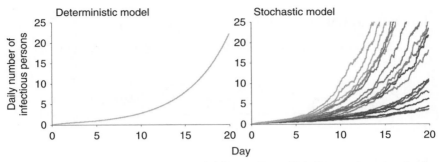

Fig. 2.4 Comparison between predictions of the number of infectious persons per day for influenza obtained using a deterministic model and a stochastic model using 20 'runs', with the rate at which individuals are infected being allowed to vary with each run.

Therefore, the model can provide the range in which an outcome, such as the number of cases over time or the probability that a given outcome (e.g. an epidemic) will occur (see Figure 2.4).

This particular feature of a stochastic model is usually appealing for decision-making purposes. For example, the output from the stochastic model in Figure 2.4 suggests that by day 10, the daily number of infectious individuals should be between 1 and 10, which is perhaps more helpful for planning purposes than the prediction from the deterministic model, which says that there should be about 3 infectious persons per day by day 10.

We will return to the methods for setting up stochastic models in Chapter 6. In the rest of this chapter, we will focus on deterministic models.

Influenza example

In the interests of simplicity, to answer our influenza problem we will develop a deterministic model.

2.6 **Setting up deterministic models**

The majority of deterministic models are so-called 'compartmental' models. The term 'compartmental' comes from the fact that the model population is stratified into broad subgroups (compartments), such as those who are susceptible, pre-infectious, infectious or immune, and the model describes the transmission of the infection using the total number of individuals in these categories. Panel 2.1 discusses some of the main types of models.

Deterministic compartmental models can be set up using either 'difference' equations or 'differential' equations. We will first describe the approach based on difference equations and we will discuss differential equations in the next chapter.

Difference equations describe the transitions between different disease categories using discrete (e.g. daily) time steps by expressing the number of individuals at a given time $t+1$ (e.g. tomorrow), in terms of the number at an earlier time t, (e.g. today).

We will use our influenza model to illustrate how we would write down these equations.

Influenza example

For our influenza example, we have decided to use the following SEIR model structure:

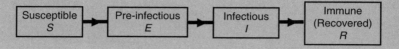

Panel 2.1 The classification of models

The classification of models into stochastic and deterministic models is over-simplistic because some deterministic models also incorporate stochastic elements and most stochastic models incorporate some deterministic elements.[20, 27] Stochastic models tend to be used when modelling transmission in small populations or when it is important to provide estimates of the range in which an outcome, such as the number of cases, might occur (see Chapter 6).

The following are other categories of models:

♦ *Compartmental*: individuals in the population are subdivided into broad subgroups ('compartments') and the model tracks the infection process for these individuals collectively. These models can be either deterministic or stochastic (see also Chapter 6).

♦ *Individual-based or microsimulation model*: the model tracks the infection process for every individual in the population. Many individual-based models are also stochastic (see also Chapter 6).

♦ '*Transmission dynamic*' or '*dynamic transmission*' *model*: the model incorporates contact (and therefore transmission) between individuals. The risk or force of infection therefore depends on the number of infectious individuals in the population (see section 2.7.1 and Panel 2.5) and will therefore change over time if the number of infectious individuals changes.

♦ *Static*: the model does not explicitly describe contact (and therefore transmission) between individuals. The risk or force of infection therefore takes predetermined values. These models are typically used when the risk of infection is known, as was the case for tuberculosis in some Western settings during the twentieth century.[28] However, static models are not reliable for looking at the effect of interventions involving reductions in the prevalence of infectious individuals, e.g. vaccination, treatment etc., which can lead to reductions in the infection risk (see Chapter 5).

♦ *Network*: A model in which the network of contacts between individuals is explicitly modelled, e.g. individual A forms a sexual partnership with individual B, who has a partnership with individual C, etc. The risk of infection for an individual in a network model depends on the person to whom they are connected. Network models have been used extensively for describing the transmission of sexually transmitted infections (see Chapter 8).

2.6.1 **Equation for the number of susceptible individuals at time $t+1$:**

Considering the susceptible individuals, the equations need to specify the fact that:

(Number of susceptible individuals at time $t+1$) =

(Number of susceptible individuals at time t)

−

(Number of individuals who are newly infected between t and $t+1$)

The number of individuals who are newly infected between t and $t+1$, in turn, is just the product of the risk that a susceptible individual is infected between time t and $t+1$ (conventionally denoted by the symbol λ_t) and the number of susceptible individuals at time t (denoted using the notation S_t), i.e. $\lambda_t\, S_t$.

For example, if 5 per cent ($= \lambda_t$) of susceptible individuals are newly infected between today and tomorrow, and 200 (S_t) susceptible individuals are present today, then the number of individuals who are newly infected between today and tomorrow equals $0.05 \times 200 = 10$.

Note that 'λ' has 't' as a subscript, reflecting the fact that it changes over time, e.g. as a result of changes in the number of infectious individuals. Parameters that do not have this subscript are assumed to be constant over time.

We can now write down the difference equation for the number of susceptible individuals at time $t+1$ as:

$$S_{t+1} = S_t - \lambda_t\, S_t \qquad\qquad 2.1$$

2.6.2 **Equation for the number of pre-infectious individuals at time $t+1$**

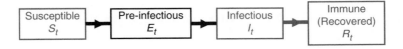

As reflected in our model diagram, the equations for individuals in the pre-infectious category need to specify the fact that:

Number of pre-infectious individuals at time $t+1$ =

(Number of pre-infectious individuals at time t)

+

(Number of individuals who are newly infected between time t and $t+1$)

−

(Number of individuals who become infectious between time t and $t+1$)

The second term in this equation is equal to the number of individuals leaving the susceptible category between time t and $t+1$ (i.e. $\lambda_t S_t$); since they are entering the pre-infectious category, the sign in front of this term is '+' rather than '−'.

The number of individuals who become infectious between time t and $t+1$, in turn, is just the product of the proportion of pre-infectious individuals who become infectious between time t and $t+1$ (we will denote this proportion by 'f') and the number of pre-infectious individuals at time t (denoted by E_t), i.e. fE_t. For example, if 20 per cent of pre-infectious individuals become infectious between today and tomorrow, and 800 pre-infectious individuals are present today, then the number of pre-infectious individuals who become infectious between today and tomorrow equals $0.2 \times 800 = 160$.

Here we are assuming that the proportion of pre-infectious individuals who become infectious in each time step is the same over time—we will return to this assumption later.

We can now write down the equations for the number of pre-infectious individuals at time $t+1$ as follows:

$$E_{t+1} = E_t + \lambda_t S_t - f E_t \qquad 2.2$$

2.6.3 Equations for the number of infectious individuals at time $t+1$

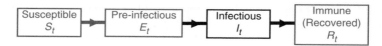

As reflected in our model diagram, the equations for the number of infectious individuals need to specify the fact that:

(Number of infectious individuals at time $t+1$)

=

(Number of infectious individuals at time t)

+

(Number of individuals who become infectious between time t and $t+1$)

−

(Number of individuals who cease being infectious between time t and $t+1$)

As we saw above, the number of individuals who become infectious between time t and $t+1$ is given by the expression fE_t.

By an analogous argument to that used above, the number of individuals who stop being infectious between time t and $t+1$ is just the product of the proportion of infectious individuals who cease being infectious between time t and $t+1$ (we will denote this proportion by r for now) and the number of infectious individuals at time t (denoted by the symbol I_t), i.e. rI_t. We will return to the definition and derivation of r later in this chapter.

We can now write down the equation for the number of infectious individuals at time $t+1$ as follows:

$$I_{t+1} = I_t + f E_t - r I_t \qquad 2.3$$

2.6.4 Equations for the number of immune ('recovered') individuals at time $t+1$

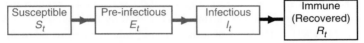

Finally, the total number of immune individuals at time $t+1$ (R_{t+1}) is given by:

(the number who were immune at time t (R_t))

$+$

(the number who became immune between time t and $t+1$ ($r I_t$))

Using mathematical notation, the equation would be written as:

$$R_{t+1} = R_t + r I_t \qquad 2.4$$

The difference equations for the model can now be summarized as:

$$S_{t+1} = S_t - \lambda_t S_t$$
$$E_{t+1} = E_t + \lambda_t S_t - f E_t$$
$$I_{t+1} = I_t + f E_t - r I_t$$
$$R_{t+1} = R_t + r I_t$$

Panel 2.2 discusses some of the technical considerations relating to these equations. Panel 2.3 discusses the notation used in equations.

These equations provide a method for predicting the numbers of individuals who are susceptible, pre-infectious, infectious, and immune over time. For example, if we know how many individuals are susceptible, pre-infectious, infectious and immune at the start (e.g. on day 0) and if we know the values for λ_t, f and r, then we can calculate the numbers of individuals in these categories on day 1. We can then substitute the values that we calculated for day 1 into the above equations to obtain the numbers of individuals who are susceptible, pre-infectious, infectious and immune on day 2 and so on. This can be done relatively easily using a computer.

Before we do this for our influenza problem, we will first discuss how the input parameters λ_t, f and r are estimated.

2.7 Specify the model's input parameters

A lack of reliable data complicates the development of models. New data sometimes need to be collected and analysed using statistical methods, or the model itself needs

Panel 2.2 Technical issues relating to models

1. Directions of the arrows

The direction of the arrows linking the different compartments in the model diagram determines whether individuals are added or taken away from the number of individuals in that compartment.

For example, there is an arrow going out of the susceptible compartment and entering the pre-infectious compartment in the SEIR model diagram described on pages 21–23, reflecting the fact that susceptible individuals are being newly infected.

Hence, there is a minus sign in front of the term for the number of individuals who are newly infected ($\lambda_t S_t$) in the equation for the number of susceptible individuals at time $t+1$ (Equation 2.1), and there is a plus sign in front of this term in the equation for the number of pre-infectious individuals at time $t+1$ (Equation 2.2).

2. Check for population size

If we add the four equations of the model for influenza to each other, we obtain the following result:

$$S_{t+1} + E_{t+1} + I_{t+1} + R_{t+1} = S_t + E_t + I_t + R_t$$

i.e. the total population size remains constant over time which is consistent with our assumption that the population is closed, or equivalently there are no births, deaths and migration into or out of the population. Summing up the numbers of individuals at time $t+1$ and comparing them against the sum at time t provides a helpful check that the assumptions have been incorporated into the model as intended.

3. Risks versus rates

Technically, the input parameters which are used in difference equations are risks since we are using, for example, the proportion of pre-infectious individuals who become infectious in each time step, the proportion of infectious individuals who recover in each time step etc.

In practice, modellers tend to work with 'rates' in difference equations, since these are easier to calculate than are risks, and they are approximately equal to the risk. For example, risks and rates are related through the following equation (see Panel 3.4 for the derivation):

$$\text{risk} = 1 - e^{-\text{rate}}$$

where 'e' is the mathematical constant 2.71828. . . (see the definition in the Basic maths section B.3). If the rate is small then the risk is approximately equal to the rate (Figure 2.5).

4. Reliability of difference equations

The reliability of difference equations depends on the time step used (see Chapter 3). For example, the number of susceptible individuals who are newly infected between

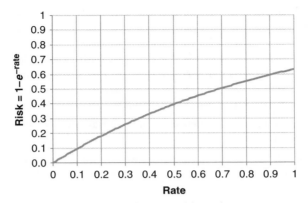

Fig. 2.5 Illustration of the relationship between risks and rates.

time t and $t+1$ (given by $\lambda_t \, S_t$) is expressed in terms of the number susceptible or infectious at time t, so if the time step used is large (three days for example), this expression may under- or overestimate the true number newly infected. More reliable estimates may then be obtained using smaller time steps, so we allow values to change more often, for example, twice a day $t + \frac{1}{2}$, $t + 1$, $t + 1\frac{1}{2}$... etc.

Taken to the limit, the differential equation approach describes the transmission dynamics in 'continuous time' (i.e. using infinitesimally small time steps δt). This is covered in the next chapter.

Panel 2.3 Notation—Greek or the Latin alphabet, lower case versus upper case?

Modellers frequently use Greek letters to write down the equations for the model, following the tradition of using Greek letters in mathematics and physics. For example, σ and γ are sometimes used to denote the rate of onset of infectiousness and the recovery rate respectively (see, for example, Anderson and May (1992)[29]).

Unfortunately, the notation used to denote the various parameters is not consistent between modellers. For example, some modellers use β, which we shall discuss in the next few pages, to denote the number of individuals effectively contacted by each person per unit time, rather than the rate at which two specific individuals come into effective contact per unit time.

To reduce potential confusion, we have minimized the use of Greek letters, using them only for terms for which their use is generally accepted. For example, we shall use λ for the force of infection and β for the transmission parameter, which we have defined to be the rate at which two specific individuals come into effective contact per unit time (see Section 2.7.1).

Following the example in previous texts,[29] we will also be using upper case letters when we refer to numbers of individuals in a given compartment, and lower case letters to refer to the *proportion* of individuals in the population that are in a given compartment.

to be fitted to the available data to estimate the input parameters. In circumstances where there is much uncertainty in the input parameters, many sets of combinations of input parameters may be assumed that lead to predictions which 'fit' the data, and each set is then used to generate predictions. We discuss these issues in further detail in later chapters.

Returning to our influenza problem, to use our difference equations to predict the number of individuals who are susceptible, pre-infectious, infectious, and immune to influenza over time, we need the following input parameters:

- λ_t—the risk that a susceptible person becomes infected between time t and $t+1$ (the 'force of infection');

- f—the proportion of infected individuals who become infectious between time t and $t+1$, or, as discussed in Panel 2.2, the rate at which pre-infectious individuals become infectious;

- r—the proportion of infectious individuals who recover (i.e. become immune) between time t and $t+1$, or the rate at which individuals recover (see Panel 2.2).

2.7.1 Calculating the risk (or force) of infection, λ_t

The risk of infection depends on the number of infectious individuals in the population and on how frequently they contact other individuals.

The simplest assumption that we could make about contact is that individuals mix randomly, i.e. the probability that two individuals meet or have contact is the same, regardless of their age or other characteristics. This assumption is similar to the 'mass action principle' that is used in the physical sciences, such that individuals contact each other in the same random way that gas molecules collide with each other. This assumption is also referred to as 'random mixing' or 'homogeneous mixing'. When mixing depends on age, social group or some other characteristic, it is said to be 'non-random' or 'heterogeneous'.

Although simple, the assumption of random mixing is useful for obtaining rough estimates of how the numbers of susceptible, infectious and immune individuals will change over time, as we shall see later. A simple method for writing down this assumption is to say that the risk of infection is proportional to the number of infectious individuals at time t, I_t, in the population as follows:

$$\lambda_t = \beta I_t$$

2.5

The precise definition of β is the per capita rate at which two specific individuals come into effective contact per unit time (see derivation below); however, for simplicity, we shall refer to it simply as the 'rate at which two specific individuals come into effective contact per unit time'.

β is also called (sometimes incorrectly) the 'transmission probability', 'transmission coefficient', 'transmission parameter', 'transmission rate' etc. An *effective contact* is defined, as by Abbey,[24] as a contact which would be sufficient to lead to infection, were it to occur between a susceptible and an infectious individual (see Panel 2.4).

Panel 2.4 The definition of an effective contact and factors affecting β

An effective contact is defined as one which is sufficient to lead to infection, were it to occur between a susceptible and an infectious individual.[24] Consequently, the definition of an effective contact depends on both the method of transmission (e.g. sexual vs respiratory vs vector-borne vs faecal–oral etc.) and the infection considered. For tuberculosis, for example, casual contact is unlikely to lead to transmission (Figure 2.6a), whereas the highly infectious nature of measles means that contact between individuals can be less intimate than that for tuberculosis in order for transmission to occur.

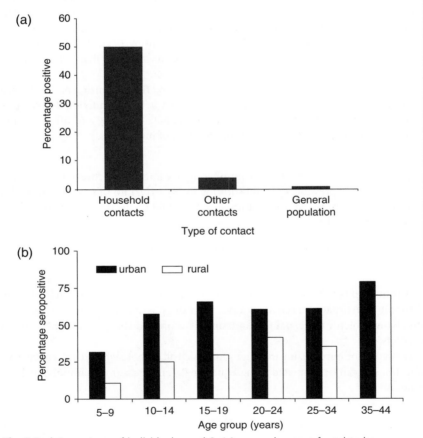

Fig. 2.6 a) Percentage of individuals aged 0–14 years who were found to be tuberculin positive (≥ 5 mm induration to tuberculin) i.e. probably infected, among household and other contacts of tuberculosis cases in Rotterdam, 1967-9.[1]
b) Comparison between the percentage of women who were seropositive for rubella antibodies in urban and rural Panama.[2]

> **Panel 2.4 The definition of an effective contact and factors affecting β** *(continued)*
>
> β depends further on other factors, such as age and setting. For example, children probably contact more individuals (who are also likely to be children) than do adults; individuals living in urban areas probably contact more individuals than do those living in rural areas. This is reflected in the higher levels of seropositivity (reflecting lifetime exposure to rubella) among urban residents in Panama, as compared with those living in rural areas (Figure 2.6b).
>
> β may also change over time: because of reductions in crowding in living conditions, individuals alive in many Western countries in the year 1900 probably contacted more individuals than did their counterparts during the late twentieth century. During the second part of the nineteenth century, ~8 per cent of the UK population lived in accommodation with more than two individuals per room, as compared with 5.5 per cent by 1901 and ~1 per cent by 1951. By 1991, only 0.25 per cent of the population lived in accommodation with more than 1.5 individuals per room.[30]
>
> Changes in behaviour or interventions may also affect β. During past influenza pandemics, for example, the amount of contact between individuals probably changed over time, with theatres and concert halls shutting and office closing hours being staggered to avoid the congregation of individuals.[31, 32]

As discussed in section 2.6.1, the number of new infections between time t and $t+1$ is given by the expression $\lambda_t S_t$. Substituting for $\lambda_t = \beta I_t$ into this expression leads to the following expression for the total number of new infections in the population between time t and $t+1$:

$$\text{Total number of new infections in the population between time } t \text{ and } t+1 = \beta I_t S_t \qquad 2.6$$

Although β is the most important parameter in transmission models, it is very difficult to estimate directly, because, with the possible exception of infections involving a vector or sexual transmission, it is often difficult to identify effective contacts.

However, for immunizing infections for which all of those who are infected become infectious, β can be estimated using Equation 2.7, if we assume that individuals mix randomly:

$$\beta = \frac{R_0}{ND} \qquad 2.7$$

where R_0 is the basic reproduction number, N is the total population size and D is the duration of infectiousness. R_0 is defined as the average number of secondary infectious persons resulting from a typical infectious person following their introduction into a totally susceptible population (see Chapter 1). Equation 2.7 can be derived heuristically by using equation 2.6 and the definition of R_0, as follows.

For example, if one infectious person enters a totally susceptible population at time $t=0$, i.e. when the number of susceptible individuals equals the total population size, or using mathematical notation, $S_0=N$, then, substituting for $S_0=N$ and $I_0=1$ into Equation 2.6 implies that βN individuals are newly infected between time $t=0$ and $t=1$. Assuming that the same number of individuals (i.e. βN) are infected on each day of the infectious period, then, by the end of the infectious period of duration D, the infectious person should have infected βND individuals. For example, if each infectious person infects two others per day, then if they are infectious for five days, they should infect $2\times5=10$ individuals during the infectious period. Stating this formally:

The total number of individuals infected by the infectious person that

was introduced into the totally susceptible population

$$= \beta ND \qquad\qquad 2.8$$

For an immunizing infection, all of those infected subsequently become infectious, and therefore the verbal definition of βND in equation 2.8 is equivalent to that of R_0. Consequently, setting βND equal to R_0 leads to the result:

$$R_0 = \beta ND \qquad\qquad 2.9$$

Dividing both sides of this equation by ND leads to Equation 2.7. Equation 2.9 is derived formally using other approaches in Chapter 4.

Note that the basic reproduction number divided by the duration of infectiousness equals the number of effective contacts made by each person *per unit time*, which we shall denote using the symbol c_e:

$$c_e = R_0 / D \qquad\qquad 2.10$$

For example, if $R_0 = 4$ (i.e. each person makes four effective contacts during their infectious period), and the average duration of infectiousness is two days, then on average, each person makes $4/2 = 2$ effective contacts each day.

By dividing c_e by the population size, N, we obtain the *per capita* number of effective contacts made by a given individual per unit time, which is given by the following equation:

$$\frac{c_e}{N} = \frac{R_0}{ND} = \beta \qquad\qquad 2.11$$

This expression is identical to that for β (Equation 2.7) which means that the precise verbal definiton of β is the '*per capita* number of effective contacts made by a given individual per unit time', or equivalently, the *per capita* rate at which two specific individuals come into effective contact per unit time.

For infections for which β cannot be measured directly or estimated using Equation 2.11, β, together with other parameters, can be obtained by fitting predictions of the numbers of infections or cases that are obtained using a model to observed data on the numbers of infections or cases respectively seen over time (see Chapter 4).

The formulation for the risk of infection in Equation 2.5 is used when we are describing infection transmission in populations which are not changing in size over time. Alternative expressions for the risk of infection, that should be used when we wish to assume that the population increases over time, are discussed in Panel 2.5. Unless stated otherwise, we will be considering models of the transmission of infections in which the population is stable over the time period that we are modelling, and we will use the notation in Equation 2.5. Other refinements to deal with small populations, where the probability of individuals contacting more than one infectious person is not negligible, or when contact is age dependent, are discussed later in this book.

Influenza example

Returning to our influenza problem, we can now calculate β using Equation 2.7. Assuming that the basic reproduction number is 2, the duration of infectiousness is 2 days and the population comprises 100,000 individuals implies that $\beta = 2/(2 \times 100,000) = 10^{-5}$ per day.

Panel 2.5 Expressions for the risk of infection: scaling parameters, density and frequency dependence

Notation, population size and scaling β parameters

As shown in Equation 2.11, β is inversely proportional to the population size. Consequently, if R_0 for an infection is identical in two populations, which have either 100,000 or 10 million individuals, β will be smallest in the population with 10 million individuals. To avoid recalculating β when using the same model in different populations, modelling studies typically replace β in the equation for the risk of infection (Equation 2.5) with the term $\dfrac{c_e}{N}$, as follows:

$$\lambda_t = \frac{c_e I_t}{N}$$

2.12

c_e reflects the number of individuals effectively contacted by a given person per unit time, although the letter β is sometimes (and confusingly) used instead of c_e.

The equation for the risk of infection used in modelling studies must therefore always be examined closely in order to obtain the correct interpretation of β. The definition of I_t should also be checked in the equation for the risk of infection, since, in the modelling literature, I_t sometimes refers to the *proportion*, rather than the *number*, of individuals in the population that are infectious.

The notation tends to differ in the STI modelling literature (see Chapter 8), where β is typically written as the product of two terms, namely the number of sexual contacts that are made per unit time and the probability of infection transmission given contact between an infectious and a susceptible person.

Frequency and density dependence ('True' and 'pseudo mass action')

When writing down expressions for the risk of infection, we also need to think about whether we want to allow the population size to change over time in the model population, and how this influences the infection risk. For example, if we are describing transmission of an infection in a city whose population size increases, we may need to have different expressions for the infection risk, depending on whether we think that, as the population grows:

1. The city boundary expands and the number of individuals effectively contacted by each person remains unchanged, so that the risk of infection remains unchanged. Transmission is said to be 'frequency-dependent' for this assumption.

2. The city boundary remains unchanged, and therefore crowding increases as the population grows, so that the risk of infection increases. In this instance, transmission is said to be 'density-dependent'.

Density dependence is plausible for animal and plant diseases. However, the amount by which the risk of infection increases with population size is not well understood, and may vary between infections. A study conducted during the late 1970s of *P muris* infection among mice[33] suggested that an increase in the number of mice in a given area leads to the same increase (i.e. there is a linear relationship) in the number of effective contacts made by each mouse. If this finding applies to human infections, then as the number of people in an area doubles, the number of individuals effectively contacted by each person per unit time (c_e) would also double. Since $\beta = \dfrac{c_e}{N}$ (Equation 2.11), this assumption means that β would remain unchanged and we can use the expression $\lambda_t = \beta I_t$ for the risk of infection (Equation 2.5), irrespective of the population size. This formulation for the infection risk was first used by Hamer in 1906[34] to describe measles transmission in London. Since that time, the term 'pseudo mass action' has been introduced to refer to this assumption,[35, 36] although, because its use has sometimes been confusing, it is discouraged.[37]

Other studies have challenged the density dependence assumption for the infection risk, hypothesizing that the number of individuals contacted by each person is better described using a power law relationship than with a linear relationship, e.g. with $c_e = \beta N^v$, where v is some number between 0 and 1, or that c_e stops increasing once the population size exceeds some value (see Chapter 12 in Anderson and May[29] and references [35, 37]).

The assumption that is used most widely for human infections is that the number of individuals effectively contacted by each person remains unchanged as the population grows. This formulation for the risk of infection is referred to as 'frequency dependence' or 'true mass action'.[35, 36] For this formulation, β changes as the population size changes, and is given by the expression $\beta = \dfrac{c_e}{N_t}$, where N_t is the population size at time t. The risk of infection is then given by the equation:

$$\lambda_t = \frac{c_e I_t}{N_t}$$

2.13

Panel 2.5 Expressions for the risk of infection: scaling parameters, density and frequency dependence (continued)

Example: the difference between using the density or frequency dependence formulations for the risk of infection

Suppose we consider a town with 10,000 (=N) individuals, of which 100 (1 per cent) were infectious with measles, with $R_0 = 13$ and $D = 7$ days.

Incorporating these values into equations 2.7 and 2.10 implies that:

$$\beta = \frac{R_0}{ND} = 13/(10,000 \times 7) = 1.86 \times 10^{-4} \text{ per day and}$$

$$c_e = R_0/D = 13/7 = 1.86 \text{ per day.}$$

Applying Equation 2.5 with $I_t = 100$ implies that the risk of infection on the given day was equal to the following:

$$\lambda_t = \beta I_t = 1.86 \times 10^{-4} \times 100 = 0.0186 \text{ per day}$$

Suppose we revisit this town several years later, when it comprises 100,000 individuals of whom 1 per cent (1000 individuals) are still infectious with measles.

If we assume frequency dependence (the number of individuals effectively contacted by each infectious person has not changed), the risk of infection would have remained unchanged at 0.0186 per day. For example, c_e would still equal 1.86 per day and so, applying Equation 2.13 with $I_t = 1000$ and $N_t = 100,000$ implies that the risk of infection equals:

$$\lambda_t = \frac{1.86 \times 1000}{100,000} = 0.0186 \text{ per day} \tag{2.14}$$

However, if we assume density-dependence (i.e. β does not change), the risk of infection would have increased to 0.186 per day. For example, $\beta = 1.86 \times 10^{-4}$ per day, and so, applying Equation 2.5 with $I_t = 1000$ implies that the risk of infection equals:

$$\lambda_t = 1.86 \times 10^{-4} \times 1000 = 0.186 \text{ per day} \tag{2.15}$$

If the population is assumed to remain unchanged over time, both the frequency and density dependent formulations for the infection risk are equivalent.

Many of the models describing the transmission of respiratory infections between humans in Western populations (see e.g. Chapters 1–12 in Anderson and May[29]) used the density dependence formulation, since the population growth over the time period that was considered in the study would not have substantially affected β. To apply the same models to a population which was different in size, then, assuming that R_0 remained unchanged, β would need to be recalculated for the new population. An advantage of using the density dependence formulation in such situations is that it simplifies the notation used in the equations, especially when we describe mixing between different age or risk groups in the population (see Chapter 7).

On the other hand, models which described the transmission of respiratory infections in developing countries (see e.g. [38, 39, 40]) in which the population increases substantially over the time period of interest, usually assumed frequency dependence. Similarly, models describing the transmission of infections among animals often (although not exclusively) use the frequency dependence formulation.[35, 37, 41]

2.7.2 Estimating the rate of onset of infectiousness, the recovery rate etc

An assumption which is often incorporated into infectious disease models is that, once infected, individuals become infectious at a constant rate, or that once infectious, individuals recover and become immune at a constant rate.

This assumption is convenient (and will be used repeatedly in this book), since the average pre-infectious and infectious periods are usually known (at least for immunizing infections), and if something occurs at a constant rate, then this rate can be calculated as 1/(average time to that event), i.e.

$$\text{rate at which something occurs} = 1 / \text{average time to the event} \qquad 2.16$$

The derivation of Equation 2.16 is discussed in Chapter 3.

For example, if we assume that the average pre-infectious period for influenza is two days, then the rate at which individuals become infectious (denoted by f in our model equations) is $1/2 = 0.5$ per day.

Similarly, the recovery rate (denoted by r in our model equations) can be obtained from the average infectious period, and the mortality rates can be calculated from the average life expectancy, as follows:

$$\text{Recovery rate } (r) = 1 / (\text{average duration of infectiousness})$$
$$\text{Mortality rate} = 1 / (\text{average life expectancy})$$

The converse of Equation 2.16 is that the average time to an event is given by 1/average rate at which the event occurs. Consequently, the life expectancy can be calculated from the average mortality rate as follows

$$\text{Average life expectancy} = 1 / (\text{average mortality rate}) \qquad 2.17$$

For example, if, on average, 1 per cent of individuals die each year, the average life expectancy is $1/0.01 = 100$ years.

The assumption that individuals become infectious or recover at a constant rate does not reflect what happens in reality, since it implies that the pre-infectious or infectious periods follow the exponential distribution (see Figure 2.7 and section 3.5.1). However, this assumption is often adequate for many modelling studies, especially those looking at the long-term dynamics of acute immunizing infections. Examples of circumstances in which this assumption may be inappropriate are provided later in the book.

If we wished to refine this assumption, for example, assume that the rate at which individuals become infectious depends on time since infection, then the pre-infectious compartment would need to be subdivided into several different compartments, with individuals progressing between compartments at some rate or after a fixed time (see, for example, Wearing *et al.* 2005).[25]

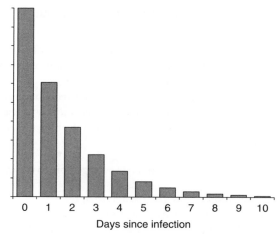

Fig. 2.7 Distribution of the time between first infection and onset of infectiousness assuming that following infection, 50 per cent of individuals become infectious each day.

2.7.3 **Time step size**

The time step size that we use in the model determines the values of our input parameters. Equations 2.1–2.4 are written assuming that the time steps in the model are of 1 unit (whatever that unit is, e.g. 1 day, 2 days, 1 month, 3 months etc.) and the units of the inputs, i.e. the rate at which susceptible individuals are infected (λ_t), the rate at which individuals become infectious (f) and the rate at which individuals recover (r) use the same time units. For example, if the equations use time steps of one day, then the rate at which individuals become infectious should be a *daily* rate. If they use a half day time step, then this rate should be the rate per half day.

If we know the rate per unit of time (e.g. per day), we can convert it to a rate for another time unit by scaling it up or down accordingly.

For example, if pre-infectious individuals become infectious (f) at a rate of 1 per cent per day, 2 per cent will become infectious every two days, 0.5 per cent will become infectious every half day etc. Note that such scaling becomes inappropriate if the difference between the time steps is large. For example, we could not say that the rate per 200 days would be $200 \times 0.01 \times 100\% = 200\%$.

Similarly, if the average life expectancy of a population is 60 years, the average mortality rate is 1/(average life expectancy) and equals 1/60 per year or 1/(60×365) per day or 0.5/(60×365) per half day.

Panel 2.6 discusses how difference equations are sometimes written using a time step size of t.

Influenza example

For our influenza problem, our β parameter was 10^{-5} per day, which is equivalent to 0.5×10^{-5} per half day. We will return to the issue of time step size in the next chapter. For now, we will just use a time step size of 1 day.

Panel 2.6 Other notation for difference equations

The following notation might also be seen in the literature for Equations 2.1–2.4:

$$S_{t+\delta t} = S_t - \lambda_t S_t \delta t \qquad\qquad 2.18$$

$$E_{t+\delta t} = E_t + \lambda_t S_t \delta t - f E_t \delta t \qquad\qquad 2.19$$

$$I_{t+\delta t} = I_t + f E_t \delta t - r I_t \delta t \qquad\qquad 2.20$$

$$R_{t+\delta t} = R_t + r I_t \delta t \qquad\qquad 2.21$$

The symbol 'δt' here symbolizes the size of a small time step. The small Greek letter δ ('delta') is traditionally used in mathematics in front of the symbol for some quantity to reflect a small change in that quantity. For example, if we used the letter 'a' to reflect 'age', we would use the notation 'δa' to reflect a small change in age.

In Equation 2.18, $S_{t+\delta t}$ reflects the number of susceptible individuals at some time $t+\delta t$, i.e. a short time of duration δt after time t. Similarly, $E_{t+\delta t}$ in Equation 2.19 reflects the number of individuals who are pre-infectious at some time $t+\delta t$, i.e. a short time of duration δt after time t etc.

Following the logic described in section 2.7.3, the terms involving λ_t, f and r include a scaling factor δt so that they reflect the number of individuals who move from one category to the next between time t and $t+\delta t$. For example, the term $\lambda_t S_t \delta t$ reflects the *number of individuals who are infected between time t and $t+\delta t$*. According to this notation, λ_t reflects the so-called 'instantaneous rate' (i.e. the rate at precisely the instant at time t) at which susceptible individuals are infected.

2.8 Setting up the model

Once all the input parameters have been specified, the model equations can be set up using a spreadsheet or a computer program and used to predict the number of susceptible, pre-infectious, infectious and immune individuals over time (Model 2.1, online).

Figure 2.8 shows predictions from this model of the number of susceptible, infectious and immune individuals over time. This highlights the fact that once a new strain of influenza enters a population, the proportion of individuals who have experienced influenza infection by the end (i.e. the proportion immune) is unlikely to be 100 per cent. We will discuss the factors which influence this proportion in Chapter 4.

2.9 Final stages in model development: model validation, optimization and prediction

Before a model is used for any serious analyses, it needs to be validated, which involves checking model outputs against independent data sets. Considering our influenza

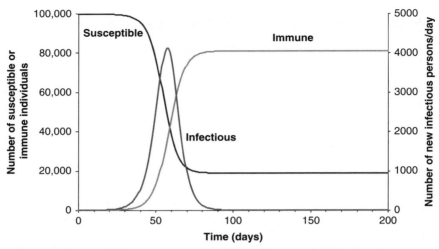

Fig. 2.8 Predictions of the number of susceptible and immune individuals and the daily numbers of infectious individuals over time following the introduction of one infectious person into a totally susceptible population comprising 100,000 individuals obtained using the difference equations for the influenza model described in this chapter (Model 2.1, online).

model, for example, we have assumed given values for the basic reproduction number and the pre-infectious and infectious periods. It would therefore be reasonable to check that the predicted proportion of individuals who are immune at the end of the epidemic is consistent with serological data collected at the end of previous pandemics. For age-stratified models, it would be appropriate to check that predictions of the proportion of individuals in different age groups who were immune at the end were consistent with the observed proportions of individuals in different age groups who were seropositive at the end of previous pandemics or the age-specific clinical attack rates.

Additionally, as described above, if given input parameters are unknown, they can be estimated using the model by fitting model predictions to the data available. For our influenza model, if the basic reproduction number, the pre-infectious and infectious periods were unknown (as might be the case during the early stages of a pandemic) they can be estimated by fitting model predictions of the weekly or daily numbers of cases to the numbers of cases seen each day or week during a pandemic (see section 4.2.5 and Panel 4.2). For this process, we use some goodness of fit statistic, which measures the distance between the model prediction and the observed data, and we vary the unknown parameters until we obtain the smallest distance and the 'best fit'.

Once the model has been validated, it may be used for detailed analyses, such as predicting the impact of control strategies. Predictions typically depend on the assumptions and the input parameters which went into the model. For example, the impact of vaccinating children against influenza or other infections will depend on contact patterns between individuals in the population. Similarly, the impact of treating the 'core group' in a model of the transmission of sexually transmitted infections will depend on contact patterns between the core group and other individuals in the population. It is therefore very important to use the model to identify the sensitivity of model prediction to different assumptions.

These issues are discussed in later chapters.

2.10 Summary

This chapter has illustrated the key steps for setting up models. Once the question to be addressed and the relevant information have been identified, the structure of the model needs to be decided. This is determined largely by the natural history of the infection (whether the infection can be classified as SI, SIS, SIRS etc.), the accuracy and time period over which the model predictions are required and the research question. Models are classified into two broad categories, namely those which are deterministic, describing what happens on average in a population, and those which are stochastic, which allow chance to influence transmission, progress or other key events in the model. Deterministic models are set up using difference or differential equations. Difference equations describe the number of individuals in a given category at some time in the future (e.g. tomorrow) in terms of the number at a previous time (e.g. today). Differential equations, which will be discussed in the next chapter, describe transmission assuming that events occur continuously.

For models which describe transmission between individuals, the infection risk is calculated at each time step using the rate at which two specific individuals come into effective contact per unit time (β) and the number of infectious individuals, with the simplest assumption being that individuals contact each other randomly. Models also require other input parameters, such as the duration of infectiousness and the rate at which individuals recover, which can be estimated from data on the pre-infectious period and the duration of infectiousness. Methods for refining these assumptions, for example, to assume that contact differs between age groups, are discussed in later chapters.

2.11 Exercises

2.1 The following shows a diagram of the Ross–Macdonald[26] model for the transmission of malaria involving humans and mosquitoes. Each of the compartments represents the proportion of individuals or mosquitoes in the population that are susceptible or infected. The dotted arrows simply reflect the fact that the prevalence of infection in humans (or mosquitoes) influences the rate at which mosquitoes (or humans) are infected. The risk of infection among humans and mosquitoes at time t are denoted by λ_t^h and λ_t^m respectively; r is the recovery rate from infection among humans, μ and b are the *per capita* death and birth rates respectively among mosquitoes.

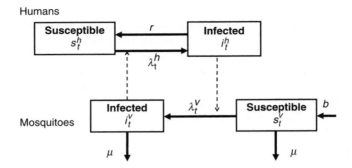

a) Write down the difference equations for this model.

b) What factors need to be accounted for when writing down the expression for the risk of infection among humans and mosquitoes?

2.2

   (a) Rewrite Equations 2.1–2.4 to incorporate the following assumptions:

      i) Susceptible, pre-infectious, infectious and immune individuals die at the same rate.

      ii) Individuals are born into the population fully susceptible to infection.

   (b) Would these assumptions be plausible if we were seeking to describe the transmission dynamics of measles or rubella? If they are implausible, how would you modify your assumptions?

   (c) Rewrite the equations in part (a) to assume that a fixed proportion (v) of newborns are immunized.

   2.3 Draw the model corresponding to the following equations:

$$S_{t+1} = S_t - \lambda_t S_t + r_1 I_t$$
$$I_{t+1} = I_t + \lambda_t S_t - r_2 I_t - r_1 I_t$$
$$R_{t+1} = R_t + r_2 I_t$$

How would you classify this model?

References

1 van Geuns HA, Meijer J, Styblo K. Results of contact examination in Rotterdam, 1967–1969. *Bull Int Union Tuberc* 1975; 50(1):107–121.

2 Dowdle WR, Ferrera W, De Salles Gomes LF *et al.* WHO collaborative study on the sero-epidemiology of rubella in Caribbean and Middle and South American populations in 1968. *Bull World Health Organ* 1970; 42(3):419–422.

3 Habbema JD, De Vlas SJ, Plaisier AP, van Oortmarssen GJ. The microsimulation approach to epidemiologic modeling of helminthic infections, with special reference to schistosomiasis. *Am J Trop Med Hyg* 1996; 55(5 Suppl):165–169.

4 Carrat F, Vergu E, Ferguson NM *et al.* Time lines of infection and disease in human influenza: a review of volunteer challenge studies. *Am J Epidemiol* 2008; 167(7):775–785.

5 Whitley RJ, Hayden FG, Reisinger KS *et al.* Oral oseltamivir treatment of influenza in children. *Pediatr Infect Dis J* 2001; 20(2):127–133.

6 Mills CE, Robins JM, Lipsitch M. Transmissibility of 1918 pandemic influenza. *Nature* 2004; 432(7019):904–906.

7 Ferguson NM, Cummings DA, Cauchemez S *et al.* Strategies for containing an emerging influenza pandemic in Southeast Asia. *Nature* 2005; 437(7056):209–214.

8 Vynnycky E, Trindall A, Mangtani P. Estimates of the reproduction numbers of Spanish influenza using morbidity data. *Int J Epidemiol* 2007; 36(4):881–889.

9 Longini IM, Jr., Halloran ME, Nizam A, Yang Y. Containing pandemic influenza with antiviral agents. *Am J Epidemiol* 2004; 159(7):623–633.

10 Chowell G, Nishiura H, Bettencourt LM. Comparative estimation of the reproduction number for pandemic influenza from daily case notification data. *J R Soc Interface* 2007; 4(12):155–166.

11 Glezen WP. Emerging infections: pandemic influenza. *Epidemiol Rev* 1996; 18(1):64–76.

12 Holmes KK, Sparling PF, Mardh P, Lemon S, Piot P, Wasserheit JN. *Sexually transmitted diseases, 3rd edn.* New York: McGraw-Hill; 1999.

13 van Boven M, de Melker HE, Schellekens JF, Kretzschmar M. Waning immunity and subclinical infection in an epidemic model: implications for pertussis in The Netherlands. *Math Biosci* 2000; 164(2):161–182.

14 van Boven M, de Melker HE, Schellekens JF, Kretzschmar M. A model-based evaluation of the 1996–7 pertussis epidemic in The Netherlands. *Epidemiol Infect* 2001; 127(1):73–85.

15 Vynnycky E, Pitman R, Siddiqui R, Gay N, Edmunds WJ. Estimating the impact of childhood influenza vaccination programmes in England and Wales. *Vaccine* 2008; 26(41):5321–5330.

16 Finkenstadt BF, Morton A, Rand DA. Modelling antigenic drift in weekly flu incidence. *Stat Med* 2005; 24(22):3447–3461.

17 Dye C, Garnett GP, Sleeman K, Williams BG. Prospects for worldwide tuberculosis control under the WHO DOTS strategy. Directly observed short-course therapy. *Lancet* 1998; 352(9144):1886–1891.

18 Murray CJL, Styblo K, Rouillon A. Tuberculosis. In Jamison DT, Mosley WH, Measham AR, Bobadilla JL, eds, *Disease control priorities in developing countries, 1st edn.* Oxford: Oxford Universty Press; 1993, pp. 233–259.

19 May RM. Uses and abuses of mathematics in biology. *Science* 2004; 303(5659):790–793.

20 Plaisier AP, van Oortmarssen GJ, Habbema JD, Remme J, Alley ES. ONCHOSIM: a model and computer simulation program for the transmission and control of onchocerciasis. *Comput Methods Programs Biomed* 1990; 31(1):43–56.

21 Longini IM, Jr., Nizam A, Xu S *et al.* Containing pandemic influenza at the source. *Science* 2005; 309(5737):1083–1087.

22 Germann TC, Kadau K, Longini IM, Jr., Macken CA. Mitigation strategies for pandemic influenza in the United States. *Proc Natl Acad Sci USA* 2006; 103(15):5935–5940.

23 Ferguson NM, Cummings DA, Fraser C, Cajka JC, Cooley PC, Burke DS. Strategies for mitigating an influenza pandemic. *Nature* 2006; 442(7101):448–452.

24 Abbey H. An examination of the Reed–Frost theory of epidemics. *Hum Biol* 1952; 24:201–233.

25 Wearing HJ, Rohani P, Keeling MJ. Appropriate models for the management of infectious diseases. *PLoS Med* 2005; 2(7):e174.

26 Macdonald G. The analysis of equilibrium in malaria. *Trop Dis Bull* 1952; 49:813–829.

27 Korenromp EL, van Vliet C, Bakker RH, De Vlas SJ, Habbema JDF. HIV spread and partnership reduction for different patterns of sexual behaviour—a study with the microsimulation model STDSIM. *Math Popul Studies* 2000; 8:135–173.

28 Sutherland I, Svandova E, Radhakrishna S. The development of clinical tuberculosis following infection with tubercle bacilli. 1. A theoretical model for the development of clinical tuberculosis following infection, linking from data on the risk of tuberculous infection and the incidence of clinical tuberculosis in the Netherlands. *Tubercle* 1982; 63(4):255–268.

29 Anderson RM, May RM. *Infectious diseases of humans. Dynamics and control.* Oxford: Oxford University Press; 1992.

30 Hunt S. Housing-related disorders. In Charlton J, Murphy M, eds, *The health of adult Britain, 1841–1994.* London: The Stationery Office; 1997, pp. 157–170.

31 Hatchett RJ, Mecher CE, Lipsitch M. Public health interventions and epidemic intensity during the 1918 influenza pandemic. *Proc Natl Acad Sci USA* 2007; 104(18):7582–7587.

32 Bootsma MC, Ferguson NM. The effect of public health measures on the 1918 influenza pandemic in U.S. cities. *Proc Natl Acad Sci USA* 2007; 104(18):7588–7593.

33 Anderson RM, May RM. Population biology of infectious diseases: Part I. *Nature* 1979; 280(5721):361–367.

34 Hamer WH. Epidemic disease in England—the evidence of variability and of persistency of type. *Lancet* 1906;(i):733–739.

35 de Jong M, Diekmann O, Heesterbeek H. How does transmission of infection depend on population size. In Mollison D, ed., *Epidemic models: their structure and relation to data.* Cambridge: Press Syndicate of the University of Cambridge; 1995, pp. 84–94.

36 Keeling MJ, Rohani P. *Modeling infectious diseases in humans and animals.* Princeton, NJ and Oxford: Princeton University Press; 2008.

37 McCallum H, Barlow N, Hone J. How should pathogen transmission be modelled? *Trends Ecol Evol* 2001; 16(6):295–300.

38 McLean AR, Anderson RM. Measles in developing countries. Part II. The predicted impact of mass vaccination. *Epidemiol Infect* 1988; 100(3):419–442.

39 McLean AR, Anderson RM. Measles in developing countries. Part I. Epidemiological parameters and patterns. *Epidemiol Infect* 1988; 100(1):111–133.

40 Vynnycky E, Gay NJ, Cutts FT. The predicted impact of private sector MMR vaccination on the burden of congenital rubella syndrome. *Vaccine* 2003; 20;21(21–22):2708–2719.

41 Heesterbeek JAP, Roberts MG. Mathematical models for microparasites of wildlife. In Grenfell BT, Dobson AP, eds, *Ecology of infectious diseases in natural populations.* Cambridge: Cambridge University Press; 1995, pp. 90–122.

Chapter 3

How are models set up?
II. An introduction to differential equations

3.1 Overview and objectives

The last chapter discussed the methods for setting models describing the transmission of infections using difference equations, which use discrete time steps, such as 1, 2, 3 days etc. This chapter discusses some limitations of difference equations and introduces the methods for setting up models using differential equations, which describe events occurring in continuous time.

By the end of this chapter you should:

◆ Understand the relationship between difference and differential equations;

◆ Be able to write down models describing the transmission dynamics of an infection using differential equations;

◆ Know when you might use differential equations;

◆ Understand how differential equations are used to make predictions;

◆ Understand the differential equations underlying the simplest models, which describe the size of a given quantity (such as population size) assuming that it changes at a constant rate over time.

3.2 How reliable are difference equations?

In the last chapter, we set up the following model describing the transmission dynamics of an immunizing infection in a closed population using the difference equations below:

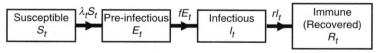

Fig. 3.1 General structure of a model describing the transmission dynamics of an immunizing infection.

$$S_{t+1} = S_t - \lambda_t S_t \qquad\qquad 3.1$$

$$E_{t+1} = E_t + \lambda_t S_t - f E_t \qquad\qquad 3.2$$

$$I_{t+1} = I_t + f E_t - r I_t \qquad\qquad 3.3$$

$$R_{t+1} = R_t + r I_t \qquad\qquad 3.4$$

Here, λ_t is the rate at which susceptible individuals are infected between time t and $t+1$, (also known as the 'force of infection'), f is the rate at which pre-infectious individuals become infectious between time t and $t+1$, and r is the rate at which infectious individuals become immune between time t and $t+1$.

A question that often arises when setting up models using difference equations is 'Does the size of the time step matter?'

To answer this question, we consider Figure 3.2, which shows how the epidemic curve that is predicted for measles or influenza following the introduction of one infectious person into a totally susceptible population, using the difference equations model described above, changes with the size of the time step.

Specifically, as the time step size increases, the predicted epidemic curve becomes less smooth, and once it becomes too large, the model predicts nonsense results. For measles, for example, it predicts that the number of infectious individuals drops below zero after the 75th day if the time step is 5 days; for influenza, the predicted number of infectious individuals fluctuates between zero and some other values once the time step is two days.

Why does the time step size influence the model predictions?

As discussed in section 2.7.3, when we change the step size in the model, we need to scale all the parameters in the equations accordingly. For example, if the rate at which two specific individuals come into effective contact per unit time (β) is 10^{-5} per day, the corresponding value per 2 days is 2×10^{-5}. Once the time step reaches a certain

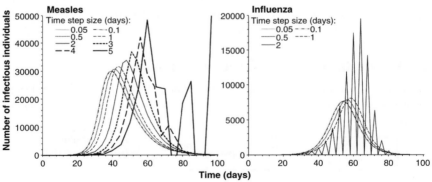

Fig. 3.2 Comparison between predictions of the numbers of infectious individuals for measles and influenza obtained using the difference equations model described in Figure 3.1, using time steps ranging between 0.05 and 5 days. For measles, $R_0 = 13$, and the average pre-infectious and infectious periods are assumed to equal eight and seven days respectively. For influenza, $R_0 = 2$, and the average pre-infectious and infectious periods are both assumed to be two days. The population comprises 100,000 individuals and 1 infectious person is introduced at the start (See Model 3.1, online).

size, β becomes so large that more individuals are predicted to be newly infected at some time step than were susceptible at the start of the time step. This, in turn eventually leads to predictions that the number of infectious individuals in the population drops below zero (see Example 3.2.1).

3.2.1 Example: The effect of the size of the time step on model predictions

The following table shows the predictions of the number of susceptible, infectious and newly infected individuals produced by the difference equations model discussed in the last chapter; the input parameters are those for measles (see Model 3.1 online). These describe predictions for the 50th–55th days after the introduction of an infectious case into a totally susceptible population, using a 1 day time step.

Table 3.1 Predictions of the number of susceptible, infectious and newly infected individuals obtained using the difference equations model described in chapter 2, using the parameter values for measles (see caption to Figure 3.2 for details). These predictions are obtained using a time step of 1 day, with $\beta = 1.86 \times 10^{-5}$ per time step.

Day	Number of individuals who are:		
	Susceptible	Infectious	Newly infected by the end of the current time step $(\beta \times S_t \times I_t)$
50	1.64	24,038	0.73
51	0.91	22,374	0.38
52	0.53	20,727	0.20
53	0.33	19,122	0.12
54	0.21	17,576	0.07
55	0.14	16,103	0.04

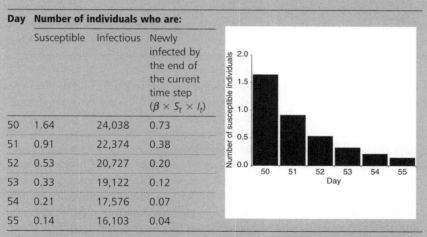

In this situation, the total number of individuals who are newly infected during the 50th–54th days is 1.50 (i.e. 0.73 + 0.38 + 0.20 + 0.12 + 0.07).

When the time step is five days, the model predicts 'nonsense' results for the 50th and 55th day, as shown in Table 3.2.

In this instance, the model predicts that 53,944 individuals are newly infected between the 50th and 55th day. This number exceeds the number of susceptible individuals who were in the population on the 50th day (50,354), which then leads to unrealistic predictions of negative numbers of susceptible individuals on day 55.

Table 3.2 Predictions of the number of susceptible, infectious and newly infected individuals obtained using the difference equations model described in chapter 2, using the parameter values for measles (see caption to Figure 3.2 for details). These predictions are obtained using a time step of 5 days, with $\beta=9.29\times10^{-5}$ per time step.

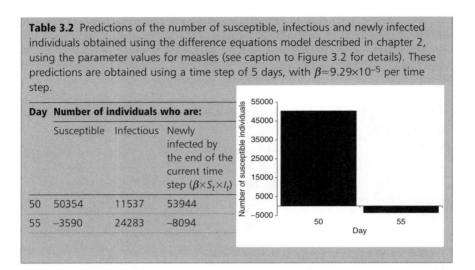

Day	Number of individuals who are:		
	Susceptible	Infectious	Newly infected by the end of the current time step $(\beta\times S_t\times I_t)$
50	50354	11537	53944
55	-3590	24283	-8094

At the other extreme, as the size of the time step *decreases*, the predicted epidemic curve becomes more and more smooth and, once the step size is sufficiently small, further decreases in the step size do not visibly affect the model's predictions. In fact, as the time step decreases, the closer the model comes to describing events which are occurring continuously, or, reality itself, given that, in reality, events occur continuously, rather than at discrete time intervals.

In general, the size of the time step in a difference equations model should be less than the shortest average duration that individuals spend in a given compartment. However, the actual size is difficult to prescribe.

For example, when the input parameters are set to be those for measles ($R_0 = 13$, average pre-infectious and infectious periods are eight and seven days respectively), the difference equations model described on page 41 predicts that there are negative numbers of susceptible individuals on day 46 if the time step is 2 days (which is <50 per cent of the duration of the infectious period). On the other hand, for influenza, if the time step is 1 day (i.e. equal to 50 per cent of the pre-infectious or infectious periods) then the number of individuals in each compartment is always positive and the model still gives sensible predictions. If we were to model the transmission of *M tuberculosis*, then since the time period between infection and disease onset can be many years, we would still get sensible predictions, even if we were to use a difference equations model which uses time steps of 1 year. Methods for avoiding problems relating to the step size are discussed in Panel 3.1.

3.3 **What are differential equations and how are they written?**

In the modelling literature, models are frequently written using differential equations. For example, the following are the differential equations which would be written for

---

Panel 3.1 Avoiding problems with the size of the time step for a model set up using difference equations

To avoid problems associated with taking time steps which are too large, checks should be included at each stage of the model's calculations to ensure that the number of individuals in any compartment do not become negative. For example, considering the difference equations model that we discussed in the last chapter, if we were to set up the model in a spreadsheet, then we might include an 'if' statement at each time step in the model, which would inform the user whenever $\beta S_t I_t$ was bigger than S_t.

Applied mathematicians and numerical analysts tend to use a different approach to determine an appropriate step size, namely they keep reducing the step size progressively until further reductions do not lead to any further changes in the key model predictions, i.e. the model predictions 'converge'. According to Figure 3.2, models of both measles and influenza transmission appear to have 'converged' once the step size has reached 0.1 day, since predictions for models with a step size of less than 0.1 day are similar to those based on a 0.1 day step size.

---

the model describing the transmission dynamics for an immunizing infection in a closed population, which is discussed in section 3.1:

$$\frac{dS(t)}{dt} = -\lambda(t)S(t)$$

$$\frac{dE(t)}{dt} = \lambda(t)S(t) - f E(t)$$

$$\frac{dI(t)}{dt} = f E(t) - rI(t)$$

$$\frac{dR(t)}{dt} = rI(t)$$

Differential equations provide a means for avoiding the issues regarding the size of the time step by describing events occurring continuously, rather than at discrete time intervals. Before describing how differential equations are written, we first discuss what differential equations represent.

Differential equations are very closely related to difference equations, although they represent slightly different things. Using difference equations, for example, we can express the number of individuals in a given category (e.g. those susceptible) at a time $t+1$ in terms of the number present at a previous time t.

When describing events occurring continuously, on the other hand, it is often impossible to write down explicit expressions for the number of individuals in a given compartment at any given time in terms of other parameters or compartments in the model. For example, we normally cannot express the actual number of susceptible individuals at time t in terms of the number of infectious individuals at time t.

Instead, when we try to describe events occuring continuously, we work with a related quantity, namely the *rate of change* in the number of susceptible (or other)

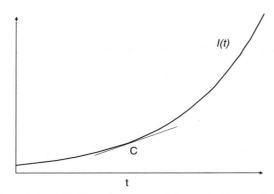

Fig. 3.3 Illustration of the definition of the rate of change in the number of infectious individuals, *I(t)*.

individuals over time, and this is written down using differential equations. The notation for the rate of change in the number of susceptible individuals over time is $\dfrac{dS(t)}{dt}$; the notation for the rate of change in the number of pre-infectious, infectious and immune individuals is $\dfrac{dE(t)}{dt}$, $\dfrac{dI(t)}{dt}$ and $\dfrac{dR(t)}{dt}$ respectively. We explain the origin of this notation later in this section.

How should we interpret differential equations?

Figure 3.3 shows how the number of infectious individuals might change over time following the introduction of infectious persons into a totally susceptible population. Since we are considering events occuring continuously, rather than at discrete time intervals, we will follow convention (see Panel 3.2) and use the notation *I(t)* rather than I_t to refer to the number of infectious persons at time *t*. Figure 3.3 also includes a line which just touches the curve of the number of infectious individuals at point C. By definition, the rate of change in the number of infectious individuals at point C is the gradient of this line.

The gradient or slope of a line (or a hill etc.) is the ratio between the amount by which the line goes up vertically and the amount by which the line goes across horizontally. If we add another point A on the line for the number of infectious persons a small distance away from C (see Figure 3.4), where A has the coordinates $(t+\delta t, I(t + \delta t))$, and draw a line between points A and C on this graph, then the slope of this line would be given by the ratio between the lengths of the lines AB and BC, i.e. $\dfrac{I(t+\delta t)-I(t)}{\delta t}$. The slope of this line, as it is currently drawn in Figure 3.4, would overestimate the gradient at point C. However, if we were to move point A closer to point C, so that the size of δt is as small as possible, then the slope of the line AC would eventually equal the gradient at point C.

This leads to the formal mathematical definition of the rate of change in the number of infectious persons, *I(t)* as 'the value of the expression $\dfrac{I(t+\delta t)-I(t)}{\delta t}$ as

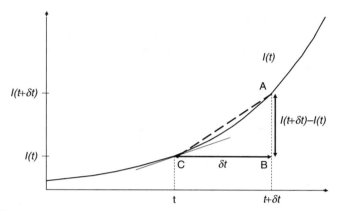

Fig. 3.4 Illustration of the definition of the rate of change in the number of infectious persons $I(t)$ over time.

the size of δt approaches zero (i.e. becomes 'very small') or, using mathematical notation,

$$\lim_{\delta t \to 0} \frac{I(t+\delta t)-I(t)}{\delta t}$$

3.5

As this expression is cumbersome to write, the rate of change is normally written as $\frac{dI(t)}{dt}$, where the '$dI(t)$' component conveys the fact that we are taking the *difference* between $I(t+\delta t)$ and $I(t)$, and the 'dt' component conveys the fact that we are taking δt to be as small and as close to zero as possible. Quite often, the 't' in parentheses is dropped altogether for convenience, so that $\frac{dI(t)}{dt}$ would be written as $\frac{dI}{dt}$. Other notation that might be used for the rate of change in the number of infectious persons is $\dot{I}(t)$ or $I'(t)$.

If the number of infectious individuals depended on something other than time, such as age ('a'), we would have used the notation $I(a)$ for the number of infectious individuals of age a, and we would be interested in calculating how $I(a)$ changes with age. In this situation, the mathematical notation for this rate of change would be $\frac{dI(a)}{da}$.

The rate of change of something is also known as 'the derivative'. If we are calculating the rate of change in, for example, the number of infectious individuals over time, we might also say that we are calculating 'the derivative of the number of infectious individuals ($I(t)$) with respect to t'.

Difference and differential equations are written using distinct notation – see Figure 3.5 and Panel 3.2 for the key distinctions.

In addition, the definitions of the parameters such as λ, f and r which are used in *differential* equations differ slightly from their definitions in *difference* equations. In difference equations, we should use risks since we are considering the proportion of

Difference equations model:

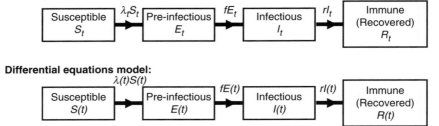

Fig. 3.5 Comparison between the notation used for difference and differential equations.

individuals that move between categories in each time step; in differential equations, we should use rates, since we are considering individuals moving between categories continuously. However, as discussed in Chapter 2, risks and rates are numerically similar if they are small (e.g. <10%—see Figure 2.5) and therefore rates are commonly used in difference equations.

The differential equations describing the rate of change in the number of individuals, over time, such as those shown in Panel 3.2, can be obtained by using an intuitive argument (see section 3.4).

Panel 3.2 A comparison between difference and differential equations

Difference equations which describe the numbers of susceptible, pre-infectious, infectious, immune individuals at time t	Differential equations which describe the rate of change in the number of susceptible, pre-infectious, infectious, immune individuals at time t
$S_{t+1} = S_t - \lambda_t S_t$	$\dfrac{dS(t)}{dt} = -\lambda(t)S(t)$
$E_{t+1} = E_t + \lambda_t S_t - f E_t$	$\dfrac{dE(t)}{dt} = \lambda(t)S(t) - f E(t)$
$I_{t+1} = I_t + f E_t - r I_t$	$\dfrac{dI(t)}{dt} = f E(t) - r I(t)$
$R_{t+1} = R_t + r I_t$	$\dfrac{dR(t)}{dt} = r I(t)$

Key definitions

Difference equation		Differential equations	
S_t	The number of susceptible individuals at time t	$\dfrac{dS(t)}{dt}$	The rate of change in the number of susceptible individuals at time t
E_t	The number of pre-infectious individuals at time t	$\dfrac{dE(t)}{dt}$	The rate of change in the number of pre-infectious individuals at time t
I_t	The number of infectious individuals at time t	$\dfrac{dI(t)}{dt}$	The rate of change in the number of infectious individuals at time t
R_t	The number of recovered (immune) individuals at time t	$\dfrac{dR(t)}{dt}$	The rate of change in the number of recovered (immune) individuals at time t
λ_t	The risk of a susceptible individual becoming infected between time t and $t+1$	$\lambda(t)$	The rate at which susceptible individuals becoming infected per unit time, at time t
f	The risk of an individual in the pre-infectious category becoming infectious between time t and $t+1$	f	The rate at which individuals in the pre-infectious category become infectious per unit time
r	The risk of an infectious individual recovering between time t and $t+1$	r	The rate at which infectious individuals recover (become immune) per unit time

Note that, when writing the number of individuals at a given time t, the t is written using a subscript if we are using difference equations and in parentheses if we are using differential equations. For example, the number of susceptible individuals at time t is represented using the notation $S(t)$ in differential equations, as compared with S_t in difference equations, reflecting the fact that we are describing events occurring continuously rather than at discrete time steps.

3.4 How do we write down differential equations?

Differential equations describe the rate of change of a given quantity relative to something else.

The rate of change in the number of individuals in a given category over time is just given by the *difference* between the number of individuals *entering* the category and the number of individuals *leaving* the category per unit time, or

+ the number entering the category per unit time

− the number leaving the category per unit time

3.4.1 Differential equations for the rate of change in the number of susceptible individuals

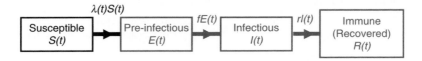

Returning to our model describing the transmission of an immunizing infection, and considering susceptible individuals, we see that, as no-one enters the susceptible class and newly infected individuals exit this category, the rate of change in the number of susceptible individuals is given by the expression:

$$\frac{dS(t)}{dt} = -\text{the number of susceptible individuals who are newly infected per unit time}$$

As discussed in section 2.6.1, the number of susceptible individuals who are newly infected per unit time is given by the product of the force of infection ($\lambda(t)$) and the number of susceptible individuals at time t (i.e. $\lambda(t)S(t)$). Using mathematical notation, the above equation would be written as:

$$\frac{dS(t)}{dt} = -\lambda(t)S(t)$$

3.6

If we assume that individuals contact each other randomly, then, by analogy with Equation 2.5, $\lambda(t)$ can be replaced by the equation

$$\lambda(t) = \beta I(t)$$

3.7

where β is the rate at which two specific individuals come into effective contact per unit time and $I(t)$ is the number of infectious individuals at time t.

3.4.2 Differential equations for the rate of change in the number of pre-infectious individuals

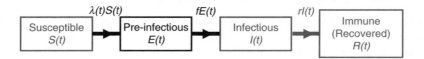

Considering individuals in the pre-infectious category in the same model, we see that newly infected individuals enter this category and infectious individuals exit this category.

The rate of change in the number of pre-infectious individuals is therefore given by the expression:

$$\frac{dE(t)}{dt} = +\text{ (the number of susceptible individuals who are newly infected}$$

per unit time) − (the number of pre-infectious individuals who become infectious per unit time).

The second term in this equation is given by the expression $fE(t)$, where f is the rate at which individuals become infectious. Using mathematical notation, the rate of change in the number of pre-infectious individuals is written as:

$$\frac{dE(t)}{dt} = \lambda(t)S(t) - f E(t)$$

3.8

3.4.3 Differential equations for the rate of change in the number of infectious and immune individuals

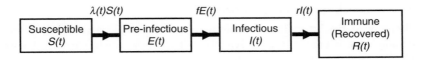

Continuing the logic in sections 3.4.1 and 3.4.2, we can write down the rate of change in the number of infectious and immune individuals as follows:

$$\frac{dI(t)}{dt} = fE(t) - rI(t)$$

3.9

$$\frac{dR(t)}{dt} = rI(t)$$

3.10

Here r is the rate at which infectious individuals recover and become immune. The expressions for the rate of change in the number of individuals in a given compartment can also be obtained by considering the formal mathematical definition of the 'rate of change' (see Appendix section A.1.1).

There are several ways of checking that the differential equations for a given model have been written correctly, as described below. Some of these methods are similar to those used for checking difference equations (Panel 2.2).

3.4.4 Methods for checking differential equations

3.4.4.1 Drawing model diagrams
We can check whether our set of differential equations have been written correctly by drawing the model diagram corresponding to those equations. To do this, we note that

the number of equations in our model should equal the number of compartments, and if there is a minus or a plus sign in front of a term in an equation, then the quantity reflected by that term leaves or enters that compartment, respectively. For example, it is impossible to draw a diagram corresponding to the following differential equations, which implies that the differential equations have been written incorrectly.

$$\frac{dS(t)}{dt} = -\lambda(t)S(t) + rR(t)$$

$$\frac{dE(t)}{dt} = \lambda(t)S(t) - fE(t)$$

$$\frac{dI(t)}{dt} = fE(t) - rI(t)$$

$$\frac{dR(t)}{dt} = rI(t)$$

3.11

The above check is closely related to that described in Section 3.4.4.3.

3.4.4.2 Check for population size

Summing up the differential equations in the model provides a helpful check that the demographic assumptions have been incorporated in the model correctly. For example, if we add the differential equations for our model describing the transmission of an immunizing infection (Equations 3.6 and 3.8–3.10) in a closed population, we obtain the following result:

$$\frac{dS(t)}{dt} + \frac{dE(t)}{dt} + \frac{dI(t)}{dt} + \frac{dR(t)}{dt} = -\lambda(t)S(t) + \lambda(t)S(t) - fE(t) + fE(t) - rI(t) + rI(t) = 0$$

Since $\frac{dS(t)}{dt} + \frac{dE(t)}{dt} + \frac{dI(t)}{dt} + \frac{dR(t)}{dt}$ represents the rate of change of the total population size, our finding that this equals zero implies that the population in the model remains unchanged over time, which is consistent with our assumption that the population is closed.

3.4.4.3 Check the number and directions of the arrows

If the differential equations for a given compartment have been written correctly, the number of terms that make up the differential equation for that compartment should equal the number of arrows that go into or out of that compartment in the model diagram. Also, the direction of the arrow determines whether or not there is a plus or minus sign in front of the term corresponding to that arrow: if an arrow goes out of the compartment, then the term for that arrow has a minus sign in front of it; otherwise, the term has a plus sign in front of it.

3.4.4.4 Example: a model describing the transmission dynamics of human respiratory syncytial virus

Human respiratory syncytial virus (RSV) is a leading cause of hospitalization among young children with infection of the respiratory tract.[1] RSV strains are divided into two broad groups, A and B. Transmission is thought to occur mainly via the hands into the nose or eyes.[1] Once infected, individuals can be reinfected, and thus older children and adults also experience morbidity associated wth RSV, although the infection in these age groups is not as well-recognized as that among young children.

Figure 3.6 shows the structure of the model describing the transmission dynamics of RSV used by White *et al.*[2] Individuals are stratified into those who are susceptible ($S(t)$), those who have been infected and are infectious for the first time ($I_s(t)$), those who have recovered from infection ($R(t)$), and those who have been reinfected and are infectious ($I_r(t)$). The rate at which recovered individuals are reinfected differs by a factor k from the rate at which susceptible individuals are infected for the first time. The rate at which infectious individuals recover to become partially immune to further reinfection (w_r) is assumed to be independent of whether they have experienced infection for the first or subsequent time. Recovered and infectious individuals can become fully susceptible to infection again at a rate (w_s) which is identical for all individuals.

The differential equations for this model are as follows:

$$\frac{dS(t)}{dt} = -\lambda(t)S(t) + w_s I_s(t) + w_s I_r(t) + w_s R(t)$$

$$\frac{dI_s(t)}{dt} = \lambda(t)S(t) - w_r I_s(t) - w_s I_s(t)$$

$$\frac{dI_r(t)}{dt} = k\lambda(t)R(t) - w_r I_r(t) - w_s I_r(t)$$

$$\frac{dR(t)}{dt} = -k\lambda(t)R(t) + w_r I_s(t) + w_r I_r(t) - w_s R(t)$$

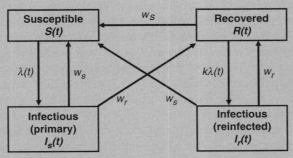

Fig. 3.6 General structure of the model describing the transmission dynamics of RSV of White *et al.*[2] The letters next to the arrows represent the rate at which individuals move from one category to the next.

The compartment for susceptible individuals has three arrows going into it (from the recovered, the infectious (primary) and the infectious (reinfected) compartments) and one arrow leaving it (reflecting susceptible individuals becoming newly infected). Consequently, the differential equation for the rate of change in the number of susceptible individuals consists of four terms, three of which have a plus sign in front of them, and the fourth has a minus sign in front of it.

Similarly, the compartment for infectious (primary) individuals has two arrows leaving it, representing infectious individuals recovering and either becoming fully susceptible, or recovering and becoming partially immune to reinfection. The compartment also has one arrow entering it, representing susceptible individuals becoming newly infected. Thus the equation for the rate of change in $I_s(t)$ has three terms, two of which have a minus sign in front of them, and the third has a plus sign in front of it.

3.5 How do we use differential equations to make predictions?

For many practical purposes, we can obtain a reasonable description of the transmission dynamics of an infection by using difference equations, with a time step which is sufficiently small (see section 3.2). Such models can be set up in a spreadsheet. However, the resulting spreadsheet can be large and too cumbersome for generating detailed long-term predictions, for example, of the number of infections occurring each day over a 100-year period (see Model 3.2, online).

At this stage, it becomes sensible to either set up the difference equations using a programming language (e.g. C, C++, Visual Basic, FORTRAN etc.) or to set up the model in a specialist modelling package. The latter normally deal with both difference and differential equations.

Several specialist packages, such as Berkeley Madonna, ModelMaker, Matlab, Mathematica, Maple and Stella are designed to manipulate differential equations. Each package converts the differential equations to difference equations using various techniques (e.g. Euler, Runge–Kutta, Bulirsch–Stoer etc.), which make special adjustments for the possible errors that are introduced during each time step. The Euler method is equivalent to setting up difference equations. An overview of one of these packages, Berkeley Madonna, which we will be using throughout the book, and which allows users to set up models using either equations or simply by drawing the model diagram, is provided online.

Note that for some simple models, as illustrated in the example below, we can get explicit expressions for the number of individuals in a given compartment in terms of the input parameters, without using specialist packages to manipulate the differential equations.

3.5.1 **A simple differential equation model: exponential decline or growth**

> **Example: calculating the size of a population assuming that individuals die at a constant rate**
>
> Suppose that we have a population with 1000 individuals who die at a rate of 0.1 per cent per year. How many of the original population of 1000 individuals will still be alive after 1, 2, 3, and 4 years?

To answer this question, we would set up a model with the following structure:

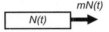

Here, $N(t)$ is the number of individuals at time t, m ($= 0.001$ per year) is the mortality rate and so $mN(t)$ is the number of individuals who die per unit time. The differential equation for this model is as follows:

$$\frac{dN(t)}{dt} = -mN(t) \qquad\qquad 3.12$$

This model belongs to the special class of models, which are used frequently in infectious disease epidemiology, biology and physics, and which we will use repeatedly in this book, that assume that the size of some quantity Q changes at a constant rate k. The rate of change in the size of quantity Q would then be written as follows:

$$\frac{dQ(t)}{dt} = -kQ(t) \qquad\qquad 3.13$$

For example, infectious disease models often make the simple assumption that newly infected individuals become infectious at a constant rate, or that infectious individuals stop being infectious at a constant rate (see Section 2.7.2).

It can be shown (see Appendix section A.1.2) that the size of quantity Q at a given time t is related to the mathematical constant e ($= 2.71828$) and k as follows:

$$Q(t) = Q(0)e^{-kt} \qquad\qquad 3.14$$

where $Q(0)$ is the size of quantity Q at the start. The size of Q is said to *decrease exponentially* over time if k is positive.

> **Example continued**
>
> Returning to the example above and applying Equation 3.14, we obtain the following expression for the size of the population at time t:
>
> $$N(t) = N(0)e^{-mt} \qquad\qquad 3.15$$

where $N(0)$ is the size of the population at the start. The corresponding expression which is obtained using difference equations is discussed in Panel 3.3.

Substituting for $N(0) = 1000$ and $m = 0.001$ per year into Equation 3.15, we obtain the following numbers of individuals (rounded to the nearest integer, i.e. whole number) in the population in years 1, 2, 3 and 4:

Year	N(t)
0	1000
1	$1000 \times e^{-0.001} = 999$
2	$1000 \times e^{-0.001 \times 2} = 998$
3	$1000 \times e^{-0.001 \times 3} = 997$
4	$1000 \times e^{-0.001 \times 4} = 996$

Panel 3.3 Derivation of the discrete-time equivalent of $N(t) = N(0)e^{-mt}$

Using difference equations notation, the size of the population at time t (N_t) would be written as follows:

$$N_{t+1} = N_t - m_r N_t \qquad 3.17$$

where m_r is the risk of dying between time t and $t+1$. Using the relationship between risks and rates (section 2.7.2), $m_r = 1 - e^{-m}$.

Substituting for $t = 0$ into Equation 3.17, we obtain the following relationship between N_1 and N_0:

$$N_1 = N_0 - m_r\, N_0 = (1 - m_r)N_0 \qquad 3.18$$

Similarly, substituting for $t = 1$ into Equation 3.17, we obtain the following relationship between N_2 and N_1:

$$N_2 = N_1 - m_r\, N_1 = (1 - m_r)N_1 \qquad 3.19$$

After substituting for $N_1 = (1 - m_r)N_0$ (Equation 3.18) into Equation 3.19, we obtain the following relationship between N_2 and N_0:

$$N_2 = (1 - m_r)N_1 = (1 - m_r)(1 - m_r)N_0 = (1 - m_r)^2 N_0 \qquad 3.20$$

Extending this logic, we obtain the following relationship between N_{t+1} and N_0:

$$N_{t+1} = (1 - m_r)^{t+1} N_0 \qquad 3.21$$

Panel 3.4 The relationship between risks and rates

As discussed in Panel 3.3, using difference equations notation, the size of the population discussed in section 3.5.1 at time t (N_t) would be written as follows:

$$N_{t+1} = N_t - m_r N_t \qquad\qquad 3.22$$

where m_r is the risk of dying between time t and $t+1$. At time $t = 1$, the number of individuals in the population is given by the expression:

$$N_1 = N_0 - m_r N_0 = (1 - m_r)N_0 \qquad\qquad 3.23$$

However, according to Equation 3.15, it is also given by the equation:

$$N(1) = N(0)e^{-m} \qquad\qquad 3.24$$

Equating Equation 3.23 to 3.24, and using the fact that N_0 must equal $N(0)$ (or 1000 in our example), we obtain the result:

$$1 - m_r = e^{-m} \qquad\qquad 3.25$$

or, equivalently:

$$m_r = 1 - e^{-m} \qquad\qquad 3.26$$

i.e. the risk$=1-e^{-\text{rate}}$.

As discussed in Panel 3.4, we can use Equation 3.15 to derive the relationship between risks and rates, i.e. risk $= 1-e^{-\text{rate}}$ (Panel 2.2). We can also use Equation 3.15 to prove the result that we use frequently throughout the text, namely that the average time to an event $=1/$(rate at which the event occurs) (see Appendix section A.1.3).

For example, the simplest models assume that individuals in the population die at a constant rate. With this assumption, the average life expectancy and the mortality rate (section 2.7.2) are related as follows:

$$\text{Average life expectancy} = 1/\text{Mortality rate} \qquad\qquad 3.27$$

Figure 3.7a shows predictions of the number of survivors in the population discussed above during the 100 years after the start, for values of the mortality rate of 0.001–0.05 per year, which according to Equation 3.27 are equivalent to values for the average life expectancy of between 20 (= 1/0.05) years and 1000 (= 1/0.001) years.

It is also worth noting that if the number of births and if the mortality rate has been the same over time for all individuals in a given population, then the age distribution in that population will be similar to that shown in Figure 3.7a. This age distribution is said to be exponential, and it is similar to one which might be seen in some developing countries (Figure 3.7b). We will be describing models using this and other kinds of age distributions later in this book.

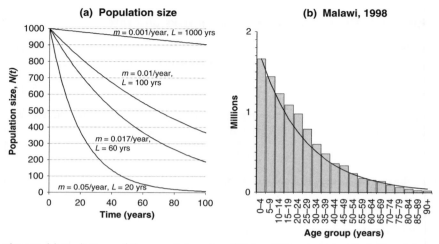

Fig. 3.7 (a) Predictions of the population size, *N(t)* for different assumptions about the annual mortality rate, *m*. The corresponding values for the life expectancy, *L*, for each value for the mortality rate are calculated using the relationship average life expectancy = 1/mortality rate (see section 2.7.2). (b) Population in Malawi (data source: National Statistical Office, Malawi and http://www.ons.gov.uk).

3.6 **Final word**

The equations discussed in this chapter are defined formally as 'ordinary differential equations', since they describe how something, such as the number of susceptible individuals changes only with respect to a single variable, i.e. time. In many models of the transmission of infections in human populations, we are also interested in how the number of susceptible, infectious, etc. individuals change with age as well.

Panel 3.5 provides a brief introduction to the methods for doing so and to partial differential equations; we will discuss methods for including age-structure into models in more detail in Chapter 5.

Panel 3.5 **Age-structured models and partial differential equations**

If we need to track the ages of individuals in our model over time we might use so-called 'partial differential equations' to describe the transmission dynamics. The equations for our model of the transmission of an immunizing infection would then be written as follows:

$$\frac{\partial S(a,t)}{\partial a} + \frac{\partial S(a,t)}{\partial t} = -\lambda(t)S(a,t)$$

$$\frac{\partial E(a,t)}{\partial a} + \frac{\partial E(a,t)}{\partial t} = \lambda(t)S(a,t) - fE(a,t)$$

$$\frac{\partial I(a,t)}{\partial a} + \frac{\partial I(a,t)}{\partial t} = fE(a,t) - rI(a,t)$$

$$\frac{\partial R(a,t)}{\partial a} + \frac{\partial R(a,t)}{\partial t} = rI(a,t)$$

The expression on the left-hand side of these equations, e.g. $\frac{\partial S(a,t)}{\partial a} + \frac{\partial S(a,t)}{\partial t}$ denotes the fact that the number of individuals in a given category changes according to age and over time. Unfortunately, these equations are more difficult to work with than are ordinary differential equations and generally require use of a programming language. For example, packages such as Berkeley Madonna cannot yet deal with partial differential equations. One method of overcoming this problem is to change the model so that individuals are stratified by the *year of birth* rather than age; the transmission dynamics within annual birth cohorts can then be described using ordinary differential equations[6] (see Chapter 5).

3.7 **Summary**

This chapter has discussed some limitations of difference equations and how the transmission dynamics of infections can be described using differential equations. These assume that individuals move between different categories (e.g. from the susceptible to the pre-infectious category) continuously, rather than at discrete time intervals. The expressions for differential equations can be obtained by considering how many individuals move into and out of each compartment per unit time. Several software packages can be used to make predictions using differential equations. These convert differential equations to difference equations and make adjustments for the error introduced by using difference equations. In many instances, predictions obtained by these packages will be very similar to those obtained using difference equations with a small time step. For the simplest models, such as those which describe the size of a population, assuming that individuals die at a constant rate, the differential equations do not need to be incorporated into software packages in order to make predictions, since it is possible to obtain an explicit expression for, for example, the population size at a given time.

In the next chapter, the differential equations describing the transmission dynamics will be studied in more detail to obtain insights into the dynamics of infections and the factors which influence the infection incidence and the course of epidemics.

3.8 **Exercises**

3.1 The following diagram shows the general structure of a model for the transmission dynamics of pertussis, which is similar to that developed by van Boven *et al.*,[3] which was intended to distinguish between individuals who were immunologically naive (i.e. those had never been infected before) and those whose immune system had been primed either through vaccination or following infection. The letters next to each arrow represent the rate at which individuals move from one category to the next.

a) Write down the differential equations for this model

b) Why might the authors have chosen to use this structure for the model, rather than a SIRS model?

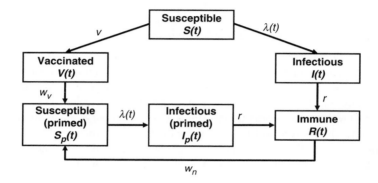

3.2

(a) Draw the model diagram corresponding to the following set of differential equations:

$$\frac{dS(t)}{dt} = -\lambda(t)S(t) - mS(t) + b(1-v)N(t)$$

$$\frac{dE(t)}{dt} = \lambda(t)S(t) - fE(t) - mE(t)$$

$$\frac{dI(t)}{dt} = fE(t) - rI(t) - mI(t)$$

$$\frac{dR(t)}{dt} = rI(t) + bvN(t) - mR(t)$$

$$N(t) = S(t) + E(t) + I(t) + R(t)$$

(b) The definitions of $\lambda(t)$, f and r for this model are provided in Panel 3.2, b is the per capita birth rate and v is the proportion of newborns that are vaccinated. How would you interpret:

(i) the parameter m?

(ii) $N(t)$?

(c) What assumption does this model make about the protection resulting from natural infection and vaccination?

3.3 The following shows a diagram of a model which tracks individuals from birth, assuming that they experience the same force of infection in each year of life. $s(t)$ and

$z(t)$ represent the proportions of individuals that are susceptible or have (ever) been infected by time t. (We will be discussing this model in detail in Chapter 5).

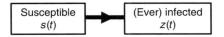

(a) Write down the differential equations for this model.
(b) Using the equations in section 3.5.1 and assuming, for simplicity, that individuals are susceptible at birth, write down the proportion of individuals of age a that:

    i) should still be susceptible;

    ii) should have ever been infected.

(c) Calculate the proportion of individuals that should have been infected by age 5, 10, 20 and 60 years in settings in which the force of infection is:

    i) 1% per year (similar to that for *M tuberculosi*s in parts of Africa[4, 5]);

    ii) 10% per year (similar to that for a low transmission setting for rubella—see Chapter 5);

    iii) 20% per year (similar to that for a high transmission setting for rubella—see Chapter 5).

Assuming that once infected, individuals are immune for life, what do you conclude about the burden of rubella infection among adults in low and high transmission settings?

References

1 Hall CB. Respiratory syncytial virus and parainfluenza virus. *N Engl J Med* 2001; 344(25):1917–1928.

2 White LJ, Mandl JN, Gomes MG *et al.* Understanding the transmission dynamics of respiratory syncytial virus using multiple time series and nested models. *Math Biosci* 2007; 209(1):222–239.

3 van Boven M, de Melker HE, Schellekens JF, Kretzschmar M. A model-based evaluation of the 1996–7 pertussis epidemic in The Netherlands. *Epidemiol Infect* 2001; 127(1):73–85.

4 Bleiker MA, Styblo K. The annual tuberculous infection rate and its trend in developing countries. *Bull Int Union Tuberc* 1978; 53:295–299.

5 Fine PE, Bruce J, Ponnighaus JM, Nkhosa P, Harawa A, Vynnycky E. Tuberculin sensitivity: conversions and reversions in a rural African population. *Int J Tuberc Lung Dis* 1999; 3(11):962–975.

6 Schenzle D. An age-structured model of pre- and post-vaccination measles transmission. *IMA J Math Appl Med Biol* 1984; 1(2):169–191.

Chapter 4

What do models tell us about the dynamics of infections?

4.1 **Overview and objectives**

In this chapter, we focus on acute infections and discuss the insights that are provided by models, such as those developed in the last two chapters, into the short and long-term dynamics of both immunizing and non-immunizing infections in the absence of interventions.

By the end of this chapter you should:

- Understand what determines whether or not the incidence of an infection increases;
- Understand the factors underlying the shape of epidemic curves;
- Be able to calculate the basic reproduction number of an infection from the growth rate of an epidemic (or outbreak) or the final epidemic (or outbreak) size;
- Understand how R_0 and other parameters can be estimated by fitting transmission models to data;
- Understand the mechanism which leads to cycles in the incidence of immunizing infections and understand the factors that influence these cycles;
- Be able to calculate the inter-epidemic period for an immunizing infection;
- Understand how the long term patterns in incidence that are associated with acute non-immunizing infections differ from those for immunizing infections.

4.2 **The short-term dynamics of infections**

4.2.1 **The theory of epidemics**

Figure 4.1 shows epidemic curves for three acute infections following their introduction into totally susceptible populations. The similarity between the general shapes of these curves, and those predicted using the models describing the transmission of immunizing infections that we discussed during the last two chapters, has led to extensive research on the properties of these models.[1, 2, 3]

This work, in turn, has led to insights into factors affecting the size, rate of increase and timing of epidemics. These insights remain useful today for interpreting data on outbreaks both for new infections or re-emergent infections (e.g. SARS or pandemic influenza) and established infections (e.g. measles and rubella). This section provides an introduction to some of the theory and its applications, using the models which we

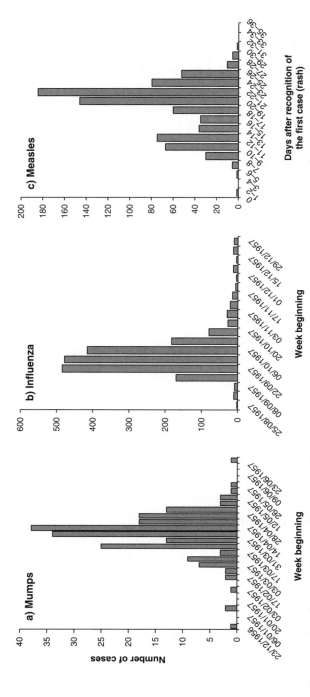

Fig. 4.1 Epidemic curves for three infections following their introduction into 'totally susceptible' populations. (a) Mumps in an Eskimo population in St Lawrence (near Alaska) in 1957;[4, 5] (b) 1957 (Asian) influenza in a General Practice population in Wales;[6] (c) Measles in Julianehåb, Southern Greenland, 1951.[7]

have developed so far. Much of the discussion in this chapter focuses on acute infections, for which the time interval between successive cases is measured in days, weeks or months. We will discuss infections with long serial intervals in Chapters 8 and 9.

4.2.2 Factors influencing trends in incidence

4.2.2.1 The basic reproduction number

In Chapter 1, we introduced the concept of the basic reproduction number, R_0, defined as the average number of infectious persons resulting from a typical infectious person following their introduction into a totally susceptible population (Section 1.3). In infectious disease modelling, the condition $R_0 > 1$ is considered to be an important 'threshold' condition that must be satisfied for the number of infectious persons to increase once an infection is introduced into a totally susceptible population.

For the models of the transmission of simple immunizing infections discussed in Chapters 2 and 3, R_0 is given by the expression:

$$R_0 = \beta ND \qquad 4.1$$

where β is the rate at which two specific individuals come into effective contact per unit time, D is the duration of infectiousness and N is the population size (Section 2.7.1). This equation is equivalent to the following, assuming that the rate at which individuals recover from being infectious (r) and the average duration of infectiousness are related through the equation $D=1/r$ (see Section 2.7.2).

$$R_0 = \frac{\beta N}{r} \qquad 4.2$$

Expressions for R_0 can be derived heuristically by considering the verbal definition of R_0. For example, βN is the number of individuals effectively contacted by a given infectious person per unit time, and therefore βND is the number of individuals effectively contacted by a given infectious person during the entire infectious period (see also Section 2.7.1).

Expression 4.1 for R_0 can also be derived using elementary logic by using the difference or differential equations for a SIR or SEIR model to show that, for the number of infectious persons to increase following the introduction of an infectious person into a totally susceptible population, the quantity βND has to be bigger than one. We reproduce the logic below (with apologies to those who find it too elementary!), since similar logic is often applied to obtain the expression for R_0 for other more complicated infections (Chapter 8).

Derivation of the result that, for the number of infectious persons with an immunizing infection to increase following the introduction of an infectious person into a totally susceptible population, $\beta ND > 1$

For simplicity, we will use the equations for a Susceptible–Infectious–Recovered (SIR) model, whereby individuals become infectious immediately after infection, before becoming immune for life (Figure 4.2). Appendix section A.2.2 provides the proof obtained using an SEIR model. The effects of births into and deaths out of the population are not considered here, but will be discussed later in this chapter.

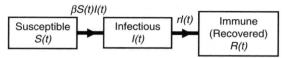

Fig. 4.2 General structure of a susceptible–infectious–immune (SIR) model. The letters above the arrows reflect the number of individuals who move from one category to the next per unit time.

For the number of infectious persons to increase at any given time point, the number of individuals who become infectious per unit time ($\beta S(t)I(t)$) must exceed the number of infectious individuals who stop being infectious per unit time ($rI(t)$):

$$\beta S(t)I(t) > rI(t) \qquad 4.3$$

If an infectious person is introduced into a totally susceptible population, the number of individuals that are susceptible to infection at the start just equals the population size (i.e. $S(t) = N$). Substituting for $S(t) = N$ into expression 4.3, implies that the following must hold for the number of infectious persons to increase after an infectious person enters the population:

$$\beta NI(t) > rI(t) \qquad 4.4$$

Cancelling both sides of this equation by the number of infectious persons at time t ($I(t)$), and then dividing both sides of this expression by the rate at which individuals recover (r) implies that the following must hold:

$$\frac{\beta N}{r} > 1 \qquad 4.5$$

Substituting for $D = 1/r$ into expression 4.5, implies that for the number of infectious persons to increase following the introduction of an infectious person into a totally susceptible population, $\beta ND > 1$.

The derivation of this threshold condition does not account for the fact that pre-infectious or infectious individuals may die during the pre-infectious or infectious periods. Anderson and May[1] (Chapters 1–4) provide details of expressions which take this into account. For most common immunizing infections, the pre-infectious and infectious periods are generally a few days (see Table 1.2), whereas the life expectancy (at least in industrialized populations) is about 70 years. As a result, since the mortality rate is much smaller than the rate at which infectious individuals recover, the effects of these adjustments to the above expression for R_0 are so small as to be negligible.

4.2.2.2 The epidemic and herd immunity thresholds and the net reproduction number

In Chapter 1 we discussed the following relationship between the proportion of the population that is susceptible (s), R_0 and the net reproduction number (R_n), which is defined as the average number of secondary infectious persons resulting from each infectious person in any specified population:

$$R_n = R_0 s \qquad\qquad 4.6$$

In general, the following holds for infections with short serial intervals (see Chapter 1):

- if each infectious person leads to *more than one* secondary infectious person (i.e. $R_n > 1$), the incidence of infectious persons *increases*;
- if each infectious person leads to *less than one* secondary infectious person (i.e. $R_n < 1$), the incidence of infectious persons *decreases*;
- if each infectious person leads to *exactly one* secondary infectious person (i.e. $R_n = 1$), the incidence of infectious persons remains *unchanged*.

The implication of Equation 4.6 is that if the proportion of the population that is susceptible exceeds the so-called 'epidemic threshold' of $1/R_0$, then R_n is greater than 1 and the incidence increases (see also Section 1.3); if it is less than $1/R_0$, then R_n is less than 1 and the incidence decreases; if it equals $1/R_0$, then R_n equals 1 and the incidence remains unchanged. For completeness, Appendix A.2.1 gives a formal derivation, using differential equations, of the result that when the number of infectious persons is at a peak, the proportion of the population that is susceptible equals $1/R_0$.

This relationship between the trend in incidence, R_n and the proportion of the population that is susceptible is illustrated in Figure 4.3 for measles and influenza, using predictions from the SEIR model discussed in the last two chapters. For simplicity, this and subsequent figures show the daily number of new infectious persons per 100,000 population, rather than the incidence (defined as the number of new infectious persons per unit time in the population at risk - see the glossary), since this is comparable to the statistic which might be reported in routine notifications and its trend mimics that in the incidence.

For example, R_0 values for influenza and measles are about 2 and 13 respectively (see Table 1.2). Thus the number of infectious persons who are infected with the influenza or measles virus should increase until the susceptible population has been depleted so much that the proportion of the population that is susceptible has decreased to 0.5 and 0.08 ($= 1/R_0$) for influenza and measles respectively, and $R_n = 1$. Transmission eventually ceases if the proportion of individuals who are susceptible remains below 0.5 and 0.08 ($= 1/R_0$) for influenza and measles respectively.

As discussed in Chapter 1, the epidemic threshold ($1/R_0$) is related to the herd immunity threshold, which is defined as the proportion of the population which should be immune for the incidence to be stable, or equivalently, for the net reproduction number to equal 1, as follows:

$$\text{Herd immunity threshold} = 1 - 1/R_0 \qquad\qquad 4.7$$

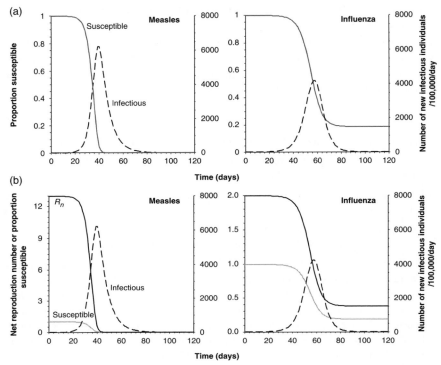

Fig. 4.3 Comparison between the daily number of new of infectious persons per 100,000 with measles or influenza, as predicted using an SEIR model and (a) the proportion of the population that is susceptible to infection and (b) the net reproduction number. The assumed parameter values for measles are: $R_0 = 13$, average pre-infectious and infectious periods are 8 and 7 days respectively. Those for influenza are $R_0 = 2$, pre-infectious period = infectious period = 2 days. One infectious person is introduced into a population comprising 100,000 susceptible individuals at the start (See Model 4.1, online).

Based on this equation, the herd immunity threshold for measles is about 0.92 (i.e. $1-1/13$) and that for influenza is about 0.5 ($= 1-1/2$). When the proportion of the population that is immune is above or below these values the incidence, and therefore the number of new infectious persons occurring per unit time, decreases and increases respectively (Figure 4.4). For example, the predicted daily number of new infectious persons per 100,000 population for influenza decreases if the proportion of the population that is immune exceeds 0.5. Note that the peak in the daily number of new infectious persons does not occur at exactly the same time that the proportion of the population that is immune equals the herd immunity threshold because of the time lag between infection and onset of infectiousness.

In general, vaccination programmes aim to achieve a coverage which is above the herd immunity threshold, since, if the proportion of the population that is immune is above this value, substantial outbreaks are unlikely to occur. As shown in Figure 4.5, for example, our model predicts that no epidemic will occur if we introduce one infectious person with measles into a population, if the basic reproduction number is 13 and the

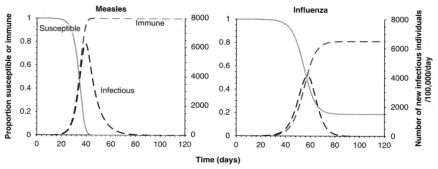

Fig. 4.4 Comparison between the proportion of individuals who are susceptible or immune to measles and influenza and the daily number of new infectious individuals per 100,000. See the caption to Figure 4.3 and Model 4.1, online, for details of parameter values.

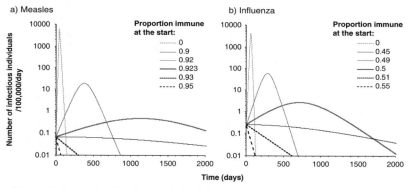

Fig. 4.5 Predictions of epidemic curves for (a) measles and (b) influenza, following the introduction of an infectious person into populations in which different proportions of individuals are immune at the start, e.g. because of vaccination. The y axis has been changed to a log10 scale to show more detail. See the caption to Figure 4.3 and Model 4.1, online, for details of parameter values.

proportion of individuals who are immune at the start exceeds 0.92 (=1–1/13). For influenza, no epidemic is predicted if this proportion exceeds 0.5 (= 1–1/2). Note that these predictions are based on the simplifying assumption that individuals mix randomly; we discuss alternatives to this assumption in Chapter 7. We will revisit these issues in Chapter 6, when we discuss the effect of chance in determining the occurence of outbreaks.

We shall discuss other features of the epidemic curve, such as the proportion of the population that is immune at the end, and extensions to the theory to explain long-term patterns in the incidence of immunizing infections later in this chapter.

4.2.3 What can we learn from the early stages of an epidemic?

Among the insights from the simple theory of epidemics[1] is that, using data on the number or incidence of infectious individuals during the early stages of an epidemic of a new or re-emergent infection, we should be able to estimate the basic reproduction number for that infection. This may be helpful in guiding the public health response to a new infection.

This was the situation in February 2003, when news of the SARS virus emerged. Two studies of the numbers of cases reported each day during the early stages of the epidemic in Hong Kong and Singapore,[8, 9] which were published in June 2003, provided some reassurance. These studies suggested that the basic reproduction number of SARS was low, i.e. <3, in comparison with that of other infections, such as measles or mumps,[1] suggesting that the SARS virus was not very transmissible. This, in combination with other features of the epidemiology of the infection, such as the fact that the peak infectiousness of cases occurred after onset of symptoms, indicated that SARS might be controllable.[10]

There are several formulae for calculating R_0 using data from the early stages of an epidemic (Table 4.1). Each of them require estimates of something which is often referred to as the 'growth rate of the epidemic', sometimes denoted by the Greek capital letter Λ (lambda). Before discussing the equations and illustrating how they can be applied to estimate R_0, we first consider what this growth rate is.

4.2.3.1 What is the growth rate in an epidemic and how do we calculate it?

In theory, during the early stages of an epidemic, the number of infectious individuals increases at an approximately constant rate (see Appendix Section A.2.4). This rate is referred to as the growth rate of an epidemic. We can obtain this growth rate graphically, as follows.

As we saw in Section 3.5.1, when something changes at a constant rate, we can write down an expression for the amount of that quantity at a given time t in terms of the rate at which it changes and the mathematical constant 'e'. Applying this result, we obtain the following expression for the number of infectious individuals at time t ($I(t)$) during the early stages of an epidemic:

$$I(t) \approx I(0)e^{\Lambda t} \qquad 4.8$$

where $I(0)$ is the number of infectious individuals at the start.

If we take the natural log of both sides of Equation 4.8 (see Basic maths section B.4 to revise logs), we obtain the following expression relating the number of infectious individuals and Λ:

$$\ln(I(t)) = \ln(I(0)) + \Lambda t \qquad 4.9$$

This equation is equivalent to that of a straight line with a gradient of Λ (see Basic maths section B.2), suggesting that if we plot the natural logarithm of the number of infectious individuals against time, we should obtain a straight line and the gradient of that line is Λ. This is illustrated in Figure 4.6 using model predictions for measles and influenza. This figure also shows that the growth rates in the number, cumulative number and daily number of new infectious individuals are very similar, since the natural log of these statistics, when plotted against time, leads to a straight line.

These observations suggest that we can estimate the *actual* growth rate in an epidemic using observed empirical data simply by plotting the natural log of the observed number of infectious individuals and calculating the gradient of the resulting line. If (as in most circumstances) data on the numbers of infectious individuals are not available, we can use data on the cumulative number of cases instead, since this increases at a similar rate to that of the number of infectious individuals during the early stages of an epidemic (see Figure 4.6).

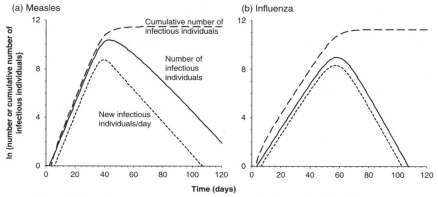

Fig. 4.6 Predictions of the natural log of the number, daily number and cumulative number of infectious individuals for (a) measles and (b) influenza, following the introduction of one infectious person into a totally susceptible population comprising 100,000 individuals. See caption to Figure 4.3 and Model 4.1 (online) for details of the parameter values.

4.2.3.1.1 Example: Estimates of the growth rate of the SARS epidemic in Hong Kong Figure 4.7 summarizes the cumulative numbers of SARS cases reported each day in Hong Kong from 17– 28 March in 2003, which were used in analyses by Lipsitch *et al.*[8] to estimate the basic reproduction number. No control measures had been introduced in Hong Kong during this period.

As shown in Figure 4.7, the line passing through the points of the log of the cumulative numbers of cases increases by about 1 unit every 8 days, or about 1/8 per day, giving a value for Λ of 0.12 per day. This line can be drawn either crudely by eye through the data points, or more formally by using linear regression.

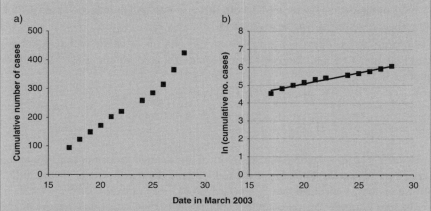

Fig. 4.7 (a) Cumulative and (b) natural log of the cumulative numbers of suspect and probable SARS cases reported in Hong Kong during 17–28 March 2003.[11]

4.2.3.2 Equations for the basic reproduction number

Each of the equations in Table 4.1 relating the basic reproduction number and the growth rate in an epidemic result from different assumptions about the average durations and distributions of both the pre-infectious and infectious periods or serial intervals (Table 4.1).

For example, for infections for which the pre-infectious period is very short in comparison with the infectious period (e.g. HIV), the equation for the basic reproduction number is:

$$R_0 = 1 + \Lambda D \qquad 4.10$$

where D is the average infectious period. The derivation of this equation is discussed in Appendix section A.2.5.

If neither the pre-infectious nor infectious periods is short, relative to the other (and therefore an SEIR model best describes the natural history), the equation for R_0 is as follows:

$$R_0 = (1 + \Lambda D)(1 + \Lambda D') \qquad 4.11$$

where D' is the average pre-infectious period.

Note that if some individuals are immune at the start of the epidemic, e.g. through vaccination or previous infection, these equations lead to estimates of the *net* reproduction number at the start of the epidemic.

4.2.3.2.1 Practical application: estimating R_0 for the SARS epidemic in Hong Kong During the early stages of the SARS epidemic, relatively little was known about the average infectious and pre-infectious periods, which made it difficult to apply several of the equations in Table 4.1. Instead, Lipsitch et al.[8] used Equation 4.16, which just required input on:

1) *The serial interval (T_s).* This was estimated directly from data on the first 205 probable cases in Singapore, which suggested that the average serial interval was about eight days.

2) *The ratio between the infectious period and the serial interval (denoted by f_r).* This was not known; however to deal with this uncertainty, Lipsitch et al. used the full range of values for f_r of between 0 and 1.

Substituting our estimate for the growth rate and the serial interval of eight days into Equation 4.16, and, assuming that f_r equals 0.3, gives a point estimate for R_0 of about 2.5:

$$R_0 = 1 + \Lambda T_s + f_r (1 - f_r)(T_s \Lambda)^2$$
$$= 1 + 0.12 \times 8.4 + 0.3 \times (1 - 0.3) \times (8.4 \times 0.12)^2$$
$$= 2.5$$

Lipsitch et al. also explored the sensitivity of this estimate to assumptions about the serial interval, e.g. assuming that it was as high as 12 days, and, after exploring different values for f_r, concluded that R_0 was likely to be in the range 2.2–3.6.[8]

The next example illustrates another application of these equations to estimate the net reproduction number.

Table 4.1 Summary of the equations relating the basic reproduction number to Λ, the 'growth rate in an epidemic'. D' and D are the average durations of the pre-infectious and infectious periods respectively, T_s is the serial interval. The equations are discussed in refs;[1, 3, 8, 20, 22] the first four equations can be derived from Equation 4.17. See section A.2.5 for the derivation of Equation 4.12.

Equation for R_0		Assumptions and further details
$1+\Lambda D$	4.12	This expression assumes that the pre-infectious period is very short in comparison with the infectious period, or individuals are infectious immediately after they are infected, as might be the case for HIV. The infectious period is assumed to follow the exponential distribution. See Appendix section A.2.5 for a derivation.
$(1+\Lambda D)(1+\Lambda D')$	4.13	The pre-infectious and infectious periods follow the exponential distribution.
$1+\Lambda T_s$	4.14	This expression is typically used when the pre-infectious and/or infectious periods are not known but are assumed to follow the exponential distribution. It can be shown that if the pre-infectious and infectious periods follow the exponential distribution, then the serial interval equals $D+D'$.
$1+\dfrac{\ln 2}{T_d}D$	4.15	This equation can be derived from Equation 4.12, using the fact that the time until the number of infectious persons doubles relative to that at some other time (T_d) is related to the growth rate through the equation $\Lambda = \dfrac{\ln 2}{T_d}$ (see Panel 4.1). Equation 4.15 is most commonly seen in the following form in the HIV literature: $T_d = \dfrac{D\ln 2}{R_0 - 1}$ (see also Chapter 8).
$1+\Lambda T_s$ $+f_r(1-f_r)(T_s\Lambda)^2$	4.16	This expression is a more detailed version of Equation 4.14 and is typically used when the pre-infectious and/or infectious periods are poorly understood but are assumed to follow the exponential distributions. f_r is the ratio between the infectious period and the serial interval.[8] Note that the values for R_0 which are obtained when $f_r = 0$ and $f_r = 1$ are identical; the highest value for R_0 is obtained when $f_r = 0.5$.
$\dfrac{\Lambda D\left(\dfrac{\Lambda D'}{m}+1\right)^m}{\left(1-\left(\dfrac{\Lambda D}{n}+1\right)^{-n}\right)}$	4.17	The expressions above can be derived from this expression. In this expression, the pre-infectious and infectious periods are assumed to follow the Gamma distribution whose shape is illustrated in Figure 4.8, with mean values D' and D respectively. m and n reflect the tightness of the distributions for the pre-infectious and infectious periods respectively. The value m (or n) $=1$ corresponds to the assumption that the distribution is exponential. See Wearing et al.[20] for further details.

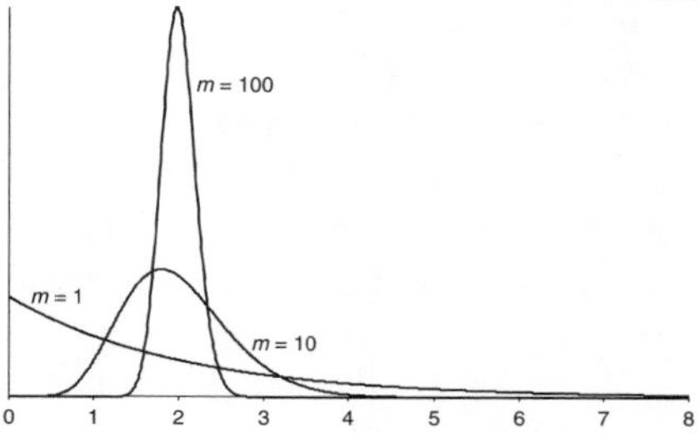

Fig. 4.8 Examples of the Gamma distribution with a mean of 2.

Panel 4.1 The relationship between the growth rate and the doubling time

Equation 4.9 can be used to obtain the relationship between the growth rate and the doubling time of an epidemic, which is defined as the time until the number of cases in the population doubles, relative to that at some other time.

For example, suppose that there is only one infectious person at time $t = 0$ (i.e. $I(0) = 1$) and there are 2 infectious persons at time $t = T_d$, i.e. $I(T_d) = 2$. Substituting for $I(0) = 1$ and $I(T_d) = 2$ into Equation 4.9, we obtain the result:

$$\ln(2) = \ln(1) + \Lambda T_d \qquad\qquad 4.18$$

Noting that $\ln(1) = 0$ (see Basic maths section B.4) we obtain the following result for the growth rate after rearranging Equation 4.18:

$$\Lambda = \frac{\ln(2)}{T_d} \qquad\qquad 4.19$$

4.2.3.2.2 Example: calculating the net and basic reproduction numbers for an influenza pandemic The emergence of the avian influenza virus among poultry during the early 2000s and the threat of an influenza pandemic led to many studies estimating the basic reproduction number of the strains which caused previous influenza pandemics.[12, 13, 14, 15]

Figure 4.9a summarizes the numbers and cumulative numbers of influenza cases per 100,000 population reported each week in Cumberland, a community with 5,234 individuals in Maryland, USA, during the 1918 (Spanish) influenza pandemic. Cases were ascertained actively through house to house surveys.[16]

As for the SARS data from Hong Kong, data on the number of infectious individuals were not available and we can use the *cumulative* numbers of cases instead to calculate the growth rate in the epidemic. The line passing through the points in Figure 4.9b increases by about 1.00 unit per week, implying that Λ was about 1/7 per day.

Given reports of a 'herald' wave of influenza during April–May 1918,[17] some individuals were probably immune to the strain which caused the pandemic by autumn 1918. Therefore applying the expressions in Table 4.1 to our estimated growth rate from autumn 1918 will provide estimates of the *net* rather than of the basic reproduction number at this time.

Assuming that the average pre-infectious and infectious periods for influenza were each two days (see Chapter 1) and using Equation 4.13, implies that the net reproduction number at the start of the pandemic in Cumberland equalled:

$$R_n = (1 + \Lambda D)(1 + \Lambda D')$$
$$= (1 + (1/7) \times 2) \times (1 + (1/7) \times 2) = 1.6 \qquad\qquad 4.20$$

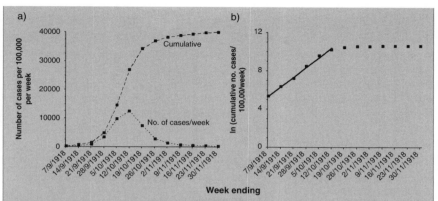

Fig. 4.9 (a) Numbers and cumulative numbers of influenza cases each week in Cumberland (Maryland, USA) during the 1918 Spanish influenza pandemic; (b) natural log of the cumulative numbers of cases in Cumberland, together with the best-fitting regression line.

The proportion of individuals who were still susceptible to infection after the herald wave in 1918 is unknown, although studies have sometimes assumed a lower limit of 70 per cent.[13, 14] This is consistent with the level of seroconversion found after the first wave of the Hong Kong influenza pandemic[18] and the influenza incidence seen during a typical season.[19]

Assuming further that, because of the herald wave in spring 1918, approximately 70 per cent of individuals were still susceptible to the pandemic strain of influenza by September, and using the relationship $R_0 = R_n/s$, which is obtained by rearranging Equation 4.6, implies that the basic reproduction number equals $1.65/0.7 = 2.4$.

4.2.3.3 Practical application of the growth rate equations

The equations in Table 4.1 have several limitations, namely:

1) The simplest expressions assume that the pre-infectious and infectious periods follow the (unrealistic) exponential distributions. This assumption may lead to an under– or overestimate in R_0.[20] Considering the example described in section 4.2.3.2.2, if we apply the most detailed Equation 4.17 and assume realistic distributions for the pre-infectious and infectious periods (see Figure 4.8), we obtain estimates of the net and basic reproduction numbers of about 1.5 and 2.2 respectively.

2) The equations can only be applied to data from the early stages of an epidemic, since they rely on the assumption that the susceptible population has not been depleted substantially by the infectious individuals (see Appendix sections A.2.4 and A.2.5).

One key advantage of the expressions in Table 4.1 is that they are independent of the proportion of cases that are reported in the population, if this is constant over time. For example, the growth rates estimated using data representing 100 or 10 per cent of

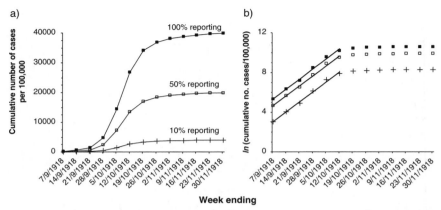

Fig. 4.10 Comparison between (a) the cumulative numbers of cases and (b) the natural log of the cumulative numbers of cases which would have been seen for the Cumberland 1918 (Spanish) influenza data, if 10, 50, and 100 per cent of cases had been reported. Figure (b) illustrates that the gradient of the best-fitting line passing through the points of the natural log of the cumulative numbers of cases is identical irrespective of the proportion of cases which are reported. See Appendix section A.2.6 for the mathematical details.

all cases in the population should be similar (see Figure 4.10 and Appendix section A.2.6). However, if the *proportion* of cases in the population who are reported increases over time (e.g. as individuals become more aware of the infection), the growth rate in the epidemic and hence the reproduction number(s) may be overestimated.

The growth rate can also be calculated using either the cumulative numbers of deaths or of infections, assuming that the case fatality or the proportions of infected individuals who are infectious remain constant over time. Use of mortality data during an epidemic will be complicated, however, by delays before deaths reach the official statistics.

4.2.3.4 Beyond the growth rate equations—estimating the reproduction numbers in real time

The emergence of the SARS virus in 2003 and the threat of an influenza pandemic has led to increasing interest in improving on the growth rate equations, and being able to track how the net reproduction number changes, for example, daily during the course of an epidemic in real time. Methods for obtaining such real-time estimates of the net reproduction number were published in 2004 by Wallinga and Teunis.[21] The methods use data on the distributions of the serial interval for cases affected in an outbreak, to estimate possible sources of infection and secondary cases from the epidemic curve.

Such estimates of the net reproduction number should provide insight into whether interventions are having an impact on transmission. Retrospective analyses of the epidemic curves for SARS in Hong Kong, Vietnam, Singapore, and China (Figure 4.11), for example, indicated that before the introduction of control, the net reproduction number was similar in all settings (i.e. ~3), and that control measures

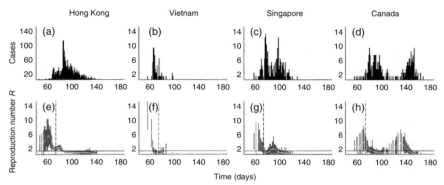

Fig. 4.11 Epidemic curves (numbers of cases by date of symptom onset) for SARS in (a) Hong Kong, (b) Vietnam, (c) Singapore, and (d) Canada and the corresponding net reproduction numbers (R) for (e) Hong Kong, (f) Vietnam, (g) Singapore, and (h) Canada, 2003. Markers (white spaces) show mean values; accompanying vertical lines show 95 per cent confidence intervals. The vertical dashed line indicates the issuance of the first global alert against SARS on March 12, 2003; the horizontal solid line indicates the threshold value $R = 1$, above which an epidemic will spread and below which the epidemic is controlled. Days are counted from January 1, 2003, onwards. Reproduced with permission from Wallinga and Teunis, 2004.[21]

introduced from the middle of March—indicated by the vertical dashed line in figures (e) and (f)—had an impact, since the net reproduction number went down and eventually reached <1. The increases in the net reproduction number in each setting during the early stages of the epidemic are attributable to 'super-spreader' events, whereby one individual led to 10 or more infections.[21]

4.2.4 What is likely to be the size of an epidemic?

Once a new or re-emergent infection appears in a population, it can be useful to predict the likely epidemic size, e.g. for planning scarce resources. According to theory,[3] which assumes random mixing, the proportion of individuals who have been infected by the end of an epidemic for an immunizing infection depends only on the basic reproduction number (see Figure 4.12 and Table 4.2).

In general, as shown in Figure 4.13, if an infection for which $R_0 > 3$ enters a population, the theory suggests that on average, everyone should eventually get infected, irrespective of the pre-infectious or infectious period and the epidemic curve (Figure 4.13). By chance, as discussed in Chapter 6, it is also possible for <100 per cent of individuals to have been infected by the end.

The final epidemic size can, in principle, also be used to estimate the basic reproduction number for an infection retrospectively, i.e. once the epidemic has occurred, using the expressions in Table 4.2. Assuming that estimates of the proportion of individuals who are infected are correct, such estimates are reliable only if the basic reproduction number is small (e.g. <3), given that the final epidemic size for all immunizing infections with a basic reproduction number of over 3 is similar.

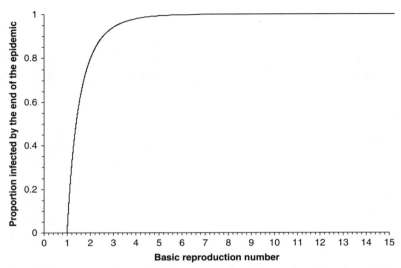

Fig. 4.12 Predicted proportion of individuals who have been infected by the end of an epidemic following the introduction of an infection with different values of R_0 into a totally susceptible population (see Table 4.2 for the equations).

Table 4.2 Summary of the key equations relating the basic reproduction number to the proportion of individuals who have been infected (or are still susceptible) by the end of an epidemic, based on the SEIR model, assuming that individuals mix randomly.

Equation		Definitions and assumptions
$R_0 = -\dfrac{\ln(1-z_f)}{z_f}$	4.21	z_f is the proportion of the population which has been infected by the end of the epidemic. All individuals are assumed to be susceptible at the start of the epidemic. See Diekmann and Heesterbeek[3] for further details.
$R_0 = \dfrac{\ln(s_f) - \ln(s_0)}{s_f - s_0}$	4.22	s_0 and s_f are the proportion of the population which is susceptible at the start and at the end of the epidemic respectively. See Diekmann and Heesterbeek[3] for further details. This equation is equivalent to Equation 4.23.
$R_0 = \dfrac{N-1}{C} \sum\limits_{j=S_f+1}^{S_0} 1/j$ $\approx \dfrac{N-1}{C} \ln\left\{ \dfrac{S_0 + \frac{1}{2}}{S_f - \frac{1}{2}} \right\}$	4.23	N is the population size, C is the number of cases (i.e. individuals who have been infected) by the end of the epidemic. S_0 and S_f are the numbers of individuals who are susceptible at the start and the end of the epidemic respectively. See Becker[24] for further details. The standard error on the estimated R_0 is as follows: $$SE(R_0) = \frac{N-1}{C} \sqrt{ \sum_{j=S_f+1}^{S_0} 1/j^2 + \frac{CR_0^2}{(N-1)^2} }$$

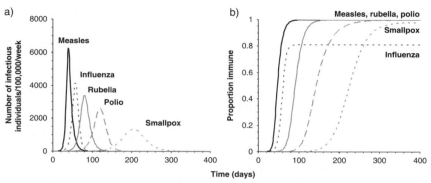

Fig. 4.13 Comparison between the epidemic curves predicted for measles, influenza, rubella, polio, and smallpox, following the introduction of an infectious person into a totally susceptible population, assuming that individuals mix randomly. See Model 4.1, online.

A further drawback of these expressions is that they assume that individuals mix randomly, although they have generally been found to be robust to assumptions about contact.[23] In addition, they do not correct for any control measures which might have been introduced during the epidemic and so the resulting estimates may underestimate the true R_0 of the infection.

4.2.4.1 Example: calculating R_0 of an infection using the epidemic size

Considering the influenza pandemic in Cumberland, a community comprising 5,234 individuals, discussed in section 4.2.3.2.2, approximately 70 per cent of individuals were probably susceptible at the start of the epidemic (i.e. $s_0 = 0.7$).

During the epidemic, there were 2,085 cases, which implies that the proportion of individuals who were susceptible at the end equals $s_f = 0.7 - 2,085/5,234 = 0.7 - 0.398 = 0.302$ (i.e. the difference between the proportion susceptible at the start and the proportion who developed disease during the pandemic). This assumes that only individuals who developed clinical symptoms were immune, which may be unrealistic.

Applying Equation 4.22 in Table 4.2, we see that:

$$R_0 = \frac{\ln(0.302) - \ln(0.7)}{0.302 - 0.7} = 2.1$$

Application of Equation 4.23 in Table 4.2, using the value $S_0 = 3,664$ (=5,234 × 0.7) and $S_f = 1,579$ (= 3,664–2,085) leads to the same estimated value for R_0.

4.2.5 Estimating R_0 or other unknown parameters by fitting models to data

R_0 and other unknown parameters can also be estimated by formally fitting model predictions to observed data. According to this process, the parameters that are being estimated are varied until the smallest distance, as reflected by some goodness of fit statistic, between the model prediction and the observed data is obtained (Figure 4.14). This approach has been used to estimate R_0 and other parameters for several infections, including pandemic influenza, Ebola, and smallpox.[12, 25, 26]

There is a vast literature on approaches for fitting models to data.[27, 28, 29, 30] These are beyond the scope of this book, and we therefore just highlight two of the most widely known approaches and provide a few further details in Panel 4.2.

The most widely known approach is that of 'least squares' whereby parameter values are found which lead to the smallest value for the 'sum of squares of the difference between the model prediction and the observed data'.

Another widely-applied approach is that of 'maximum likelihood' whereby the best-fitting parameter values are those which lead to the largest value for the expression for the so-called likelihood (or probability) of observing the data. The expression for the likelihood takes account of measurement error in the data points themselves (see Hillborn and Mangel[29], Model 4.2 (online) and the online files associated with Chapter 5). According to statistical theory, when fitting by maximum likelihood to data considered to be normally distributed (as might be the case for 'count' data involving many individuals) the parameter values are the same as those which would be obtained by using least squares.

Most mathematical model-building packages provide an 'optimize' routine which allows users to find parameter values which lead to the minimum or maximum value of some expression specified in the model. For example, at the time of writing, Excel has the 'Solver' routine and Berkeley Madonna has the 'optimize' function.

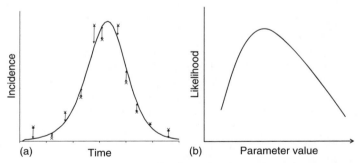

Fig. 4.14 Illustration of the fitting process. (a) When fitting a model describing the transmission dynamics of an infection to data, the size of the unknown parameters are varied until the smallest distance between the observed data and the model prediction is achieved. (b) An example of how the likelihood may change for different values for the parameter being estimated. The best-fitting parameter value is the one which leads to the maximum value for the likelihood. Note that it is possible for more than one combination of parameters to lead to a plausible fit to the data; in such instances, it would be reasonable to accept the combination which is biologically plausible and leads to the best overall likelihood.

Panel 4.2 Fitting models and sensitivity analyses

A statistic that is often used when fitting models by maximum likelihood is the 'log likelihood deviance'. The deviance calculates how far, for a given set of parameters, predictions from the model *deviate* from those of the 'saturated' model, which is defined as the best possible model, whose predictions pass through every single point in the dataset. The formal definition of the log-likelihood deviance is:

$$2 \times (\text{Log-likelihood of the saturated model}$$

$$-$$

$$\text{Log-likelihood of observing the data set})$$

Finding parameter values which lead to the smallest log-likelihood deviance is the same as finding parameters which lead to the maximum likelihood of observing the data. Examples of deviance calculations are provided in Model 4.2 (online) and with the files associated with Chapter 5.

The deviance is convenient to use since it follows the chi-square distribution with degrees of freedom given by the difference between the number of data points used to fit the model and the number of parameters.[27, 28, 29, 30] This can be used to assess whether the fit of the model is adequate: the p value, which is obtained by referring the optimal deviance to the chi-square distribution with the appropriate degrees of freedom, gives the probability of observing the data set or one with a lower likelihood, given that the model is correct. If only one parameter is being estimated, its lower and upper 95 per cent confidence limits are given by the values which lead to a deviance which differs by 3.84 from the optimal deviance.

Where more than one parameter is being estimated, 95 per cent confidence intervals are often calculated using the profile likelihood approach, whereby the values for all the parameters, except for one, are fixed at their optimal values, and the lower and upper 95 per cent confidence limits of the remaining parameter are given by the values which lead to a deviance which differs by 3.84 from the optimal deviance. Other approaches, which can be computationally-demanding, include working out a confidence region for the unknown parameters.

During the last decade, with improvements in computational speed, Markov Chain Monte Carlo (MCMC) methods have been increasingly applied to estimate parameters,[68] especially if the model has many unknown input parameters. These identify best-fitting parameter values using various algorithms, such as Metropolis–Hastings or Gibbs sampling. An advantage of this approach is that 95 per cent confidence (or credibility) intervals for the parameter values, together with their full multivariate distributions, are obtained at the same time as the best-fitting parameter values. Estimates of the correlations between the different parameter values are important for many applications, such as forecasting future numbers of cases or calculating the cost effectiveness of given interventions.

In practice, it is often difficult to reliably fit models which have many (20 or more) unknown input parameters. In such instances, instead of fitting models to data, modellers often try to make predictions using a wide range of plausible parameter values, for example, generated using the technique of 'Latin Hypercube Sampling'.[69]

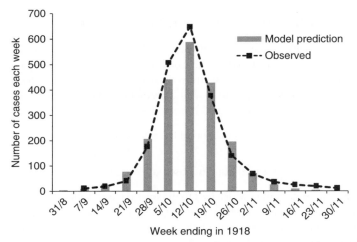

Fig. 4.15 Comparison between predictions of the numbers of cases each week in Cumberland, obtained using the best-fitting SEIR model, and the observed data (Model 4.2 (online)).

4.2.5.1 Example: estimating R_0 for the 1918 influenza pandemic in Cumberland (USA) by fitting a transmission model to the data

Figure 4.15 compares the numbers of cases each week during the 1918 influenza pandemic in Cumberland (Section 4.2.3.2.2) against the best-fitting predictions obtained using an SEIR model. The average pre-infectious and infectious periods were both assumed to be 2 days, 30 per cent of individuals were assumed to be immune at the start and a fixed proportion of those who were infectious had symptoms. For simplicity, symptomatic and asymptomatic individuals were assumed to be equally infectious.

In total, three parameters were fitted, namely: R_0, the proportion of infectious persons who were reported and the number of people who were infectious at the start of the outbreak. The best-fitting values were as follows: R_0: 2.57 (95% CI: 2.56–2.59); proportion of infectious persons that were reported: 0.77 (95% CI: 0.74–0.80); number of infectious individuals at the start: 0.80 (95% CI: 0.74–0.86), with an overall deviance of 146 (10 degrees of freedom).

As illustrated in this example the estimate of R_0 obtained by fitting the model to data is generally consistent with that obtained using the final epidemic size and the growth rate in the epidemic (see Sections 4.2.3.2.2 and 4.2.4.1).

4.3 The long-term dynamics of acute infections

4.3.1 Why does the incidence of immunizing infections cycle over time?

Figure 4.16 shows the mortality and notification rates for several infections over time. This highlights the fact that the incidence of immunizing infections typically cycles

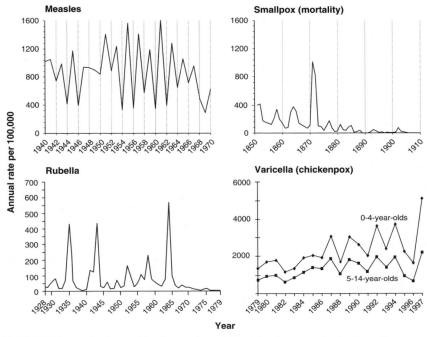

Fig. 4.16 Patterns in the notification and mortality rates for several infectious diseases, before the introduction of vaccination into the routine schedule. The data for measles and smallpox are the crude notification and mortality rates respectively for England and Wales.[31] The data for rubella reflect the notification rates in ten selected US areas (Maine, Rhode Island, Connecticut, New York City, Ohio, Illinois, Wisconsin, Maryland, Washington, Massachusetts), 1928–1979. Reproduced with permission from Preblud et al, 1980.[32] The data for chickenpox are physician consultation rates for 0–4 and 5–14-year-olds for Manitoba, Canada, extracted with permission from Brisson et al, 2001.[33]

over time with the frequency of the cycles differing between infections. Epidemics of measles, for example, occurred every two years in England and Wales, whereas those for smallpox used to occur every five years.

As shown in Figure 4.17, similar cycles are predicted by an SEIR model of the transmission of a simple immunizing infection which incorporates individuals being born into the population and dying (Model 4.3 (online) and Panel 4.3).

Why do these cycles occur?

The answer to this question lies with changes in the proportion of the population which is susceptible, the net reproduction number and the birth rate. We first explore how the proportion of the population that is susceptible or immune and the net reproduction number change whilst the incidence, and therefore, the number of new infectious persons per unit time, increases or decreases during an epidemic cycle.

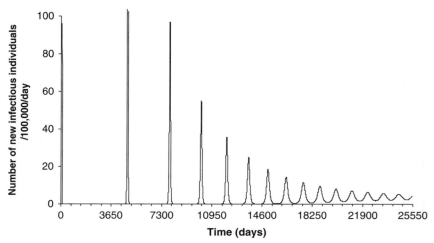

Fig. 4.17 Predictions of the daily number of new infectious persons with measles per 100,000 population following the introduction of one infectious person into a totally susceptible population comprising 100,000 individuals, obtained using the model described in Panel 4.3. The pre-infectious and infectious periods are eight and seven days respectively, $R_0 = 13$ and the mortality rate = birth rate = 3.92×10^{-5} per day (see Panel 4.3 and Model 4.3 (online)), which is equivalent to an average life expectancy of 70 years.

Panel 4.3 Incorporating births and deaths into a model describing the transmission dynamics of an immunizing infection

Figure 4.18 shows the general structure of a model of the transmission of an immunizing infection which incorporates births into and deaths out of the population.

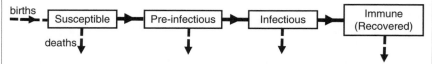

Fig. 4.18 General structure of a model describing the transmission of an immunizing infection, incorporating births into and deaths out of the population.

The differential equations for the model are as follows:

$$\frac{dS(t)}{dt} = bN(t) - \lambda(t)S(t) - mS(t)$$

4.24

$$\frac{dE(t)}{dt} = \lambda(t)S(t) - fE(t) - mE(t)$$

4.25

$$\frac{dI(t)}{dt} = fE(t) - rI(t) - mI(t)$$

4.26

$$\frac{dR(t)}{dt} = rI(t) - mR(t)$$

4.27

The definitions are as follows:

$S(t)$, $E(t)$, $I(t)$, $R(t)$ equal the total number of individuals who are susceptible, pre-infectious, infectious and immune respectively at time t;

b is the per capita birth rate;

m is the per capita mortality rate;

$N(t)$ is the total population size at time t and equals $S(t)+E(t)+I(t)+R(t)$;

f is the rate at which individuals become infectious, calculated as 1/average pre-infectious period;

r is the rate at which individuals recover from being infectious, calculated as 1/ infectious period.

If the population size remains unchanged over time, the birth rate equals the mortality rate, and the mortality rate is calculated as 1/average life expectancy. The force of infection, (t), can be calculated using the expression:

$$\lambda(t) = \beta I(t)$$

where β is the rate at which two specific individuals come into effective contact per unit time, and is calculated as (see Section 2.7.1):

$$\beta = \frac{R_0}{ND}$$

Here, D is the duration of infectiousness and 't' has been dropped from the notation for the population size, since we assume that the latter remains unchanged over time.

If we wished to assume that the population increases over time (birth rate>death rate), then we would need to use the following expression for the force of infection (see Panel 2.5):

$$\lambda(t) = \frac{c_e I(t)}{N(t)}$$

where c_e is the number of individuals effectively contacted by each person per unit time, and calculated using the expression $c_e = \frac{R_0}{D}$.

According to the formulation used in Equations 4.24–4.27, individuals are born susceptible and the mortality rate is identical for all individuals. In reality, the mortality rate is likely to differ between infectious and other individuals. This model also assumes that individuals die at a constant rate and implicitly assumes that the population has an exponential age distribution (see Section 2.7.2). To incorporate an age-dependent mortality rate, each of the compartments would need to be subdivided by age (see Chapter 5).

As we saw in section 4.2.2, during the course of an epidemic for an acute infection, these different statistics follow the pattern shown in Table 4.3.

Figure 4.19 shows predictions of these statistics during an epidemic cycle, using the model described in Panel 4.3, which incorporates births into and deaths out of the population (see also Model 4.3, online). In general, the changes in these statistics during an epidemic cycle are analogous to those summarized in Table 4.3. Appendix section A.2.7

Table 4.3 Summary of changes in R_n and the proportion of the population that is susceptible and immune at different stages in an epidemic

Incidence or no. of new infectious persons per unit time	R_n	Proportion susceptible	Proportion immune
Increasing	>1	>$1/R_0$	<$1-1/R_0$
Decreasing	<1	<$1/R_0$	>$1-1/R_0$
Constant (at a peak)	1	=$1/R_0$	=$1-1/R_0$ = herd immunity threshold

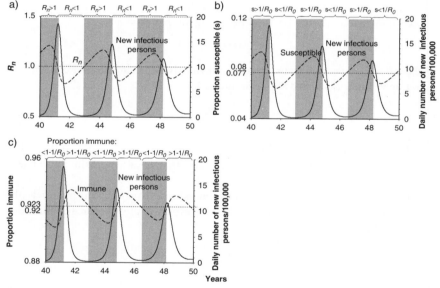

Fig. 4.19 Comparison between the daily number of new infectious persons with measles per 100,000 population predicted using the model described in Panel 4.3, and (a) the net reproduction number; (b) the proportion of the population which is susceptible; (c) the proportion of the population which is immune. R_0 is assumed to equal 13; see the caption to Figure 4.17 for the other parameter values. The shaded portions correspond to the periods when the daily number of new infectious persons is increasing, and therefore all of the following hold: R_n >1, proportion susceptible >$1/R_0$ and the proportion of the population that is immune is below the herd immunity threshold ($1-1/R_0$). The x axis shows the number of years since the introduction of one infectious person into a population comprising 100,000 susceptible individuals. Note that the short pre-infectious period for measles (8 days) means that the plot of the daily number of new infections per 100,000 population will be very similar to that of the daily number of new infectious persons per 100,000 population. See Model 4.3, online.

provides the mathematical proof that when the incidence is at a peak or a trough for the model described in Panel 4.3, the proportion of the population that is susceptible equals $1/R_0$.

A particularly interesting feature of the epidemic cycle shown in Figure 4.19 is that the peaks in the proportion of the population that is susceptible, and therefore the daily number of new infectious persons depend on the birth rate. For the predictions shown in Figure 4.19, the daily birth rate was approximately equal to 4 per 100,000, and we see the following occurs (Figure 4.20):

1) whilst the daily number of new infectious persons is *bigger than the birth rate*, the proportion of individuals who are susceptible *decreases;*

2) whilst the daily number of new infectious persons is *less than the birth rate*, the proportion of the population that is susceptible *increases;*

3) whilst the daily number of new infectious persons *equals the birth rate*, the proportion of individuals who are susceptible is *at a peak or a trough* (i.e. it is neither increasing nor decreasing).

This relationship between the birth rate, the daily number of new infectious persons and trends in the proportion of the population that is susceptible follows from the fact that the daily number of new infectious persons reflects the rate at which susceptible individuals are *being removed* from the population, and the birth rate reflects the rate at

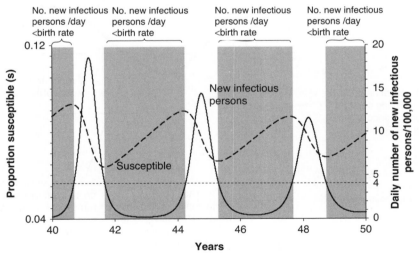

Fig. 4.20 Comparison between the daily number of new infectious persons with measles per 100,000 population, obtained using the model described in Panel 4.3, and the proportion of the population which is susceptible. The shaded areas correspond to the periods when the proportion of the population that is susceptible is increasing and therefore when the daily number of new infectious persons is less than the birth rate (= mortality rate = 1/life expectancy = $1/(70 \times 365) \approx 4$ per 100,000 per day). See the caption to Figure 4.17 for the parameter values. The x axis shows the number of years since the introduction of one infectious person into a population comprising 100,000 susceptible individuals.

which susceptible individuals *are added* to the population. The number of new infectious persons per day must therefore *decrease* if more individuals are being removed from the population than the number being added, i.e. number of new infectious persons per day>birth rate. As discussed extensively by previous authors, including Hamer in 1906[34] (see the historical review on pages 155–159 of Keeling and Rohani),[35] the effect of births entering the population on the proportion of the population that is susceptible also helps to answer why, for immunizing infections, the numbers of new infectious persons cycle at all.

For example, once an epidemic has peaked, then, without susceptible newborns entering the population, the proportion of individuals who are susceptible would remain below the threshold level of $1/R_0$ and transmission would eventually cease (see section 4.2.2.2).

With susceptible newborns continuously entering the population, however, the following sequence of events (see Figure 4.21) generate the cycles in the numbers of new infectious persons per unit time:

1) The susceptible population increases once the rate at which susceptible newborns entering the population exceeds the rate at which susceptible individuals are being removed from the population, i.e. the number of new infectious persons per unit time drops below the birth rate.

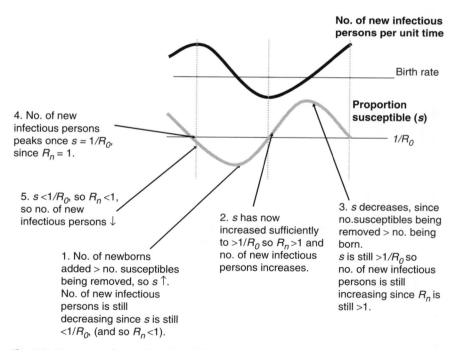

No. of new infectious persons per unit time

Birth rate

Proportion susceptible (s)

$1/R_0$

4. No. of new infectious persons peaks once $s = 1/R_0$, since $R_n = 1$.

5. $s < 1/R_0$, so $R_n < 1$, so no. of new infectious persons ↓

1. No. of newborns added > no. susceptibles being removed, so s ↑. No. of new infectious persons is still decreasing since s is still $< 1/R_0$, (and so $R_n < 1$).

2. s has now increased sufficiently to $> 1/R_0$ so $R_n > 1$ and no. of new infectious persons increases.

3. s decreases, since no. susceptibles being removed > no. being born. s is still $> 1/R_0$ so no. of new infectious persons is still increasing since R_n is still > 1.

Fig. 4.21 Summary of the effect of individuals being born into the population on the proportion of individuals who are susceptible (s) and the number of new infectious persons per unit time for an immunizing infection, at different stages of the epidemic cycle. The stages are numbered in the same order that they are numbered in the main text.

2) Some time after the susceptible population starts to increase, the proportion of individuals who are susceptible exceeds the threshold level, $1/R_0$. At this point, the number of new infectious persons per unit time starts to increase, since $R_n > 1$ (because $R_n = R_0 s > 1$).

3) Shortly after the number of new infectious persons per unit time starts to increase, the number of infectious persons in the population is so large that the former exceeds the birth rate (i.e. the rate at which susceptible individuals leave the population exceeds the rate at which they enter it). This causes the susceptible population to decrease.

4) The number of new infectious persons per unit time peaks once the proportion of the population which is susceptible equals the threshold level of $1/R_0$, since R_n now equals 1.

5) Once the proportion of the population which is susceptible has decreased to below the threshold level of $1/R_0$, the number of new infectious persons per unit time starts to decrease since R_n is now <1.

6) The continuing entry of susceptible newborns means that eventually the susceptible population increases and we reach step 1 in the cycle.

Changes in the susceptible population do not fully explain the cycles in incidence of immunizing infections. This is illustrated by the fact that, apart from a few exceptions (Panel 4.4), the simplest models predict that the size of the peaks in the number of new infectious persons per unit time should become progressively smaller over time and eventually disappear (i.e. 'damp out') (Figure 4.17). A detailed mathematical explanation for this damping (which is beyond the scope of the book, as it relies on use of so-called 'imaginary numbers') is provided in Anderson and May[1] and Keeling and Rohani.[35] In practice, many factors influence these cycles; we discuss the main ones below.

4.3.2 Factors influencing the cycles in incidence of immunizing infections

4.3.2.1 Seasonal contact

Several studies have explored the effect of seasonal contact on the incidence of immunizing infections.[36, 37, 38] Contact between individuals, especially children, can vary greatly during a year because of school holidays, as discussed in Panel 4.5 (Figure 4.23b). This shows findings from analyses by Fine and Clarkson[36] demonstrating that the transmission parameter for measles was lowest during the periods when schools were closed. As shown in Figure 4.24, models of the transmission of measles which incorporate changes in contact because of school holidays predict cycles which are reasonably consistent with those observed and do not damp out (Model 4.5, online).

Other studies have also highlighted the importance of contact between children at schools in transmission of infections. For example, a study in Israel during a brief period when teachers were on strike in the year 2000 found that diagnoses of respiratory infections among children were 42 and 20 per cent lower during the period when schools were closed, as compared with those seen before and after the strike respectively.[39] Another study in France concluded that during the school holidays, influenza transmission to children was reduced by 20–29 per cent as compared with that during term time.[40]

Panel 4.4 The Hamer model—the model whose predictions never damp out

Figure 4.22 shows predictions from the following model (Model 4.4, online), which is implicit in Hamer (1906)[34] and aimed to describe the transmission of measles in London.

$$S_{t+1} = S_t - C_{t+1} + B_{t+1} \qquad\qquad 4.28$$

$$C_{t+1} = kS_tC_t \qquad\qquad 4.29$$

According to Equation 4.28 the number of individuals who are susceptible to infection at a given time $t+1$ (S_{t+1}) equals the number who were susceptible at a previous time t (S_t), after subtracting the number who became cases between time t and $t+1$ (C_{t+1}), and adding in the number of individuals who were born between time t and $t+1$ (B_{t+1}). According to Equation 4.29, the number of cases at time $t+1$ is proportional to the number of susceptible individuals and cases at time t (denoted by S_t and C_t respectively); the factor k is analogous to the β parameter used in the models discussed in Section 2.7.1, and can be interpreted as the fraction of contacts between a susceptible and a case which resulted in the susceptible person becoming a case.[36]

The cycles in the numbers of cases predicted by this model do not damp out (Figure 4.22). In contrast with the model described in Panel 4.3, whose predictions of the number of new infectious persons per unit time do damp out (Figure 4.17), Hamer's model takes time steps of one serial interval (approximately two weeks for measles). Consequently, all of those effectively contacted in each time step become infectious and recover at the same time, and different generations of cases are not present in the population at the same time. Interestingly, predictions from Hamer's model do damp out, if the equations are modified slightly so that the generations of cases overlap (see pages 138–9 in Anderson and May[1] for further discussion).

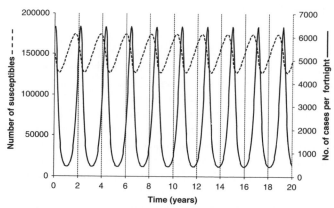

Fig. 4.22 Predictions of the number of susceptible individuals and cases obtained using Hamer's model. $S_0 = 150,000$, $C_0 = 6,400$ (the number of measles cases estimated at the peak of an epidemic in London during the early 1900s), $k = 6.667 \times 10^{-6}$ per serial interval, $B_t = 2,200$ per serial interval. See Model 4.4, online.

Panel 4.5 Evidence for seasonal transmission of infections

Fine and Clarkson (1982)[36] estimated how the transmission parameter for measles changed each week in England and Wales using the Hamer model described in Panel 4.4 and weekly numbers of notifications during the period 1950–1965. Rearranging Equation 4.29, the authors calculated the transmission parameter k using the expression:

$$k = C_{t+1} / (S_t C_t) \qquad\qquad 4.30$$

C_t was taken to equal the average number of measles cases which were reported each week during the period 1950–1965, which typically increased during the week after the summer holidays (Figure 4.23a). The average number of susceptible individuals in each week during this period (S_t) was calculated using data on the number of individuals notified each year and assumptions about undernotification (Figure 4.23c). According to these analyses, the transmission parameter was lowest during the school holidays (Figure 4.23b). Analyses of these data using other approaches have found similar patterns in the transmission parameters.[46]

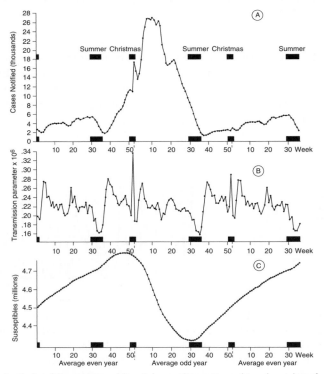

Fig. 4.23 Analysis of the average biennial measles pattern, based on data from 1950 to 1965 in the UK.[36] (a) Average number of cases notified per week; (b) calculated weekly transmission parameters; (c) estimated numbers of susceptibles. Shaded blocks indicate school summer and Christmas holiday periods. Reproduced with permission from Fine and Clarkson, 1982.[36]

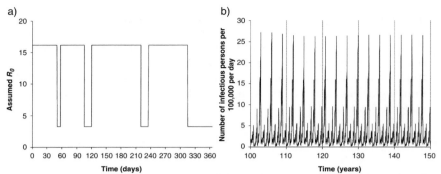

Fig. 4.24 (a) Possible pattern in R_0 for measles, during the course of a school year in the UK, assuming that the average value is 13. The lowest values correspond to school-holidays (Model 4.5, online). The lowest value for R_0 is 20 per cent of the highest value; the average is about 13. (b) Predictions of the daily number of infectious persons per 100,000 population using the model described in Panel 4.3, assuming that R_0 changes over time in the manner shown in (a). See the caption to Figure 4.17 for all other parameter values. The x axis shows the time since the introduction of an infectious person into a totally susceptible population comprising 100,000 individuals.

Changes in contact patterns during the course of a year may also occur because of climatic factors. In some developing countries, studies have linked measles outbreaks to the timing of the rainy season, for example, to the end of the rainy season in Niger[41] or to the period of early rains, when migration of individuals from rural areas to urban areas is likely to be at its greatest[42] (Figure 4.25).

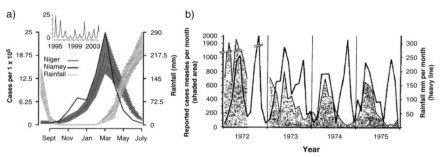

Fig. 4.25 (a) Comparison between the mean monthly number of reported measles cases per 100,000 population in Niamey (the capital of Niger) and Niger during the period 1995–2004 and the mean monthly rainfall. The shaded areas reflect ± 2 standard deviations of the mean; the inset figure shows the monthly numbers of cases per 10,000 population in Niger. Reproduced with permission from Ferrari et al, 2008.[41] (b) Comparison between the mean monthly rainfall in Yaounde, Cameroon (shaded area), during the period 1972–75 and the monthly numbers of reported measles cases (heavy line). Reproduced with permission from Guyer and McBean, 1981.[42]

4.3.2.2 Basic reproduction number

As shown in Figure 4.16, the inter-epidemic period differs between infections and, in the absence of vaccination, is shorter for measles than it is for smallpox. The main reason for these differences is that the basic reproduction number for measles is greater than it is for the other infections. As a result, the proportion of the population that must be susceptible for a measles epidemic to occur ($1/R_0$) is lower for measles than the proportion that must be susceptible for epidemics of other infections to occur. Considering smallpox, for example, for which R_0 is about 5, the proportion of the population that must be susceptible for an epidemic to occur is about $1/5 = 0.2$, whereas that for measles is about $1/13 = 0.08$. It therefore takes less time for the susceptible population to grow, through the continuous entry of newborns, to the size required for a measles epidemic to occur, than it does for a smallpox epidemic.

It has been shown[1] that without interventions such as vaccination, the inter-epidemic period, T, and R_0 are related through the following approximation:

$$T \approx 2\pi \sqrt{\frac{L(D + D')}{R_0 - 1}}$$

4.31

where L is the average life expectancy, D' and D are the average pre-infectious and infectious periods respectively and π is the universal constant 3.14... The derivation of this result is beyond the mathematical scope of this book, although readers can find a detailed proof in Appendix C of Anderson and May[1] or on pages 30–31 of Keeling and Rohani.[35] As we shall see in Chapter 5, R_0 is related to the life expectancy (L) and the average age at infection (A) through the expression $R_0 = 1 + L/A$. Substituting this expression for R_0 into Equation 4.31 leads to the following expression for the inter-epidemic period:

$$T \approx 2\pi \sqrt{A(D + D')}$$

4.32

Methods for calculating the average age at infection are discussed in Chapter 5.

In general, predictions of the inter-epidemic period based on Equation 4.31 have been found to be roughly consistent with those observed for different infections.[1] Exercise 4.2 discusses some applications and limitations of these equations.

4.3.2.2.1 Example: calculating the inter-epidemic period for rubella Substituting for $R_0 = 7$, a pre-infectious period (D') of 10 days and an infectious period (D) of 11 days for rubella (see Table 1.2),[43] and a life expectancy of 70 years ($= 70 \times 365$ days) into Equation 4.31 leads to an estimate of the inter-epidemic period of five years:

$$T \approx 2\pi \sqrt{\frac{70 \times 365 \times (10 + 11)}{7 - 1}} \approx 1{,}879 \, \text{days} \approx 1{,}879 / 365 = 5 \, \text{years}$$

4.33

This estimate is compatible with that observed in Western populations (Figure 4.16).

4.3.2.3 Birth rate

Extending the arguments described in section 4.3.1, the inter-epidemic period for a given infection should decrease as the birth rate increases. For example, in a population with a high birth rate, the susceptible population grows to the size required for an epidemic to occur sooner than in populations in which the birth rate is low. As shown in Figure 4.26a, for settings in which the birth rate is high (e.g. 25 or 40 per 1000 per year, similar to those seen in parts of Asia or sub Saharan Africa during the early 2000s[44]), model predictions suggest that the inter-epidemic period for measles could be much shorter than two years (Model 4.6, online).

These predictions are consistent with the (limited) data available to date from developing countries, where annual cycles in measles notifications have been reported (see e.g. Figure 4.25a (inset) and Figure 4.25b). The interpretation of such annual cycles is complicated by the fact that the national data are composed of data from different regions, and epidemics do not always occur at regular intervals in each region.[41, 45]

On the other hand, the annual cycles in the notifications of measles which were observed in England and Wales during the period 1945–1950 (Figure 4.26b), before they settled into a two-year cycle, have been attributed to a temporary post-war increase in the birth rate, i.e. a 'baby boom'.[46]

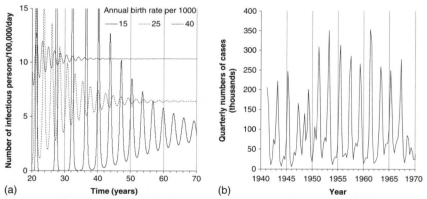

(a)   Time (years)   (b)   Year

Fig. 4.26 (a) Predictions of the daily number of infectious persons per 100,000 population with measles for different values of the birth rate, obtained using the model described in Panel 4.3, assuming that the birth rate exceeds the death rate (Model 4.6, online). The average life expectancy is assumed to be 60 years; the annual birth rates of 15, 25, 40 per 1000 are similar to those seen in the USA, South Central Asia and sub-Saharan Africa during the early 2000s.[44] All other parameter values in the model are identical to those described in the caption to Figure 4.17. The x axis shows the time since the introduction of one infectious person into a totally susceptible population comprising 100,000 persons. (b) Observed notifications of measles in England and Wales during the period 1940–1970.[47]

4.3.2.4 Age-dependent contact

Work by Schenzle[48] has illustrated that if the model described in Panel 4.3 is adapted so that individuals are stratified by age and contact between individuals is strongly 'with-like' (assortative), with most contacts occurring between individuals in the same annual birth cohorts (corresponding to annual school year cohorts), then it predicts that the cycles in incidence persist. On the other hand, studies have argued that, as hypothesized previously,[1] models can recreate the cycles in measles incidence without incorporating age-dependent mixing, and therefore age-dependent contact is not the key factor influencing the cycles.[49] Methods for incorporating age-dependent mixing are described in Chapter 7.

4.3.2.5 Stochastic effects

So far, we have used models that allow transmission to continue even if only 'fractions' of individuals are present in the population. Models which deal with only whole (integer) numbers of individuals, and allow chance to determine contact between individuals (i.e. are stochastic) typically predict regular cycles in the number of new infectious persons, as long as the population size is sufficiently large.[50, 51, 52] In small populations, the cycles typically fade out due to the depletion of susceptible individuals, although they may resume if imported cases enter the population (Figure 4.27).

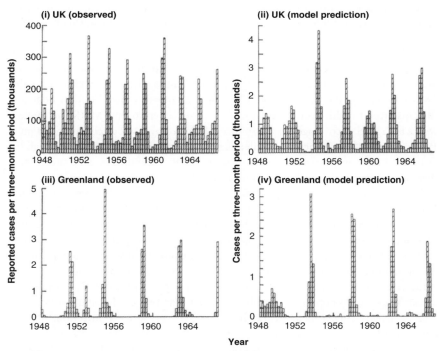

Fig. 4.27 Comparison between observed notifications of measles in (i) the UK and (iii) Greenland against those predicted using a stochastic model. Reproduced with permission from Anderson and May, 1986.[50]

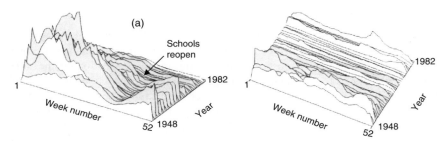

Fig. 4.28 Seasonal patterns in measles and pertussis notifications (left and right-hand figures respectively), based on weekly case reports in England and Wales, 1948–82. Reproduced with permission from Anderson *et al*, 1984.[54]

The effect of seasonal contact patterns and chance events (e.g. influx of new cases) may differ between infections.[53] For example, the time until the cycles in incidence settle down after a slight perturbation in models is predicted to be longer for pertussis than for measles.[53] The reason for this prediction is not yet fully understood, although the relatively long infectious period (15 days) for pertussis may make the cycles sensitive to any changes.[53] Such a sensitivity to small changes may help to explain why the peaks in measles notifications occur at the same time each year, whereas those for pertussis occurred at different times of the year in England and Wales (Figure 4.28).

4.3.2.6 Vaccination

Increases in the inter-epidemic period following the introduction of vaccination have been seen for several infections. For example, epidemics of measles occurred roughly every two years in the UK before vaccination of infants was introduced in 1968, and then occurred roughly every three years until 1988, when routine MMR vaccination, with a high level of coverage, was introduced, followed by a MR catch-up campaign in 1994[55] (Figure 4.29a). The inter-epidemic period is currently very long, although the estimates of the proportion of the population that is susceptible in 2008 suggest that there is potential for an outbreak of up to 100,000 measles cases to occur.[56]

These increases in the inter-epidemic period are consistent with model predictions. For example, extending the intuitive argument in section 4.3.2.3, the introduction of vaccination reduces the number of susceptible individuals entering the population per unit time; it therefore takes longer for the susceptible population to grow to the size required for the epidemic to occur, as compared with the situation in unvaccinated populations. As shown in Figure 4.29b, this reasoning is consistent with model predictions.

Interestingly, the increase in the inter-epidemic period for measles from about 2 years to 2–3 years appears to have been smaller than that predicted using Equation 4.32 (3–4 years), given theoretical estimates of the average age at infection.[1, 54] This has been attributed to several factors, including the fact that the equation implicitly assumes that individuals contact each other randomly. As we shall see in Chapter 7, contact between individuals is strongly age-dependent. Since the introduction of a routine vaccination programme at a sufficiently high coverage leads to an increase in

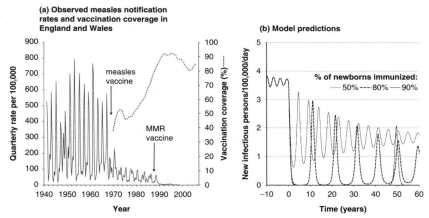

Fig. 4.29 (a) Quarterly notification rates of measles and vaccination coverage in England and Wales. Data sources: Office for Population Censuses and Surveys[47] and the Health Protection Agency.[58] (b) Predictions of the daily number of new infectious persons with measles per 100,000 population following the introduction of vaccination of newborns in year 0, obtained using the model described in Panel 4.3, after adapting it to deal with vaccination (Model 4.7, online). The parameter values are identical to those described in the caption to Figure 4.17.

the average age at infection (Chapter 5), it may reduce the amount of ongoing transmission by a smaller amount than expected, if transmission is pushed into the age group which is most efficient at transmitting.

As shown in Figure 4.29b, the incidence may fall to a very low level following the introduction of vaccination at a high level of coverage, before the epidemic cycles resume. This period following the introduction of vaccination, when there is little ongoing transmission, has been referred to as the 'honeymoon period'[57] and reflects the time until the susceptible population grows to the threshold level required for an epidemic to occur. Such periods of low incidence have been observed in several settings following the introduction of vaccination.[57]

4.4 The dynamics of acute non-immunizing infections

Figure 4.30 shows notification data over a 40-year period for gonorrhoea and syphilis from four cities in the US presented in a study by Grassly *et al.*[59] As discussed in detail in Chapter 8, both infections are transmitted sexually and the duration of infectiousness is typically less than 6 months.[60] Despite their similarities, the long-term dynamics of the infections differ, with notifications of syphilis appearing to cycle every 10 years, whereas those for gonorrhoea did not cycle at all (Figure 4.30).

These differences have been attributed to differences in the duration of immunity provided by the two infections.[59] Once individuals recover from gonorrhoea infection, for example, they appear to be fully susceptible to reinfection; for syphilis, previous

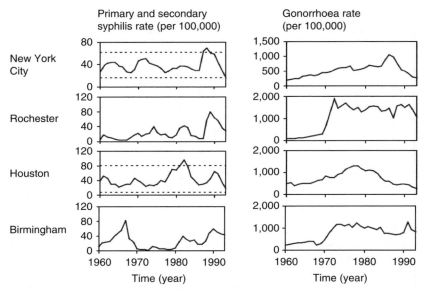

Fig. 4.30 Numbers of cases of syphilis and gonorrhoea per 100,000 population reported in four cities in the US after 1960. Reproduced with permission from Grassly *et al*, 2005.[59]

infection may provide some immunity, although its duration is not fully understood.[61]

Predictions of the effect of different durations of immunity on the long-term dynamics are illustrated in Figure 4.31, for assumptions for R_0 and the average duration of infectiousness which were used by Grassly *et al*.[59] For example, a susceptible–infectious–susceptible (SIS) model, which assumes that, once recovered from infection, individuals become fully susceptible to reinfection, predicts that the number of new infectious persons per 100,000 per month in the long-term should remain stable (Figure 4.31a and Model 4.8, online). However, a susceptible–infectious–recovered–susceptible (SIRS) model which assumes that the duration of immunity is 8–12 years predicts that this would cycle over time, with an inter-epidemic period of 10–15 years, which is compatible with that observed for syphilis (Figure 4.31b and Model 4.8 (online)).

In general, all other assumptions being identical, the inter-epidemic period is predicted to decrease if the average duration of immunity decreases. A short duration of immunity is associated with an increased number of individuals entering the susceptible population per unit time; consequently, the threshold value for the proportion of the population that should be susceptible ($1/R_0$) for an epidemic to occur is reached sooner when the duration of immunity is short than when the duration of immunity is long.

The long term dynamics of several other non-immunizing infections appear to be consistent with predictions from an SIRS model. For example the dynamics of RSV

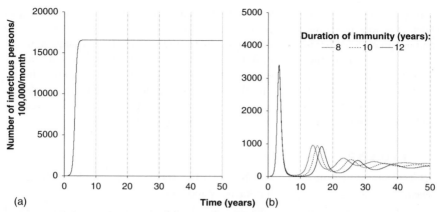

Fig. 4.31 Comparison between predictions of the long-term number of new infectious persons per 100,000 per month assuming that (a) infection does not provide any immunity (an SIS model) and (b) infection provides immunity lasting 8–12 years to reinfection (SIRS model). Individuals enter and leave the population at a rate of 1/30 per year (obtained as 1/(average duration that individuals are sexually active), $R_0 = 1.5$ and the average duration of infectiousness is 2 months (Model 4.8, online).

transmission are compatible with previous infection providing partial or waning immunity to reinfection.[62, 63] Also, antigenic drift in seasonal influenza in humans has been described using SIRS models.[64, 65, 66] These have modelled single strains belonging to each of the influenza subtypes (H1N1, H3N2 and flu B) circulating in the population; the effect of antigenic drift has been incorporated by assuming that previously infected individuals lose their immunity and become susceptible to the circulating strain at a constant rate, depending on the subtype. [64, 65, 66]

4.5 **Summary**

This chapter has illustrated several insights into the properties of epidemics for acute infections that are provided by the models which were discussed during the last two chapters. The basic reproduction number determines whether or not the number of infectious persons increases following the introduction of an infection into a totally susceptible population. It also determines the proportion of the population that must be susceptible for the incidence to increase. For example, if the proportion of the population which is susceptible is greater than $1/R_0$, the net reproduction number is greater than 1 and the incidence increases for acute infections. The basic reproduction number also determines the growth rate of an epidemic and the final epidemic size, and can be estimated from these statistics and the serial interval or generation time, or by fitting transmission models to data.

This chapter has also illustrated how the cycles in the incidence of immunizing infections result from changes in the proportion of the population that is susceptible, which stem from the entry of susceptible newborns into the population and the removal of susceptible individuals, after they contact infectious individuals and become immune. Further factors, including changes in contact during the course of a year, the birth rate and vaccination further influence the frequency of these cycles. For the acute non-immunizing infections, the long-term dynamics depend on the duration of immunity provided by the infection: for infections which confer no immunity (e.g. gonorrhoea), the incidence is unlikely to cycle; for those conferring partial immunity (e.g. syphilis), the incidence is likely to cycle over time, with the inter-epidemic period decreasing with the duration of protection associated with the infection.

4.6 **Exercises**

4.1 Table 4.4 shows the weekly numbers of influenza cases reported in Gothenberg, Sweden, during the 1918 Spanish influenza pandemic.[67]

a) Calculate the growth rate in the epidemic during the first and second waves and use this to estimate the net and basic reproduction numbers for each wave, assuming that 30 and 50 per cent of individuals were immune at the start of the first and second waves respectively, and that the average pre-infectious and infectious periods were both 2 days.

b) Calculate R_0 using the final epidemic size.

c) Which estimate of R_0 is likely to be most reliable?

d) What do your answers tell us about changes in the transmissibility of the influenza virus between successive waves of a pandemic?

Table 4.4 The weekly numbers of influenza cases reported in Gothenberg during the 1918 Spanish influenza pandemic.[67] The population comprised about 196,943 individuals in 1918.

Week beginning	No of cases reported	Week beginning	No of cases reported	Week beginning	No of cases reported
06/07/1918	1	14/09/1918	181	23/11/1918	752
13/07/1918	18	21/09/1918	464	30/11/1918	727
20/07/1918	573	28/09/1918	1,181	07/12/1918	630
27/07/1918	1,084	05/10/1918	2,196	14/12/1918	573
03/08/1918	1,120	12/10/1918	3,287	21/12/1918	430
10/08/1918	815	19/10/1918	2,555	28/12/1918	368
17/08/1918	517	26/10/1918	1,606	04/01/1919	466
24/08/1918	344	02/11/1918	1,297	11/01/1919	440
31/08/1918	185	09/11/1918	907	18/01/1919	317
07/09/1918	155	16/11/1918	737	25/01/1919	215

4.2

a) The inter-epidemic period for measles was about two years in England and Wales during the period 1950–1968 (Figure 4.16). Assuming an average life expectancy of 70 years, pre-infectious and infectious periods of eight and seven days respectively, use Equation 4.31 to calculate R_0 during this time.

b) The inter-epidemic period for measles was about three years during the period 1968–1988 (i.e. after the introduction of measles vaccination). Suggest possible values for the average age at infection during this time. What are the limitations of this estimate?

References

1 Anderson RM, May RM. *Infectious diseases of humans. Dynamics and control.* Oxford: Oxford University Press; 1992.

2 Bailey NTJ. *The mathematical theory of epidemics.* New York: Hafner Publishing Company; 1957.

3 Diekmann O, Heesterbeek JA. *Mathematical epidemiology of infectious diseases: model building, analysis and interpretation.* Chichester: John Wiley; 2000.

4 Philip RN, Reinhard KR, Lackman DB. Observations on a mumps epidemic in a virgin population. *Am J Hyg* 1959; 69(2):91–111.

5 Philip RN, Reinhard KR, Lackman DB. Observations on a mumps epidemic in a 'virgin' population. 1958. *Am J Epidemiol* 1995; 142(3):233–253.

6 Ministry of Health. *The influenza pandemic in England and Wales 1957–58.* 1960. 100. London, Her Majesty's Stationery Office. Reports on Public Health and Medical Subjects.

7 Christensen PE, Schmidt H, Bang Ho, Andersen V, Jordal B, Jensen O. An epidemic of measles in southern Greenland, 1951; measles in virgin soil. II. The epidemic proper. *Acta Med Scand* 1953; 144(6):408–429.

8 Lipsitch M, Cohen T, Cooper B *et al.* Transmission dynamics and control of severe acute respiratory syndrome. *Science* 2003; 300(5627):1966–1970.

9 Riley S, Fraser C, Donnelly CA *et al.* Transmission dynamics of the etiological agent of SARS in Hong Kong: impact of public health interventions. *Science* 2003; 300(5627): 1961–1966.

10 Anderson RM, Fraser C, Ghani AC *et al.* Epidemiology, transmission dynamics and control of SARS: the 2002–2003 epidemic. *Philos Trans R Soc Lond B Biol Sci* 2004; 359(1447):1091–1105.

11 http://www.who.int/csr/sars/country/en/index.html. Cumulative number of reported probable cases of Severe Acute Respiratory Syndrome (SARS). 2008. 17–5–2008.

12 Chowell G, Nishiura H, Bettencourt LM. Comparative estimation of the reproduction number for pandemic influenza from daily case notification data. *J R Soc Interface* 2007; 4(12):155–166.

13 Mills CE, Robins JM, Lipsitch M. Transmissibility of 1918 pandemic influenza. *Nature* 2004; 432(7019):904–906.

14 Vynnycky E, Trindall A, Mangtani P. Estimates of the reproduction numbers of Spanish influenza using morbidity data. *Int J Epidemiol* 2007; 36(4):881–889.

15 White LF, Pagano M. Transmissibility of the influenza virus in the 1918 pandemic. *PLoS ONE* 2008; 3(1):e1498.

16 Frost W, Sydenstricker E. Influenza in Maryland. Preliminary statistics of certain localities. *Public Health Rep* 1919; 34(11):491–504.

17 Olson DR, Simonsen L, Edelson PJ, Morse SS. Epidemiological evidence of an early wave of the 1918 influenza pandemic in New York City. *Proc Natl Acad Sci USA* 2005; 102(31):11059–11063.

18 Stuart-Harris C. Epidemiology of influenza in man. *Br Med Bull* 1979; 35(1):3–8.

19 Monto AS, Koopman JS, Longini IM, Jr. Tecumseh study of illness. XIII. Influenza infection and disease, 1976–1981. *Am J Epidemiol* 1985; 121(6):811–822.

20 Wearing HJ, Rohani P, Keeling MJ. Appropriate models for the management of infectious diseases. *PLoS Med* 2005; 2(7):e174.

21 Wallinga J, Teunis P. Different epidemic curves for severe acute respiratory syndrome reveal similar impacts of control measures. *Am J Epidemiol* 2004; 160(6): 509–516.

22 Wallinga J, Lipsitch M. How generation intervals shape the relationship between growth rates and reproductive numbers. *Proc Biol Sci* 2007; 274(1609):599–604.

23 Ma J, Earn DJ. Generality of the final size formula for an epidemic of a newly invading infectious disease. *Bull Math Biol* 2006; 68(3):679–702.

24 Becker N. *Analysis of infectious disease data.* Chapman and Hall; 1989.

25 Chowell G, Hengartner NW, Castillo-Chavez C, Fenimore PW, Hyman JM. The basic reproductive number of Ebola and the effects of public health measures: the cases of Congo and Uganda. *J Theor Biol* 2004; 229(1):119–126.

26 Gani R, Leach S. Transmission potential of smallpox in contemporary populations. *Nature* 2001; 414(6865):748–751.

27 Armitage P, Berry G. *Statistical methods in medical research, 3rd edn.* Oxford: Blackwell Scientific Publications; 1994.

28 Clayton D, Hills M. *Statistical methods in epidemiology.* Oxford: Oxford University Press; 1993.

29 Hillborn R, Mangel M. *The ecological detective. Confronting models with data.* Princeton: Princeton University Press; 1997.

30 Wetherill GB. *Intermediate statistical methods.* London: Chapman and Hall; 1981.

31 Registrar General. *Annual report of the Registrar General of births, deaths and marriages in England and Wales.* 1939. London, England, Her Majesty's Stationery Office.

32 Preblud SR, Serdula MK, Frank JA, Jr., Brandling-Bennett AD, Hinman AR. Rubella vaccination in the United States: a ten-year review. *Epidemiol Rev* 1980; 2: 171–94.

33 Brisson M, Edmunds WJ, Law B *et al.* Epidemiology of varicella zoster virus infection in Canada and the United Kingdom. *Epidemiol Infect* 2001; 127(2):305–314.

34 Hamer WH. Epidemic disease in England – the evidence of variability and of persistency of type. *Lancet* 1906;(i):733–739.

35 Keeling MJ, Rohani P. *Modeling infectious diseases in humans and animals.* Princeton and Oxford: Princeton University Press; 2008.

36 Fine PE, Clarkson JA. Measles in England and Wales—I: An analysis of factors underlying seasonal patterns. *Int J Epidemiol* 1982; 11(1):5–14.

37 London WP, Yorke JA. Recurrent outbreaks of measles, chickenpox and mumps. I. Seasonal variation in contact rates. *Am J Epidemiol* 1973; 98(6):453–468.

38 Yorke JA, London WP. Recurrent outbreaks of measles, chickenpox and mumps. II. Systematic differences in contact rates and stochastic effects. *Am J Epidemiol* 1973; 98(6):469–482.

39 Heymann A, Chodick G, Reichman B, Kokia E, Laufer J. Influence of school closure on the incidence of viral respiratory diseases among children and on health care utilization. *Pediatr Infect Dis J* 2004; 23(7):675–677.

40 Cauchemez S, Valleron AJ, Boelle PY, Flahault A, Ferguson NM. Estimating the impact of school closure on influenza transmission from Sentinel data. *Nature* 2008; 452(7188):750–754.

41 Ferrari MJ, Grais RF, Bharti N *et al.* The dynamics of measles in sub-Saharan Africa. *Nature* 2008; 451(7179):679–684.

42 Guyer B, McBean AM. The epidemiology and control of measles in Yaounde, Cameroun, 1968–1975. *Int J Epidemiol* 1981; 10(3):263–269.

43 Heymann DL. *Control of communicable diseases manual, 18th edn.* Washington, DC: American Public Health Association; 2004.

44 World Population Prospects. *The 2006 Revision and World Urbanization Prospects: The 2005 Revision.* Population Division of the Department of Economic and Social Affairs of the United Nations Secretariat. 2005.

45 Cummings DA, Moss WJ, Long K *et al.* Improved measles surveillance in Cameroon reveals two major dynamic patterns of incidence. *Int J Infect Dis* 2006; 10(2):148–155.

46 Finkenstadt BF, Grenfell BT. Time series modelling of childhood diseases: a dynamical systems approach. *Appl Statist* 2000; 49(2):187–205.

47 Office for Population Censuses and Surveys. *The Registrar General's statistical review of England and Wales. Part I. Tables, Medical.* 1970. London, Her Majesty's Stationery Office.

48 Schenzle D. An age-structured model of pre- and post-vaccination measles transmission. *IMA J Math Appl Med Biol* 1984; 1(2):169–191.

49 Earn DJ, Rohani P, Bolker BM, Grenfell BT. A simple model for complex dynamical transitions in epidemics. *Science* 2000; 287(5453):667–670.

50 Anderson RM, May RM. The invasion, persistence and spread of infectious diseases within animal and plant communities. *Philos Trans R Soc Lond B Biol Sci* 1986; 314(1167):533–570.

51 Bartlett MS. Measles periodicity and community size. *J R Statist Soc* 1957; A120:48–70.

52 Bartlett MS. The critical community size for measles in the United States. *J R Statist Soc* 1960; 123:37–44.

53 Rohani P, Keeling MJ, Grenfell BT. The interplay between determinism and stochasticity in childhood diseases. *Am Nat* 2002; 159(5):469–481.

54 Anderson RM, Grenfell BT, May RM. Oscillatory fluctuations in the incidence of infectious disease and the impact of vaccination: time series analysis. *J Hyg (Lond)* 1984; 93(3):587–608.

55 Ramsay M, Gay N, Miller E *et al.* The epidemiology of measles in England and Wales: rationale for the 1994 national vaccination campaign. *Commun Dis Rep CDR Rev* 1994; 4(12):R141–R146.

56 Choi YH, Gay N, Fraser G, Ramsay M. The potential for measles transmission in England. *BMC Public Health* 2008; 8:338.

57 McLean AR. After the honeymoon in measles control. *Lancet* 1995; 345(8945):272.

58 Office for Population Censuses and Surveys. *Communicable disease statistics.* Series MB2 no 6. 1979. London, Her Majesty's Stationery Office.

59 Grassly NC, Fraser C, Garnett GP. Host immunity and synchronized epidemics of syphilis across the United States. *Nature* 2005; 433(7024):417–421.

60 Holmes KK, Sparling FP, Stamm WE *et al. Sexually transmitted diseases.* New York: McGraw-Hill Professional; 2008.

61 Garnett GP, Aral SO, Hoyle DV, Cates W, Jr., Anderson RM. The natural history of syphilis. Implications for the transmission dynamics and control of infection. *Sex Transm Dis* 1997; 24(4):185–200.

62 Weber A, Weber M, Milligan P. Modeling epidemics caused by respiratory syncytial virus (RSV). *Math Biosci* 2001; 172(2):95–113.

63 White LJ, Mandl JN, Gomes MG *et al.* Understanding the transmission dynamics of respiratory syncytial virus using multiple time series and nested models. *Math Biosci* 2007; 209(1):222–239.

64 Dushoff J, Plotkin JB, Levin SA, Earn DJ. Dynamical resonance can account for seasonality of influenza epidemics. *Proc Natl Acad Sci USA* 2004; 101(48):16915–16916.

65 Finkenstadt BF, Morton A, Rand DA. Modelling antigenic drift in weekly flu incidence. *Stat Med* 2005; 24(22):3447–3461.

66 Vynnycky E, Pitman R, Siddiqui R, Gay N, Edmunds WJ. Estimating the impact of childhood influenza vaccination programmes in England and Wales. *Vaccine* 2008; 26(41):5321–5330.

67 Ministry of Health. *Report on the pandemic of influenza, 1918–19.* 1920. 4. His Majesty's Stationery Office. Reports on Public Health and Medical Subjects.

68 Gilks WR, Richardson S, Spiegelhalter DJ. *Introducing Markov chain Monte Carlo.* London: Chapman and Hall; 1996.

69 Blower S, Dowlatabadi H. Sensitivity and uncertainty analysis of complex models of disease transmission: an HIV model, as an example. *International Statistical Review* 1994; 62(2):229–243.

Chapter 5

Age patterns

5.1 Overview and objectives

In this chapter, we discuss age patterns in the proportion of the population that is susceptible and the number of new infections per unit time and how they are affected by the basic reproduction number and the force of infection. We also discuss how vaccination programmes can lead to changes in the force of infection, which, besides having the beneficial effect of reducing the overall number of new infections occurring in the population, can also lead to increases in the proportion of individuals that are susceptible and the number of new infections in some age groups.

By the end of this chapter you should:

+ Know how R_0 can be calculated, assuming random mixing, from the average force of infection and the proportion of the population that is susceptible;

+ Be able to analyse age-specific serological data for immunizing and non-immunizing infections to estimate both the crude and age-specific force of infection;

+ Know what is meant by herd immunity;

+ Understand the effect of vaccination on the force of infection and how, besides leading to reductions in the overall number of new infections per unit time, it can lead to increases in the proportion of individuals that are susceptible and in the number of new infections per unit time in older age groups;

+ Understand the differences between predictions from a dynamic transmission model and a static model.

5.2 Age patterns—analysing cross-sectional data

5.2.1 The acute immunizing infections

So far in this book, we have mainly discussed patterns in the *overall* proportion of a population that is susceptible or the number of new infections or infectious persons per unit time. In practice, these patterns vary greatly with age. For example, a larger proportion of children than adults are likely to be susceptible to immunizing infections, given that children have had fewer years of exposure to the infection than adults.

Consequently, if we take a cross-section of the population and measure the proportion of individuals who have antibodies or some marker of previous infection (assuming that no individuals have been vaccinated), we are likely to see patterns similar to those in Figure 5.1: the proportion of individuals with antibodies and who are presumably immune to infection increases with increasing age. In addition, the proportion of

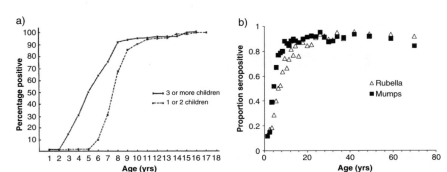

Fig. 5.1 (a) Data on the age-specific proportion of individuals in large and small families who were seropositive to measles in New Haven, Connecticut in 1957.[3] Reproduced with permission from Black, 1959.[3] (b) Data on the age-specific proportion of individuals who were seropositive to mumps and rubella in 1988 in England and Wales.[4] The data for rubella were collected among males only.

individuals that were seropositive to mumps increased more rapidly with age than for rubella in England and Wales, indicating that mumps was more infectious than rubella (Figure 5.1b). The proportion of individuals that have antibodies is also likely to vary between settings, depending on crowding (Figure 5.1a).

These age patterns are determined by the average force of infection (average rate at which susceptible individuals are infected) which, as shown below, can be estimated using data such as those shown in Figure 5.1. These patterns, in turn, can be used to calculate the basic reproduction number and other helpful epidemiological statistics, such as the average age at infection and the proportion of the population that is susceptible.

5.2.2 **Estimating the average force of infection**

What do we mean by the average force of infection for an endemic immunizing infection? As we saw in Chapters 2 and 3, if we assume that individuals contact each other randomly, the force of infection ($\lambda(t)$) and the number of infectious individuals ($I(t)$) at time t are related through the expression:

$$\lambda(t) = \beta I(t) \qquad\qquad 5.1$$

where β is the rate at which two specific individuals come into effective contact per unit time (Section 2.7.1). For immunizing infections the number of infectious individuals cycles over time and therefore the force of infection must also cycle over time. However, in the absence of vaccination or other interventions, the *average* value of the force of infection remains approximately constant (Figure 5.2). We will use the symbol λ (dropping the 't' in parentheses) to refer to this average value.

We can predict the proportion of individuals in each age group that should be susceptible by using the following simple model, which tracks individuals from birth

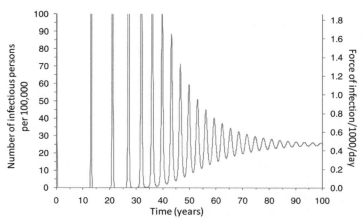

Fig. 5.2 Predictions of the number of infectious persons per 100,000 population with measles, assuming $R_0 = 13$, following the introduction of one infectious person into a totally susceptible population, obtained using the model described in Panel 4.3. The pre-infectious and infectious periods are eight and seven days respectively, $R_0 = 13$ and the per capita mortality rate = birth rate = 3.92×10^{-5} per day, which is equivalent to an average life expectancy of 70 years. One infectious person is introduced into the population comprising 100,000 individuals at the start.

and uses the average annual force of infection for the rate at which susceptible individuals are infected:

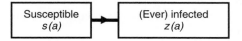

Note that the '(Ever) infected' compartment comprises all those who are not susceptible, i.e. it includes those who have been infected have recovered and are immune, those who have been infected but are not yet infectious, and those who are infectious. We will use the notation $z(a)$ to refer to this group of individuals collectively, who are of age a. This model implicitly assumes that the mortality rates are identical for susceptible individuals and those (ever) infected.

Predictions from this model are shown in Figure 5.3, assuming that all individuals are susceptible at birth: if the average force of infection is high, e.g. about 25%/year, which is similar to that seen for measles in Ethiopia during the early 2000s,[5] then, on average, 50 per cent of individuals should have been infected by age 4–5 years, and most have been infected by age 10 years. If it is low, e.g. 5%/year, on the other hand, about 40 per cent of individuals are still susceptible at age 20 years.

This model is known as a 'simple catalytic model'. Panel 5.1 discusses the origin of the name for this model. It belongs to the class of models for which we can express the size of a given compartment in terms of the mathematical constant 'e' (see Section 3.5.1).

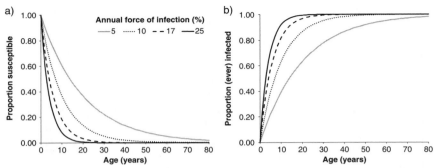

Fig. 5.3 Predictions of the proportion of individuals that a) should still be susceptible or b) have (ever) been infected by the time they reach different ages, assuming that the average annual force of infection is between 5 and 25 per cent (see Model 5.1 online).

In our case, the proportion of individuals that are susceptible at age a, $s(a)$, equals the expression:

$$s(a) = e^{-\lambda a} \qquad\qquad 5.2$$

The proportion of individuals who have ever been infected by age a ($z(a)$) is given by 1–proportion susceptible at age a, i.e.

$$z(a) = 1 - e^{-\lambda a} \qquad\qquad 5.3$$

The force of infection is typically estimated by formally fitting predictions from the catalytic model to the data, whereby the value of the force of infection is varied until the smallest distance, as reflected by some goodness of fit statistic, between the model prediction and the observed data is obtained. Methods for fitting models to data are discussed in section 4.2.5.

Factors relating to the data which need to be considered when fitting models are discussed in section 5.2.5. Figure 5.4 compares the best-fitting simple catalytic model against the rubella and mumps data for England and Wales (see Figure 5.1). The best-fitting average annual force of infection is 11.6 per cent (95% CI: 11.1–12.1%) and 19.8 per cent (95% CI: 19.1–20.5%) for rubella and mumps respectively. Methods for refining these estimates to account for maternally-derived immunity and age-dependencies in the force of infection are discussed in section 5.2.3.5.

Methods for obtaining crude estimates for the force of infection, which are useful for verifying estimates obtained by fitting models to data, are discussed below.

5.2.2.1 Quick and approximate methods for estimating the force of infection

5.2.2.1.1 The median age at infection The average force of infection can be estimated by using the equation $\lambda \approx 1/A$ (see section 5.2.3.1 for the derivation), substituting the median age at infection for A in this equation. The median age at infection is defined as the age by which 50 per cent of individuals have been infected and can be

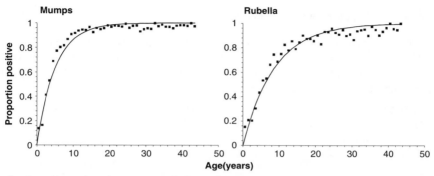

Fig. 5.4 Comparison between predictions of the age-specific prevalence of mumps and rubella seropositivity for England and Wales obtained using the best-fitting catalytic model and the observed data from Figure 5.1. See Model 5.2, online.

Panel 5.1 What is a catalytic model?

Catalytic models are identical to SI, SIR and SIRS models (see Figure 2.2), except that they do not explicitly describe transmission between individuals, i.e. the force of infection is not expressed in terms of a transmission parameter 'β' and the number of infectious persons. Instead, individuals are assumed to become infected at some constant age- or time-dependent rate. Thus, catalytic models simply aim to describe the data, without explicitly modelling the mechanism (i.e. contact between susceptible and infectious individuals) by which they arise.

The term 'catalytic model' stems from Münch,[16] who used an analogy from chemistry. At the time, it was thought that in a typical reaction, the molecules from the catalyst exerted a constant force on some substance (S_1), changing it into another substance (S_2), as described in the following diagram:

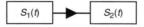

The rate of change in the proportion of the mixture which is made up by substance S_1 (denoted by $s_1(t)$) would be written as follows (see section 3.5.1), where λ is the force exerted by the catalyst per unit time:

$$\frac{ds_1}{dt} = -\lambda s_1(t)$$

By analogy, in real life, susceptible individuals are exposed to a 'force of infection' from birth resulting from exposure to infectious individuals, converting them into infected individuals.

Panel 5.1 What is a catalytic model? *(continued)*

Table 5.1 summarizes the difference and differential equations for this model. Note that both types of equations are written with respect to age, rather than time, since we are describing how the proportion of individuals that are susceptible or (ever) infected changes as individuals age.

Table 5.1 Summary of the difference and differential equations for the simple catalytic model describing the proportion of individuals of age *a* that are susceptible or (ever) infected

	Difference equations	**Differential equations**
Proportion susceptible (s_a and $s(a)$)	$s_{a+1} = s_a - \lambda s_a$	$\dfrac{ds}{da} = -\lambda s(a)$
Proportion ever infected (z_a and $z(a)$)	$z_{a+1} = z_a + \lambda s_a$ or,: $z_{a+1} = z_a + \lambda(1 - z_a)$, (obtained after substituting for $s_a = 1 - z_a$ into the above equation, assuming that the proportion susceptible = 1–proportion ever infected.)	$\dfrac{dz}{da} = \lambda s(a)$

If λ is identical for all ages, s_a and z_a can be rewritten as follows:

$$s_a = (1 - \lambda)^a \qquad\qquad 5.4$$

$$z_a = 1 - (1 - \lambda)^a \qquad\qquad 5.5$$

Equation 5.4 is derived by using the fact that the risk of escaping infection in 1 year of life is $1-\lambda$, and so the proportion of individuals who escape infection in 2 years of life ($= s_2$) is $(1-\lambda) \times (1-\lambda)$. The proportion who escape infection in 3 years of life ($= s_3$) equals $(1-\lambda) \times (1-\lambda) \times (1-\lambda) = (1-\lambda)^3$. Extending this logic to *a* years of life gives the result $s_a = (1-\lambda)^a$.

We obtain Equation 5.5 by substituting for $s_a = 1-z_a$ into Equation 5.4 and rearranging the resulting equation.

read off from a plot of the data. It is about five years for the mumps data in Figure 5.1, implying that the force of infection was about 20%/year.

5.2.2.1.2 The age-specific risk of infection Equation 5.6 gives a method for estimating the risk of infection experienced between age groups *a* and *a*+1 (λ_a), where s_a is the estimated proportion of individuals in age group *a* who are susceptible.

$$\lambda_a = 1 - \frac{s_{a+1}}{s_a} \qquad\qquad 5.6$$

This equation is obtained by rearranging the difference equation $s_{a+1} = s_a - \lambda_a s_a$ (see Table 5.1). Risks and rates are related through the expression: $risk = 1 - e^{-rate}$, or equivalently, $rate = ln(1-risk)$ (see Panel 2.2); the force of infection can therefore be calculated by using the equation $ln(1-\lambda_a)$.

5.2.2.1.3 The average annual risk of infection The average risk of infection experienced in each year of life by the time individuals reach a years can be estimated by using Equation 5.7, which is obtained by rearranging the difference equation $s_a = (1 - \lambda)^a$ (see Equation 5.4).

$$\lambda = 1 - s_a^{1/a} \qquad\qquad 5.7$$

This equation has been applied to estimate the average annual risk of M $tuberculosis$ infection in different settings using tuberculin survey data.[6] Whilst useful for obtaining quick estimates, its main disadvantage is that it provides no insight into when this risk occured.

5.2.2.1.4 Example: estimating the risk of mumps infection The proportions of 5–9 and 10–14 year olds who were seronegative to mumps in England and Wales during the 1980s[4] was $s_{5-9} = 0.21796$ and $s_{10-14} = 0.06873$. Applying Equation 5.6, the risk of infection between the ages 5–9 and 10–14 years is given by:

$$\lambda = 1 - \frac{0.06873}{0.21796} = 0.68467$$

This risk is interpretable as a five-year risk, i.e. as the proportion of uninfected 5–9-year-olds who were infected by age 10–14 years. Note that $1-0.68467$ is interpretable as the proportion of individuals who stay susceptible between the ages 5–9 and 10–14 years. We can therefore apply Equation 5.7 to estimate the average annual risk of infection experienced between the ages 5–9 and 10–14 years as $\lambda = 1 - (1 - 0.68467)^{1/5} = 0.206$ per year.

This value is very similar to the average annual risk of infection for 10–14-year-olds estimated using Equation 5.7, i.e. $\lambda = 1 - 0.06873^{1/12} = 0.20$ per year, assuming that the average age of 10–14-year-olds is 12 years.

5.2.3 Applying estimates of the average force of infection

5.2.3.1 The average age at infection

As discussed in section 2.7.2, if we assume that something occurs at a constant rate, then the average time to the event and the average rate at which it occurs are related through the equation:

average time to event $= 1 /$ (average rate at which the event occurs)

Using this equation, the average time to infection (i.e. the average age at infection) and the average force of infection are related through the equation:

$$A \approx 1 / \lambda \qquad\qquad 5.8$$

Table 5.2 Summary of the main equations for the average age at infection.
See Exercise 5.7 for the derivations of equations 5.10 and 5.11.

Type of population	Equation	Equation number
All populations (general equation)	$A = \dfrac{\int_0^\infty a\lambda(a)S(a)da}{\int_0^\infty \lambda(a)S(a)da}$	5.9
Exponential age distribution	$A = \dfrac{1}{\lambda + 1/L} \text{ or } \dfrac{1}{\lambda + m}$	5.10
Rectangular age distribution	$A = \dfrac{1}{\lambda}\left(\dfrac{1-(1+\lambda L)e^{-\lambda L}}{1-e^{-\lambda L}}\right)$	5.11

$S(a)$ is the number of individuals of age a who are susceptible, $\lambda(a)$ is the force of infection among individuals of age a, L is the average life expectancy and m is the average mortality rate.

This relationship is approximate, since the average age at infection depends on how many individuals die before being infected and hence on the mortality rate (see below). It also assumes that the force of infection is independent of age and that individuals mix randomly. Table 5.2 summarizes the main equations for the average age at infection for a population with an exponential age distribution (i.e. similar to that in some developing countries—see Figure 3.7), and for populations with a rectangular age distribution. The latter are similar to those in Western populations, in which few (in theory, no) individuals die until they reach some life expectancy, L.

These expressions and the expression $A = 1/\lambda$ give very similar estimates for realistic values for the life expectancy and a force of infection of >5%/year (Figure 5.5

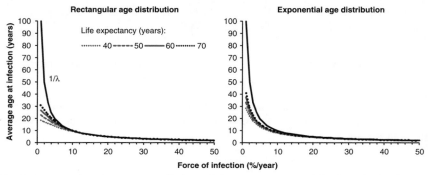

Fig. 5.5 Comparison between predictions of the average age at infection obtained using the expression $1/\lambda$ (solid black line) and the exact equations (Equations 5.10 and 5.11) (dotted or grey lines) for populations with rectangular and exponential age distributions respectively, for different values for the life expectancy.

and exercise 5.4). Consequently, the expression $A = 1/\lambda$ is often used to calculate the average age at infection; taking account of maternally derived immunity, this expression would be written as:

$$A \approx 1/\lambda + 1/\mu \qquad\qquad 5.12$$

where $1/\mu$ is the average duration of protection resulting from maternally-derived antibodies.

Equation 5.9 is often evaluated using estimates of the age-specific *proportion* rather than the actual *number* of individuals who are susceptible at age a, if the latter is not available. This expression reflects the average age at infection among individuals who ultimately experience infection (see [4]), i.e. it excludes those who are never infected. Alternative expressions accounting for such individuals are discussed in refs.[4, 7]

5.2.3.1.1 Example: the average age at mumps infection The average force of mumps infection in England and Wales during the 1980s was about 19.8 per cent per year. Applying Equation 5.8, this implies that the average age at infection was about $1/0.198 \approx 5.05$ years; assuming a life expectancy of 70 years and applying Equation 5.11 implies that the average age at infection was very similar, i.e.

$$\frac{1}{0.198}\left(\frac{1-(1+0.198\times70)e^{-0.198\times70}}{1-e^{-0.198\times70}} \right) \approx 5.05 \text{ years.}$$

5.2.3.2 The proportion of the population that is susceptible

It can be shown (Appendix section A.3.1 and A.3.2 and ref [9]) that for populations with exponential or rectangular age distributions, and assuming that individuals mix randomly, the average proportion of the population that is susceptible (s), the average force of infection and the average life expectancy (L) are related through the following equation:

$$\text{Exponential age distribution:} \quad s = \frac{1}{\lambda L + 1} \qquad\qquad 5.13$$

$$\text{Rectangular age distribution:} \quad s \approx \frac{1}{\lambda L} \qquad\qquad 5.14$$

Substituting the relationship $\lambda \approx 1/A$ into Equations 5.13 and 5.14 leads to the following equations for the proportion of the population that is susceptible:

$$\text{Exponential age distribution:} \quad s \approx \frac{A}{A+L} \qquad\qquad 5.15$$

$$\text{Rectangular age distribution:} \quad s \approx A/L \qquad\qquad 5.16$$

Figure 5.6b provides an intuitive derivation for Equation 5.16.

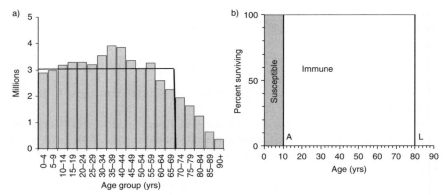

Fig. 5.6 (a) Example of a population with a rectangular age distribution: England, 2004. Data sources: http://www.ons.gov.uk (b) Intuitive explanation for the expression $s = A/L$. For a population with a rectangular age distribution, we can assume that everyone is susceptible until the average age A, when they become immune, and everyone dies at age L. The proportion susceptible is therefore given by the area of the grey rectangle in figure b) divided by the area of the entire rectangle between the ages 0 and L. In this example, $A = 10$ years, $L = 80$ years and therefore the proportion of the population that is susceptible equals $10/80 = 0.125$.

5.2.3.2.1 Example: the proportion of the population that is susceptible to mumps infection The average age at mumps infection in England and Wales during the 1980s was about five years (section 5.2.3.1.1). Assuming an average life expectancy of 70 years, and applying Equation 5.16 implies that the proportion of the population that was susceptible was about $5/70 \approx 0.07$.

The proportion of the population that is susceptible can also be estimated directly from the data without using estimates of the average force of infection, using the following equation:

$$s = \sum_a p_a \frac{S_a}{N_a}$$

5.17

assuming that the individuals who are negative to the biological test for infection are susceptible to infection. Here p_a is the proportion of the population that is in age group a (obtained from life tables) and S_a is the number of susceptibles among the N_a individuals of age a who were tested. This expression is interpretable as the age-weighted average of the proportion of individuals that are susceptible.

If the population has a rectangular age distribution, p_a can be calculated using the following expression:

$$p_a = \frac{width\ of\ age\ group\ a}{Life\ expectancy}$$

5.18

5.2.3.2.2 Example: calculating the proportion of the population that is susceptible directly from data Columns 2–4 of the following table show data on the number of individuals in different age groups who were positive, negative (S_a) and tested (N_a) for mumps antibodies in England and Wales during the 1980s;[4] the proportion that were negative (S_a/N_a) is provided in column 5.

Age group (years)	Number			S_a/N_a	p_a	$p_a \times S_a/N_a$
	Positive	Negative (S_a)	Total (N_a)			
1–4	436	963	1,399	0.68835	4/70	0.03933
5–9	1,263	352	1,615	0.21796	5/70	0.01557
10–14	1,477	109	1,586	0.06873	5/70	0.00491
15–19	754	38	792	0.04798	5/70	0.00343
20–29	1,651	46	1,697	0.02711	10/70	0.00387
30–39	825	27	852	0.03169	10/70	0.00453
40+	234	4	238	0.01681	30/70	0.0072

The values for p_a are provided in column 6, assuming a life expectancy of 70 years. For example, the width of the age group 10–14 years equals 5 years. If the life expectancy is 70 years, $p_{10-14} = 5/70 = 0.071$. The final column provides the values for $p_a \times S_a/N_a$. Summing these values for all age groups leads to the following estimate for the proportion of the population that is susceptible:

$$s = 0.03933 + 0.01557 + 0.00491 + 0.00343$$
$$+ 0.00387 + 0.00453 + 0.0072$$
$$= 0.0788$$

5.2.3.3 The basic reproduction number

As discussed in section 4.3.2, for an endemic immunizing infection, and assuming that individuals mix randomly, the average proportion of the population that is susceptible, s, is related to the basic reproduction number through the expression:

$$s = 1/R_0 \tag{5.19}$$

After rearranging this expression, we obtain the following expression for R_0:

$$R_0 = 1/s \tag{5.20}$$

Substituting for $s = \dfrac{1}{\lambda L + 1}$ and $s \approx \dfrac{1}{\lambda L}$ (Equations 5.13 and 5.14) into Equation 5.20, assuming further that individuals mix randomly, leads to the following equations for R_0 for populations with exponential and rectangular age distributions:

$$\text{Exponential age distribution:} \quad R_0 = 1 + \lambda L \tag{5.21}$$

$$\text{Rectangular age distribution:} \quad R_0 \approx L\lambda \tag{5.22}$$

Equation 5.22 predicts that, if the average life expectancy is 70 years and R_0 is up to 20, the maximum force of infection that would be seen is about 28 per cent per year, assuming that individuals mix randomly (Figure 5.7). In reality, the force of infection often differs between different age groups and can be greater than 28 per cent per year (Section 5.2.3.5). Methods for estimating R_0 which account for age-dependent mixing are discussed in Chapter 7.

After substituting $\lambda \approx 1/A$ (Equation 5.8) into Equations 5.21 and 5.22, we obtain the following expressions for R_0 in terms of the average age at infection, A:

$$\text{Exponential age distribution: } R_0 \approx 1 + L/A \qquad 5.23$$

$$\text{Rectangular age distribution: } R_0 \approx L/A \qquad 5.24$$

Equations 5.21–5.24 are useful for obtaining quick and approximate estimates of R_0 from the force of infection estimated from serological or other data.

5.2.3.3.1 Example: estimating the basic reproduction number for mumps and rubella

1) The proportion of the population that was susceptible to mumps infection during the 1980s in England and Wales was about 0.07 (section 5.2.3.2.1). Applying the equation $R_0 = 1/s$ implies that the basic reproduction number was about $1/0.07 \approx 14$.

2) The average force of rubella infection in England and Wales during the 1980s was about 11.6 per cent (section 5.2.2). Assuming an average life expectancy of 70 years and applying Equation 5.22 implies that the basic reproduction number was about $70 \times 0.116 \approx 8$.

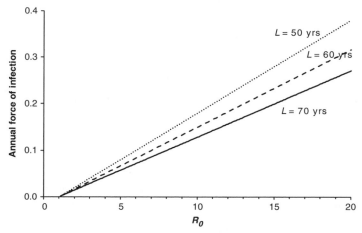

Fig. 5.7 Relationship between the average annual force of infection and R_0, as predicted using Equation 5.22.

5.2.3.4 The effect of the force of infection and R_0 on the age-specific proportion of individuals that are susceptible and the number of new infections per unit time

The number of new infections which occur in specific age groups is of particular interest for infections which are associated with adverse outcomes, if they occur at certain ages. For example, individuals who are infected with measles or mumps as adults face an increased risk of encephalitis; likewise, adults infected with poliovirus face an increased risk of developing paralytic polio. For rubella, infection during the first trimester of pregnancy can result in a child being born with Congenital Rubella Syndrome (CRS) which is associated with significant disability. Similarly, infection with cytomegalovirus or toxoplasma during pregnancy is associated with an increased risk of a child being born with congenital problems.

The number of new infections per unit time is given by the expression (sections 2.6.1 and 3.4.1):

$$\lambda(t)S(t) \tag{5.25}$$

where $S(t)$ is the number of susceptible individuals at time t. Extending this logic, the average number of new infections per person per unit time among individuals of age a is given by the expression:

$$\lambda(a,t)s(a,t)$$

where $\lambda(a,t)$ is the average force of infection among individuals of age a at time t and $s(a,t)$ is the proportion of individuals of age a who are susceptible to infection at time t. Substituting for $s(a)=e^{-\lambda a}$ (i.e. equation 5.2) into this expression and assuming that the force of infection does not depend on age, leads to the following expression for the number of new infections per person per unit time:

$$\lambda e^{-\lambda a} \tag{5.26}$$

Figure 5.8 shows predictions of the average age-specific number of new infections per 100,000 population for rubella (or another infection) in which the force of infection ranges between 5 and 25 per cent per year, obtained using Equation 5.26. This shows that, if the force of infection is high in the absence of vaccination, most individuals are immune by the time they are adults (Figure 5.3), so that few adults (and therefore pregnant women) should be experiencing infection for the first time. Therefore, in such settings the burden of CRS should be low. Methods for extending Equation 5.26 to calculate the actual burden of CRS are discussed in[8–10].

These age patterns strongly determine the impact of introducing rubella-containing vaccine (section 5.3.3).

5.2.3.5 Refining estimates of the force of infection

5.2.3.5.1 Maternally derived immunity For some infections, a high proportion of infants have maternally-derived antibodies which last for the first 6–9 months of life

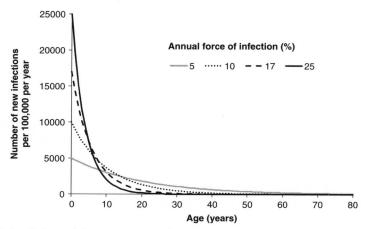

Fig. 5.8 Predictions of the average annual number of new infections per 100,000 population in different age groups, obtained by using Equation 5.26.

and provide protection against infection (see Figure 5.9a). The following shows an adaptation of the simple catalytic model to include maternal immunity:

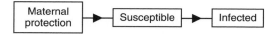

Maternal immunity is typically incorporated in models using one of two assumptions (Model 5.3, online):

a) Individuals are immune to infection during the first, e.g. six months of life, depending on the infection, and are susceptible thereafter. The expression for the proportion of individuals who are susceptible at a given age a is analogous to that for the simple catalytic model, i.e. $e^{-\lambda(a-0.5)}$. In this expression, 'a–0.5' reflects the number of years during which individuals were susceptible to infection.

b) Maternal immunity is lost at a constant rate, e.g. μ, which equals 1/(average duration of protection provided by maternal antibodies). It can be shown (Exercise 5.6a) that the expression for the proportion of individuals that are susceptible at a given age a is

$$\frac{\mu(e^{-\mu a} - e^{-\lambda a})}{\lambda - \mu}$$

The duration of maternally-derived immunity, relative to the force of infection, is important for designing vaccination strategies, since vaccinating infants who still have maternal immunity means that many doses of vaccine will be 'wasted'. However, if the force of infection is high, vaccinating older children may scarcely affect morbidity, as many children will have been infected before they have had the chance to be vaccinated.[9]

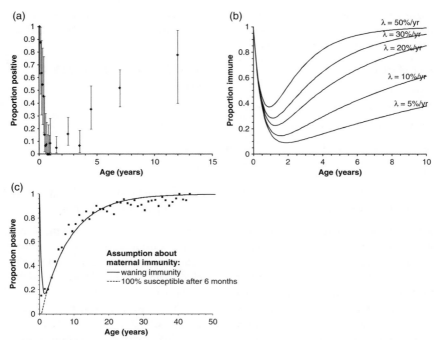

Fig. 5.9 (a) Proportion of individuals found to be positive for rubella antibodies in Caieiras, São Paulo State, Brazil during the period November 1990–January 1991.[12] (b) Predictions of the age-specific prevalence of immunity for different assumptions about the annual force of infection (λ) and assuming that maternally-derived immunity lasts six months on average (see Model 5.3, online). (c) Comparison between the prediction from models which best fit the rubella data in Figure 5.1, assuming that maternally-derived immunity is either solid for the first 6 months of life, or declines, lasting for six months on average (Model 5.3 online).

The best age at vaccination is the one at which the smallest proportion of individuals is immune (either through natural infection or maternal acquisition), which is <1 and >1.5 years if the force of infection is high and low respectively (Figure 5.9b). Considering measles, for example, the first dose of vaccine is recommended for children aged 9 months in settings with high levels of transmission, and at age 12–15 months in industrialized settings, where the amount of ongoing transmission is low.[11]

In general, the force of infection that is estimated by fitting catalytic models to data should be similar irrespective of the assumption about how immunity is lost (i.e. whether it is lost at a constant rate or whether individuals have solid immunity to infection during the first six months of life) and it is higher than that obtained by fitting a simple catalytic model (Table 5.3). An explanation for this is that a simple catalytic model overestimates the number of years during which individuals are at risk of infection, as it assumes that individuals are susceptible at birth. Therefore, to match

Table 5.3 Summary of the best-fitting forces of infection obtained by fitting a catalytic model to the rubella data in Figure 5.1, for different assumptions about the protection that is derived from maternal antibodies.

Type of model	Force of infection (% per year) (95% CI)
Simple catalytic	11.6 (*11.1–12.1*)
Exponential decline in maternal immunity	12.0 (*11.1–13.0*)
100% susceptible after age 6 months	12.1 (*11.6–12.6*)

See Figure 5.9c for the model prediction. See Model 5.3, online.

the observed data, the force of infection in the model can be lower than that required when it is assumed that individuals are immune during the first year of life.

5.2.3.5.2 Age-dependency in the force of infection The assumption that the force of infection is identical for all age groups is unrealistic. Considering our rubella example, the best-fitting model predictions for 5–14-year-olds that are obtained using the simple catalytic model underestimate the observed data (Figure 5.4), suggesting that the true force of infection for children exceeded the average value. Conversely, model predictions overestimate the data among older individuals, suggesting either that the force of infection among adults was lower than the average value, or that the test was less than 100 per cent sensitive in the elderly, who were infected many years previously.

To estimate an age-dependent force of infection using catalytic models, we first need to identify if and how the force of infection changes with age. For cross-sectional data on the age-specific proportion of individuals who are negative to the test (s_a), the simplest method for doing so is to plot $-ln(s_a)$ against the mid-point of each age category[7] (Figure 5.10). It can be shown (Panel 5.2) that if the plot follows a straight line, as is the case for the Fiji dataset in Figure 5.10, then it is reasonable to assume that the force of infection is identical for all age groups, and the gradient of this line equals the force of infection.

The plot of $-ln(s_a)$ can often be broken down into several straight lines, for example, with one line passing through the data points for adults, and another line passing through those for children, as for the Chinese and UK dataset in Figure 5.10. Such plots suggest that the force of infection is age-dependent, and, in a given age group, equals the gradient of the line through the points $-ln(s_a)$ spanning that age group (Panel 5.2). Considering the plot for the UK dataset for example, the gradient of the line through the points $-ln(s_a)$ for adults is shallower than that for the line for children, suggesting that the force of infection for adults is less than that for children. This age pattern is seen for many infections and can be attributed to several factors (see Panel 5.3).

The plot of $-ln(s_a)$ needs to be interpreted cautiously. For example, the apparent change in the gradient at about age 15 years for the plot for China in Figure 5.10 reflects the fact that seropositivity was effectively 100 per cent by age 10 years. This highlights the general problem of estimating the force of infection for adults for prevalent infections.

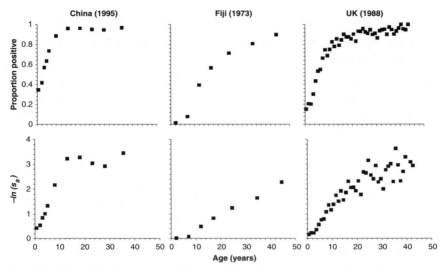

Fig. 5.10 Plots of the proportion of the population that was seropositive and −ln(observed proportion seronegative) for different settings for rubella.[4, 13, 14]

Panel 5.2 Determining whether the force of infection is age-dependent

(a) Why should a plot of −ln(s_a) be linear if the force of infection is not age-dependent?

If the force of infection is identical for all age groups, then the proportion of individuals of a given age a who are negative to the test (s_a) can be described using the expression (Equation 5.2):

$$s_a = e^{-\lambda a}$$

Taking the natural logarithms of both sides of this equation and applying that rules of logarithms (see Basic maths section B.4), we see that:

$$ln(s_a) = ln(e^{-\lambda a}) = -\lambda a$$

Rearranging this expression, we see that:

$$-ln(s_a) = \lambda a$$

which is the equation of a straight line (see Basic maths section B.2), i.e. if we plot −ln(s_a) against age, we should see a straight line, whose gradient is λ.

Panel 5.2 Determining whether the force of infection is age-dependent *(continued)*

(b) Interpreting the plot of –*ln*(s_a) if it consists of several straight lines

We consider the situation when the force of infection equals constant (but different) values λ_1 and λ_2 in the age groups 0–<15 and ≥15 years. In this instance, the following expressions describe the proportion of individuals of age a who are negative to the test:

$$s_a = \begin{cases} e^{-\lambda_1 a} & a < 15 \text{ years} & 5.27a \\ e^{-15\lambda_1} e^{-\lambda_2(a-15)} & a \geq 15 \text{ years} & 5.27b \end{cases}$$

Note that the expression for individuals aged over 15 years equals the product of:

1. The proportion of individuals who are susceptible at age 15 years (i.e. $e^{-15\lambda_1}$) and

2. The proportion of individuals who escape infection between the ages 15 and a years, i.e. $e^{-\lambda_2(a-15)}$.

Taking the natural log of both sides of Equation 5.27a for s_a, we see that:

$$-ln(s_a) = \lambda_1 a \text{ for } a < 15 \text{ years}$$

As discussed in section a) (see above), this is the equation of a straight line, and so a plot of $-ln(s_a)$ against age should be linear until age 15 years, with a gradient of λ_1.

Following the same steps using equation 5.27b for s_a for those aged ≥15 years, we see that:

$$-ln(s_a) = -ln(e^{-15\lambda_1} e^{-\lambda_2(a-15)}) \qquad \text{for } a \geq 15 \text{ years}$$

By the rules of logarithms (see Basic maths section B.4), this equation simplifies to

$$-ln(s_a) = 15\lambda_1 + \lambda_2(a-15) \qquad \text{for } a \geq 15 \text{ years}$$

This equation is also that of a straight line, with a gradient of λ_2. Consequently if a plot of $-ln(s_a)$ against the age midpoints can be broken down into several straight lines, it would be reasonable to assume that the force of infection is age-dependent, and, in a given age group, equals the gradient of the line through the plot spanning that age group.

Panel 5.3 Why might the force of infection differ between children and adults and between settings?

Differences in the force of infection between children and adults are seen for many infections. They were observed particularly for the 1957 (Asian) influenza pandemic (see Figure 5.11). Such differences can be attributable to several factors:

1. Differences in exposure to infection between children and adults, occurring because of differences in contact patterns. For example, children are most likely to contact other children, who are also most likely to be infectious.

2. Differences in susceptibility, for example, young individuals are perhaps more 'susceptible' to infection than are older individuals, since their immune system may be less developed.

3. Genetic factors. For example, those who are most susceptible to infection get infected when young, whilst the rest of the population is infected at a slow rate, which can lead to apparent age differences in the force of infection (see Chapter 8 in [9]).

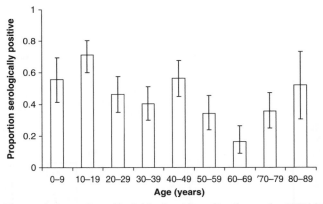

Fig. 5.11 Observed proportion of individuals with antibodies to the 1957 (Asian) influenza strain in Sheffield (UK) in 1957[1]. The high proportion of elderly individuals found to have antibodies is attributable to previous exposure to a related strain[2].

The force of infection also depends on the study population, for example, whether it is urban/rural, developed/developing etc. The high force of rubella infection for China, as compared with the UK, as implied in Figure 5.10, may be due to differences in crowding. The very high force of infection among young children in China, as compared with the UK for the study period may be attributable to intense exposure to other children, e.g. at crèches or day-care centres. Data on measles serology from New Haven, 1957[47] also suggested that there are differences in age-specific patterns between large and small families (Figure 5.1).

Table 5.4 Summary of the main types of catalytic models.

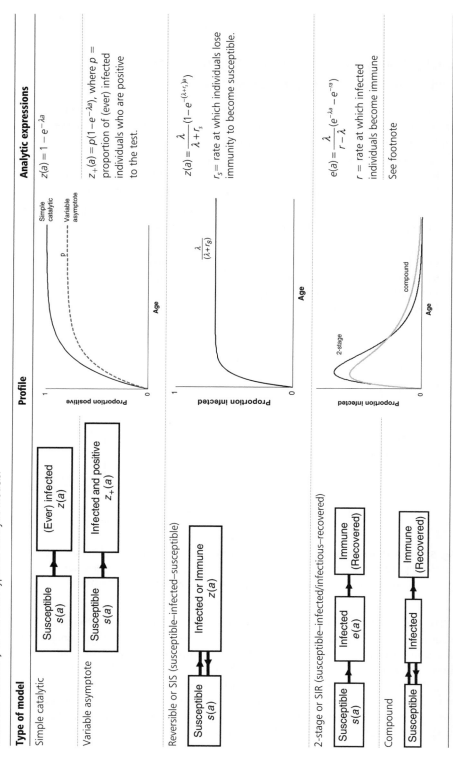

Type of model		Profile	Analytic expressions

Simple catalytic

Susceptible $s(a)$ → (Ever) infected $z(a)$

$z(a) = 1 - e^{-\lambda a}$

Variable asymptote

Susceptible $s(a)$ → Infected and positive $z_+(a)$

$z_+(a) = p(1 - e^{-\lambda a})$, where p = proportion of (ever) infected individuals who are positive to the test.

Reversible or SIS (susceptible–infected–susceptible)

Susceptible $s(a)$ ⇄ Infected or Immune $z(a)$

$z(a) = \dfrac{\lambda}{\lambda + r_s}(1 - e^{-(\lambda + r_s)a})$

r_s = rate at which individuals lose immunity to become susceptible.

2-stage or SIR (susceptible–infected/infectious–recovered)

Susceptible $s(a)$ → Infected $e(a)$ → Immune (Recovered)

$e(a) = \dfrac{\lambda}{r - \lambda}(e^{-\lambda a} - e^{-ra})$

r = rate at which infected individuals become immune

Compound

Susceptible → Infected ⇄ Immune (Recovered)

See footnote

Analytic expressions for all the compartments in the compound model can be found either by trying some possible solutions which have the general form $s(a) = Ke^{qa}$ and $e(a) = Je^{qa}$ and manipulating the differential equations (M. Vynnycky, personal correspondence), or by typing in the differential equations for the model into a mathematical package, such as Maple or Mathematica. The resulting equation is too complex to reproduce here.

Age-dependent forces of infection are usually incorporated into catalytic models assuming that the force of infection is 'piecewise' constant (i.e. constant but different) in the age groups indicated by the plot of $-ln(s_a)$ (see e.g. [15]). For the UK dataset in Figure 5.10, for example, the gradient of the plot of $-ln(s_a)$ appears to differ between the age groups 0–14 and ≥15 years, suggesting that the force of infection changes at about age 15 years. In fact, if we fit an age-dependent catalytic model through these data, we estimate that the annual force of infection is about 13 per cent and 4 per cent for children and adults respectively (Model 5.4, online). It would also be reasonable to stratify the 0–14-year-olds further, e.g. to assume that the force of infection differs between the groups <1, 1–4 and 5–14 years, since infants have different contact patterns from 1–4-year-olds, who, in turn, probably have different mixing patterns from schoolchildren.

5.2.4 Age patterns for non-immunizing infections

The catalytic models discussed so far have assumed that once individuals are immune, they remain immune for life, and that everyone would become immune if they lived for long enough. For the infections for which these assumptions are inappropriate, other kinds of catalytic models may be applied.[16] These are summarized in Table 5.4 and are discussed briefly below:

- *Variable asymptote model*: this is identical to the simple catalytic model except that it assumes that a proportion of individuals can never be infected, or some individuals do not test positive, despite having been infected, due to the poor sensitivity of the test. This model has been applied to measles and whooping cough data[16, 17].

- *Reversible or SIS (susceptible–infected–susceptible) model*: for this model, individuals are infected at a rate λ, and once infected, lose their infected status and subsequently become susceptible at a rate r_s. The age-specific proportion of individuals who are infected plateaus at a level of $\dfrac{\lambda}{\lambda + r_s}$ (Exercise 5.8). This model has been applied to cross-sectional tuberculin data,[16, 18] diphtheria, malaria[19] and filariasis.[20]

- *Two-stage or SIR (susceptible–infected/infectious–recovered) model*: for this model, evidence of infection disappears, but immunity to the infection remains. This model has been applied to yaws and histoplasmosis data;[16] it has also been extended to allow infected individuals to become susceptible again (a 'compound' model) and applied to hookworm data.[21]

The methods for estimating the unknown parameters in these models are analogous to those described in section 4.2.5.

5.2.5 Practical considerations when analysing data

Much of the emphasis in this section has been on the methods for analysing seropositivity prevalence data. However, attention should also be paid to the data which are being analysed. We conclude this section with a list of some of the key questions which should be considered before fitting the model to the data:

1) How were the data collected and what biases might be involved? For example, were the samples submitted specifically to investigate infection? Such data may lead to an overestimate in the force of infection.

2) What does a plot of the proportion positive by age suggest about the type of catalytic model which should be used (see Table 5.4)? For example, does the proportion positive increase steeply with age and towards 100 per cent? Does it reach a plateau at less than 100 per cent? Does it peak before subsequently declining?

3) Are there any outliers in the data? If so, it may be necessary to exclude them from the analyses.

4) When were the data collected? For infections for which the incidence cycles over time, the fit of a catalytic model to data collected immediately after an epidemic may be poor for the younger age groups. In this instance, the fitting should be restricted only to data from older individuals, who would have survived both epidemic and non-epidemic years. See also Whittaker and Farrington (2004).[22]

5) What does the 'infection marker' represent, e.g. past infection, current infection, recent infection, immunity, non-specific reaction etc.? The question is often complicated, since the sensitivity of the test is rarely 100 per cent.

6) Does the proportion of individuals who are positive to the marker for previous infection include vaccinated individuals? If so, such individuals should be excluded from the data, if vaccination records are available. Otherwise, if individuals have been vaccinated only at birth (or very soon thereafter), the proportion of individuals of a given age a who are naturally infected and positive to the test can be estimated using the expression $(z_a-v_a)/(1-v_a)$ where z_a is the proportion of individuals who are presumed immune (through vaccination or natural infection) and v_a is the proportion of individuals who had been vaccinated at birth.[4]

7) What is the median age at infection? This can be used to check that the force of infection estimated using formal methods is correct by using the relationship $A = 1/\lambda$ (Equation 5.8).

8) How might the force of infection change with age? (see section 5.2.3.5.2).

9) Etc...

5.3 The effect of vaccination on the dynamics of infections

5.3.1 The indirect effects of vaccination

All countries currently routinely vaccinate young children against several common childhood infections, such as measles, mumps and rubella, as well as against other infections such as diphtheria, tetanus, *Haemophilus influenzae*. As shown in Figure 5.12, the introduction of measles and pertussis vaccination in England and Wales led to substantial reductions in the notification rates for these infections. These reductions stem from both the direct and indirect effect of vaccination.

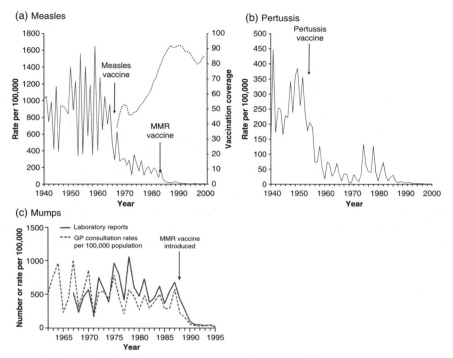

Fig. 5.12 Annual notification rates for measles (a) and pertussis (b) in England and Wales. Data source: Health Protection Agency. (c) Lab reports and GP consultation rates for mumps in England and Wales. Reproduced with permission from Gay *et al*,1997.[24]

For example, vaccination directly reduces the prevalence of infectious individuals, since those who would have become infected and infectious do not do so because they have been vaccinated and are immune. Unvaccinated individuals also benefit from such reductions, since the reduced prevalence of infectious persons means that the opportunity for them to become infected has decreased (i.e. they are 'indirectly protected'). This indirect protection is one part of 'herd immunity'.[23]

These effects of herd immunity are also predicted by models. For example, Figure 5.13 shows predictions of the effect of vaccination from a model describing the transmission of measles (see Panel 4.3): substantial reductions are predicted for the number of infectious persons and the force of infection following the introduction of vaccination with a coverage of 50 and 75 per cent among newborns. For example, the average force of infection is predicted to decrease greatly, from an average value of about 0.48 per 1000 per day to about 0.1 per 1000 per day (taken as the midpoint between the peaks and the troughs) if 75 per cent of newborns are immunized.

There is a mathematical relationship (Appendix sections A.3.3 and A.3.4 and Chapter 5 in Anderson and May[9]) between the expected average force of infection (λ') in the long term following the introduction of vaccination of a proportion, *v*, among

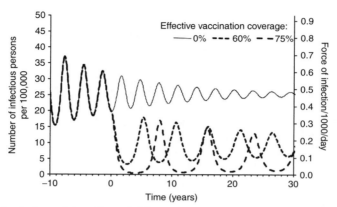

Fig. 5.13 Predictions of the effect of different levels of vaccination coverage from the year 0 among newborns on the number of infectious persons per 100,000 population (left axis) and the force of infection (right axis), obtained using the model described in Panel 4.3 (adapted to deal with vaccination of newborns) and Model 4.7, online. Vaccination is assumed to provide lifelong protection; individuals are assumed to mix randomly; $R_0 = 13$; the average pre-infectious and infectious periods are 8 and 7 days respectively, $L = 70$ years and the birth rate = death rate.

newborns, R_0 and the life expectancy, which depends on the age distribution of the population, assuming further that individuals mix randomly:

$$\text{Rectangular age distribution}: R_0 = \frac{\lambda' L}{(1-v)(1-e^{-\lambda' L})} \tag{5.28}$$

$$\text{Exponential age distribution}: R_0 = \frac{\lambda' L + 1}{(1-v)} \tag{5.29}$$

Equation 5.28 predicts that, for low levels of the vaccination coverage, the reduction in the force of infection equals the proportion of individuals that are protected by vaccination for both low and high transmission areas (Figure 5.14). For example, vaccination of 25 per cent of newborns leads to a 25 per cent reduction in the force of infection. However, in a low transmission setting ($R_0 = 7$), vaccination of 90 per cent of newborns is predicted to lead to a reduction in the force of infection which is greater than 90 per cent. We discuss the corresponding equations for the situation when individuals are vaccinated at older ages later in this chapter.

5.3.2 The effect of vaccination on the age-specific proportion of individuals that are susceptible

As discussed in Section 5.2.2, the size of the force of infection determines the proportion of individuals that are susceptible at a given age: if it is high, few adults are still susceptible to infection. Any decreases in the force of infection after vaccination is

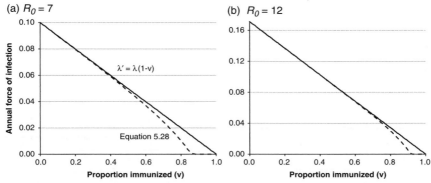

Fig. 5.14 Predictions of the average annual long-term force of infection following the introduction of vaccination, calculated using Equation 5.28 (dotted line) for different levels of the immunization coverage among newborns, in (a) a low transmission ($R_0 = 7$); and (b) a high transmission setting ($R_0 = 12$), assuming a life expectancy (L) of 70 years. The solid line shows the annual force of infection which would be seen if the force of infection was directly proportional to the proportion of individuals that are protected by vaccination (v), i.e. if $\lambda' = \lambda(1-v)$. See also Exercise 5.10.

introduced should therefore lead to increases in the proportion of unvaccinated individuals that are still susceptible by the time they are adults.

Figure 5.15 shows empirical evidence for such increases. Figure 5.15a shows data from Greece, where MMR vaccination became available in the private sector in 1975, and the proportion of women of childbearing age who did not have antibodies for rubella increased from about 10 per cent in 1975 to over 35 per cent by 1991.[25, 26]

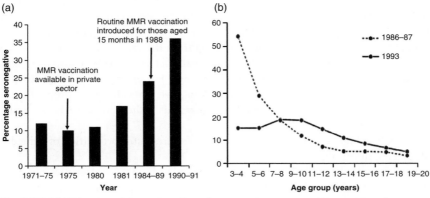

Fig. 5.15 (a) Estimates of the proportion of pregnant women and/or women of childbearing age who did not have antibodies for rubella in Greece, as measured using either haemagglutinin inhibition assays (HIA) or enzyme-linked immunosorbent assay (ELISA).[25, 26] (b) Estimates of the proportion of sera that were submitted for microbiological investigation to sentinel Public Health Laboratory Service (PHLS) laboratories in England that were negative for mumps antibodies.[24] Reproduced with permission from Gay *et al*, 1997.[24]

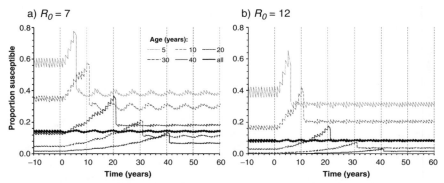

Fig. 5.16 Predictions of the effect of vaccinating 50 per cent of newborns from the year 0 against rubella on the proportion of individuals in different age groups that are susceptible in (a) a low transmission setting ($R_0 = 7$) and (b) a high transmission setting ($R_0 = 12$) obtained using the model described in Panel 5.4 (Model 5.5, online).

These increases occurred before children received MMR vaccination routinely (from 1988 and 1991 for those aged 15 months and 9 years respectively); the uptake of MMR vaccination in the private sector was unknown. Figure 5.15b shows data from England and Wales, where MMR vaccination was introduced for young children in 1988: the proportion of 9–15-year-olds (who were too old to have been vaccinated) that were seronegative to mumps increased between 1986–7 and 1993, for example, from about 12 per cent to 20 per cent for 9–10-year-olds.

As shown in Figure 5.16, these changes are predicted using age-structured models, such as that discussed in Panel 5.4. For example, after rubella vaccination is introduced among 50 per cent of newborns, the proportion of individuals that are susceptible increases initially in those age groups who escaped vaccination (i.e. they were born before vaccination was introduced), since they are benefitting from the reduced prevalence of infectious individuals resulting from the vaccination programme. As might be expected, the proportions of individuals that are susceptible stop increasing once the first cohorts of vaccinees reach that age. For example, the proportion of 5-year-olds that are susceptible stops increasing five years after the introduction of vaccination of newborns in the model because this is the first year when the first cohort of vaccinees reaches age 5 years.

Figure 5.16 highlights three other interesting features in the proportion of individuals that are susceptible.

First, fewer young children are susceptible in the long term after vaccination is introduced than before the introduction of vaccination (e.g. 56 per cent vs 40 per cent of five year olds in the low transmission setting). Such differences are intuitively reasonable because, in the model, 50 per cent of individuals had been vaccinated at birth and were no longer susceptible.

Second, Figure 5.16 suggests that vaccination of newborns does not affect the overall proportion of individuals who are susceptible, and that it simply redistributes the susceptible population into different age groups. An explanation for this prediction is

Panel 5.4 Methods for incorporating age-structure into models

The method of Schenzle[48] is commonly used to describe transmission in an age-structured population. With this approach, individuals are stratified into annual strata and remain in the same stratum until the end of the year, when they all move into the next age stratum, in the same way that children at school remain in the same class for a full year. The model is represented diagrammatically in Figure 5.17. The population described in this model is referred to as a 'realistic age structured' (RAS) population. For simplicity, the effects of maternal immunity are not included.

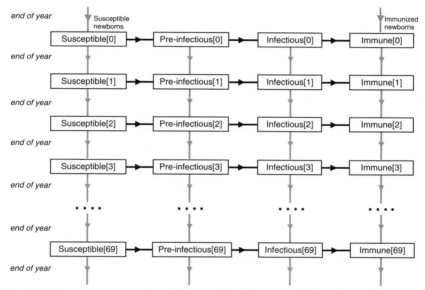

Fig. 5.17 General structure of a model describing transmission in a realistic age-structured population assuming that newborns are vaccinated.

The equations for the model can be written down using difference equations or differential equations for each age stratum. For simplicity, the above model assumes that the population has a rectangular age structure, with individuals surviving until age 70 years; however, the method can be adapted to deal with other age distributions. The difference equations are as follows:

If t is any time apart from the end of year:

$$S[a]_{t+1} = S[a]_t - \lambda_t S[a]_t$$

$$E[a]_{t+1} = E[a]_t + \lambda_t S[a]_t - fE[a]_t$$

$$I[a]_{t+1} = I[a]_t + fE[a]_t - rI[a]_t$$

$$R[a]_{t+1} = R[a]_t + rI[a]_t$$

Panel 5.4 Methods for incorporating age-structure into models *(continued)*

If *t* is the end of the year:

$$S[a]_{t+1} = S[a-1]_t - \lambda_t S[a-1]_t$$

$$E[a]_{t+1} = E[a-1]_t + \lambda_t S[a-1]_t - fE[a-1]_t$$

$$I[a]_{t+1} = I[a-1]_t + fE[a-1]_t - rI[a-1]_t$$

$$R[a]_{t+1} = R[a-1]_t + rI[a-1]_t$$

$$S[0]_{t+1} = B(1-v)$$

$$E[0]_{t+1} = 0$$

$$I[0]_{t+1} = 0$$

$$R[0]_{t+1} = Bv$$

where

$S[a]_t$ is the number of susceptible individuals of age *a* at time *t*;

$E[a]_t$ is the number of individuals of age *a* years in the pre-infectious category at time *t*;

$I[a]_t$ is the number of infectious individuals of age *a* at time *t*;

$R[a]_t$ is the number of immune individuals of age *a* years at time *t*;

B is the number of births per year

λ_t is the force of infection between *t* and *t+1*. Assuming that individuals contact each other randomly, the force of infecton is given by the expression:

$$\lambda_t = \beta \sum_{a=0}^{69} I[a]_t$$

f is the rate at which individuals become infectious;

r is the rate at which infectious individuals recover and become immune;

v is the proportion of newborns that is immunized.

For the rubella example discussed in Figure 5.16, $f = 0.1$/day and $r = 0.091$/day, corresponding to an average pre-infectious period of 10 days and an average infectious period of 11 days.

The approach of Schenzle is an efficient way of describing transmission in an age-structured population. There are other methods for setting up such models:

◆ Set up difference or partial differential equations (Panel 3.5) in both age and time. This approach can be computationally demanding, especially if daily age and time steps are used.

◆ Stratify individuals into the age groups of interest and assume that individuals age at a constant rate. This approach is not recommended, since the ageing process is applied to everyone irrespective of the time that they have spent in a compartment. It can, therefore, result in the paradox whereby a proportion of individuals can be born on one day, but will be in another age group the following day.

that, if the vaccination coverage is below the herd immunity threshold, the infection is still endemic, and so each infectious person still leads to one other infectious person, i.e. the net reproduction number (R_n) still equals one. Assuming that individuals mix randomly, then if the net reproduction number equals 1, the proportion of the population that is susceptible equals $1/R_0$, irrespective of the vaccine coverage (see section 4.2.2.2).

Analyses of measles data for England and Wales have found that the size of the susceptible population after vaccination was introduced in 1968 was very similar to that before 1968 (4–4.5 million).[27] However, the relationship $R_n = R_0 \times$ proportion susceptible does not hold if we assume that individuals do not mix randomly (see Chapter 7) and so in reality, the overall proportion of the population that is susceptible probably changes after vaccination is introduced.

Third, more adults are susceptible in the long term after vaccination is introduced than before the introduction of vaccination, if the effective vaccination coverage is below the herd immunity threshold, for example, 18 per cent vs 13.3 per cent respectively of 20-year-olds in the low transmission setting. The model assumes that vaccination provides lifelong protection to infection (Panel 5.4) and so differences between the proportion of adults that are susceptible before and after vaccination is introduced result only from the reduced force of infection because of vaccination. This reduced force of infection means that a substantial proportion of those who were not vaccinated at birth are still susceptible by the time they become adults. In fact, this proportion is so high that it outweighs the effect of removing 50 per cent of each cohort from the susceptible population at birth through vaccination (see the calculation in section 5.3.2.1).

5.3.2.1 Example: calculating the proportion of adults that are susceptible in the long term following the introduction of vaccination among newborns in the low-transmission setting ($R_0 = 7$)

The average force of infection before the introduction of vaccination among newborns with an effective coverage of v in the low transmission setting was about 10 per cent per year. This can be calculated using the equation $\lambda = R_0/L$ (obtained after rearranging Equation 5.22), and assuming a life expectancy of 70 years and $R_0 = 7$.

Applying Equation 5.2, the proportion of individuals that are susceptible by age 20 years ($s(20)$) before vaccination among newborns is introduced is given by the equation:

$$s(20) = e^{-20 \times \lambda} = e^{-20 \times 0.10} = 0.135$$

In the long term after the introduction of vaccination, the proportion of individuals of age a that are susceptible ($s(a)'$) is given by the following expression:

proportion of individuals of age a that were not
vaccinated at birth ($=1-v$)

$\times$

proportion of those who were not vaccinated at
birth who were still susceptible by age a

5.30

Applying Equation 5.2, the second term in this expression is given by $e^{-\lambda' a}$, and thus applying Equation 5.30, $(s(a)')$ is given by the following:

$$s(a)' = (1-v)e^{-\lambda' a} \qquad 5.31$$

As shown in Figure 5.14a, the long-term force of infection following the introduction of vaccination with an effective coverage of 50 per cent of newborns is $\lambda' = 4.8$ per cent per year. Substituting for $\lambda' = 0.048$ per year and $v = 0.5$ into Equation 5.31 leads to values for the proportion of 20-year-olds that are susceptible of

$$s(a)' = (1-v) \, e^{-20\lambda'} = (1-0.5) \times e^{-20 \times 0.048} = 0.194$$

i.e. the proportion of 20 year olds that is susceptible increases from 0.135 before vaccination is introduced to 0.194 in the long term, as a result of 50 per cent effective vaccination coverage among newborns.

Figure 5.18 shows that such increases in the proportion of individuals in given age groups that are susceptible do occur in practice after vaccination is introduced. For example, the proportion of 7–9-year-olds and 10–14-year-olds that appeared to be susceptible to measles in England and Wales increased between 1988 and 1991, even though the proportion of individuals in these age groups who had been vaccinated as infants had increased over time (Figure 5.12a).

To reduce the potential for increases in the proportion of individuals that are susceptible in given age groups, the introduction of a vaccine into a routine schedule is sometimes accompanied by a 'catch-up' campaign, targeting a broad range of age groups. For example, a catch-up campaign targeting preschool children aged over two years

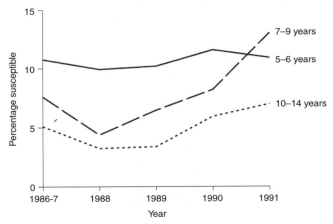

Fig. 5.18 Estimates of the percentages of 5–6, 7–9 and 10–14-year-olds who were susceptible to measles in England and Wales, as measured by the Public Health Laboratory Service serological surveillance.[28] Reproduced with permission from Ramsey et al, 1994.[28]

was conducted when routine MMR vaccination was introduced for 2-year-olds in 1988 in England and Wales.[28] Similarly, when routine meningococcal C conjugate vaccination was introduced for those aged 2, 3 and 4 months in the UK in November 1999, a catch-up campaign targeting everyone aged <25 years was also conducted. As discussed in Panel 5.5, for all of the strategies involving a catch-up campaign, the predicted annual numbers of cases of meningococcal C disease were four times less than those resulting from strategies which did not include a catch-up campaign.

We now discuss how changes in the age-specific proportion of individuals that are susceptible affect the age-specific numbers of new infections occurring per unit time.

Panel 5.5 Modelling the impact of meningococcal vaccination in the UK

Meningococcal disease is caused by infection with *Neisseria meningitidis*. There are at least 13 serogroups of meningococci, with serogroups B and C being the most common in the UK.[49] In most instances, exposure to *Neisseria meningitidis* leads to carriage, although for a small proportion of individuals, it leads to invasive disease including septicaemia and meningitis, depending on the age at which it is acquired.[50] Before the introduction of meningococcal C vaccination in the UK, epidemics of meningococcal C infection occurred approximately every year (Figure 5.19a).

The study of Trotter *et al.* used the model described in Figure 5.19b to examine the impact of several vaccination strategies against meningococcal C infection on the burden of serogroup C disease. Vaccinated individuals were stratified into those vaccinated routinely or those vaccinated during a catch-up campaign. The duration of protection provided by vaccination was generally shorter among young children than for teenagers/young adults, and those vaccinated in the catch-up campaign were older than those vaccinated routinely.[51] The compartments referring to 'Other serogroup' in Figure 5.19b reflect those who could be carriers of other serogroups or *N lactamica*. However, since the authors assumed that individuals could not be carriers of more than one serogroup, including individuals in the 'Other category' in the model simply had the effect of reducing the proportion of individuals who are susceptible to meningococcal C disease. The number of individuals with meningococcal disease is calculated as an age-dependent fraction of the total number of carriers.

As shown in Figure 5.19c, all the strategies involving a catch-up campaign were predicted to have a bigger impact on the annual numbers of cases of meningococcal disease than those which involved simply the introduction of routine vaccination among young children. For example, the model predicted that there would be 200 cases of meningococcal C disease five years after the introduction of vaccination for all strategies involving a catch-up campaign, as compared with about 800 cases if the strategy did not include a catch-up campaign.

Panel 5.5 Modelling the impact of meningococcal vaccination in the UK *(continued)*

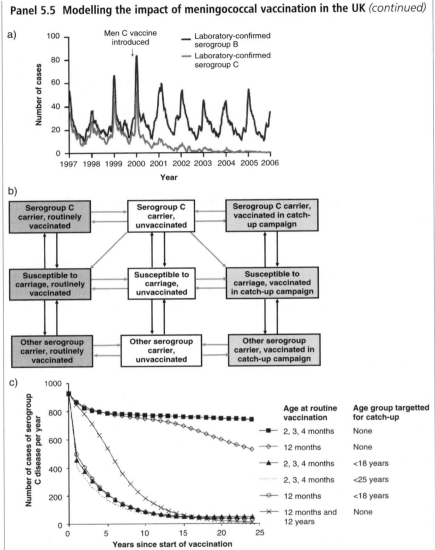

Fig. 5.19 (a) Laboratory-confirmed cases of meningococcal disease in England and Wales, five-week moving averages. Reproduced with permission from The Green Book, 2008.[49] (b) General structure of the model developed by Trotter *et al*.[40] to explore the impact of Meningococcal serogroup C vaccination in the UK. Vaccination-related arrows in the model are shaded in grey; the black arrows reflect either transmission or recovery from carriage. (c) Predictions of the impact of different vaccination strategies on the annual numbers of cases of meningococcal C disease, obtained using the model of Trotter *et al*.[40] Reproduced with permission from Trotter *et al*, 2005.[40]

5.3.3 The effect of vaccination on the age-specific numbers of new infections per unit time

In general, reductions in the force of infection after vaccination is introduced mean that the average age at infection increases. Adapting expressions 5.10 and 5.11, we obtain the following expressions for the long-term average age at infection (A') following the introduction of vaccination in terms of the post-vaccination average force of infection, λ' (see also Anderson and May[9]) and assuming further that individuals mix randomly:

$$\text{Rectangular age distribution}: A' = \frac{1-(1+\lambda'L)e^{-\lambda'L}}{\lambda'(1-e^{-\lambda'L})}$$

5.32

$$\text{Exponential age distribution}: A' = \frac{1}{\lambda'+m}$$

5.33

Equation 5.33 is equivalent to the following (Appendix section A3.5):

$$A' = \frac{A}{(1-v)}$$

5.34

where A is the average age at infection before the introduction of vaccination among newborns and v is the proportion of newborns that are immunized, assuming further that vaccination provides lifelong protection against infection. Figure 5.20 shows estimates of the average age at infection obtained using these equations. For example, with 80 per cent coverage among newborns, the average age at infection is predicted to increase from about 10 to 31 years for the low transmission setting ($R_0 = 7$) in a population with a rectangular age distribution.

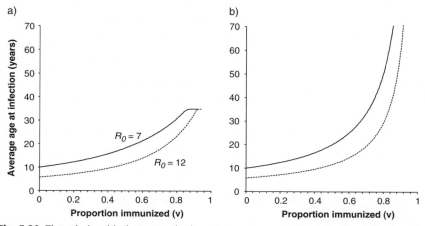

Fig. 5.20 The relationship between the long-term average age at infection following the introduction of vaccination and the proportion of newborns that are immunized for a population with a (a) rectangular age distribution and (b) exponential age distribution, as calculated using Equations 5.32 and 5.34 respectively and assuming an average life expectancy (L) of 70 years and $R_0 = 7$ or 12.

The increase in the average age at infection occurs because the number of incident infections in older age groups increases after vaccination is introduced. As we saw in Section 5.2.3.4, the following gives the number of new infections per person per unit time among individuals of age a:

$$\lambda(a)s(a) \qquad\qquad 5.35$$

where $\lambda(a)$ is the average force of infection among individuals of age a and $s(a)$ is the proportion of individuals of age a who are susceptible to infection. Combining this equation with Equation 5.31 leads to the following expression for the number of new infections per person among individuals of age a in the long-term following the introduction of vaccination:

$$\lambda'(1-v)e^{-\lambda'a} \qquad\qquad 5.36$$

If the force of infection *decreases* after vaccination is introduced among infants, but the proportion of individuals in a given age group that are susceptible *increases*, then Equation 5.26 suggests that the number of new infections per unit time in that age group can also increase, as illustrated in the following example.

5.3.3.1 Example: calculation of the long-term average number of new infections among 20-year-olds after vaccination among newborns is introduced in a high transmission setting The average force of rubella infection in the high transmission setting before the introduction of vaccination among newborns was 17.1 per cent per year (Figure 5.14), which, applying the equation $s(a) = e^{-\lambda a}$ (Equation 5.2), implies that the average proportion of 20-year-olds that were susceptible was $e^{-0.171\times20} = 0.0327$.

Applying Equation 5.26, the average annual number of new infections per 100,000 population among 20-year-olds before the introduction of vaccination among newborns would have been:

$$0.171\times0.0327\times100,000 = 559 \text{ per } 100,000 \text{ per year}$$

As shown in Figure 5.14, with 50 per cent coverage among newborns, the average force of infection in the long-term, λ' is 8.6 per cent per year.

Applying Equation 5.31, we obtain the following value for the average proportion of 20-year-olds that are susceptible in the long term after the introduction of vaccination:

$$s(a)' = (1-0.5)\times e^{-\lambda'20} = 0.5\times e^{-0.086\times20} = 0.090$$

Applying Equation 5.26, the annual number of new infections per 100,000 population among 20-year-olds becomes:

$$0.086\times0.0900\times100,000 = 770 \text{ per } 100,000 \text{ per year}$$

i.e. the average annual number of new infections for 20 year olds increases from 559 to 770 per 100,000 per year, following the introduction of vaccination with 50 per cent effective coverage among newborns.

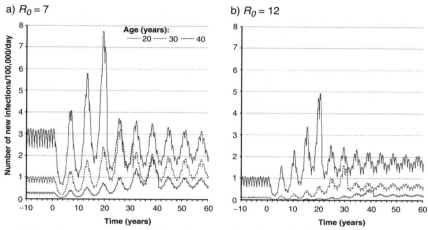

Fig. 5.21 Predictions of the daily number of new rubella infections per 100,000 population in a (a) low transmission setting ($R_0 = 7$) and (b) high transmission setting ($R_0 = 12$), assuming that vaccination of newborns is introduced in the year 0, with an effective coverage of 50 per cent, obtained using the model described in Panel 5.4 (see also Model 5.5 online).

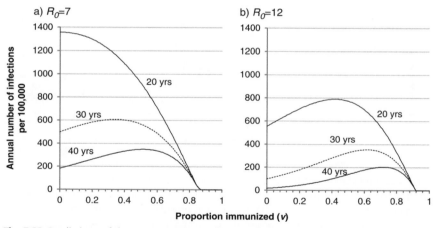

Fig. 5.22 Predictions of the average age-specific annual number of new infections per 100,000 obtained using Equation 5.36 and the long-term force of infection, as calculated using Equation 5.28 for different levels of vaccination coverage among newborns (see Figure 5.14) for a) low transmission setting ($R_0=7$) and b) high transmission setting ($R_0=12$).

Figures 5.21 and 5.22 show predictions of the number of new rubella infections per 100,000 in different age groups for high and low transmission settings for different levels of vaccination coverage among newborns. For both settings, the predicted average annual number of new infections per 100,000 increases initially in all age groups and in the long term, the greatest relative increases among adults are predicted for the high transmission settings. For example, the annual number of new rubella infections per 100,000 increased fourfold from about 100 per 100,000 to about 380 per 100,000

Panel 5.6 The impact of vaccinating individuals at different ages

Equations 5.28 and 5.29 for the long-term post-vaccination force of infection assume that individuals are vaccinated at birth. The following are the equations assuming that individuals are vaccinated at age a_v (see Appendix section A.3.3 and A.3.4 and [9]).

$$\text{Rectangular age distribution: } R_0 = \frac{\lambda' L}{1 - v e^{-\lambda' a_v} - (1-v) e^{-\lambda' L}} \tag{5.37}$$

$$\text{Exponential age distribution : } R_0 = \frac{1 + \lambda' L}{1 - v e^{-(\lambda' + m) a_v}} \tag{5.38}$$

where $m\ (= 1/L)$ is the average mortality rate. As shown in Figure 5.23, the greatest impact on the overall amount of transmission is obtained by vaccinating at as young an age as possible, although the difference between the impact resulting from vaccinating newborns, 1, or 2-year-olds is small. On the other hand, vaccinating 13-year-olds (which was the UK strategy for rubella from the 1970s until 1988) reduces the overall amount of transmission only slightly.

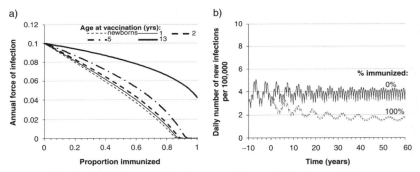

Fig. 5.23 (a) Relationship between the long-term force of infection and the proportion of newborns, 1, 2, 5, and 13-year-olds that are immunized, calculated using Equation 5.37, assuming that vaccination provides lifelong protection, and $R_0 = 7$ and $L = 70$. (b) Predictions of the overall daily number of new infections per 100,000, assuming that 100 per cent of 13-year-olds are vaccinated from year zero, as obtained using the model described in Panel 5.4. (see Model 5.6, online).

among 30-year-olds in the high transmission setting, and less than twofold in the low transmission setting (from about 500 to 600 per 100,000 per year—see Figure 5.22).

For several infections, such increases have important implications, especially if they occur among adults, and have been studied extensively[29–34] (see refs [9, 30, 31] for a detailed review). Considering rubella, they can lead to increases in the burden of congenital rubella syndrome (CRS), since infection with rubella during pregnancy may result in a child being born with CRS. Similarly, for measles and mumps they can lead to increases in the overall burden of mumps or mumps otitis and measles encephalitis. Evidence that increases occur in reality is provided by the outbreak of 25 cases of CRS in Greece in a single year, 1993, where MMR vaccination became available in the private sector in 1975 (see section 5.3.2). In contrast, only 14 cases were thought to have occurred during the period 1950–92.[25, 26] Similarly, increases in the ages of mumps cases have been seen in England and Wales in recent years, following the introduction of MMR vaccination in 1988.[35] Most of the cases were in unvaccinated cohorts, who were too old to have been vaccinated in the routine programme.

Countries have used different rubella vaccination strategies when rubella vaccine became available during the 1970s. For example, during the 1970s and 1980s, the strategy in England aimed to protect those at highest risk by providing rubella vaccine routinely to teenage girls, before they reached childbearing age. This strategy has relatively little impact on the overall amount of transmission (Panel 5.6). In the US, vaccination has routinely been provided to 1-year-olds since 1969, aiming to prevent transmission in the overall population. A sufficiently high level of vaccination coverage was, in principle, attainable, given the mandatory requirements for children to be vaccinated before enrolling at school. A detailed evaluation of the merits of these strategies using modelling techniques is provided in [30, 32].

The issues discussed above remain relevant today given the global initiatives for providing access to immunization (http://www.gavialliance.org). Because of the potential for vaccination to lead to increases in the burden of CRS, WHO currently recommends that countries which introduce rubella vaccination among infants should also vaccinate adult women.[36] In addition, it recommends that rubella vaccine should only be added to the infant immunization schedule if a coverage of over 80 per cent can be sustained in the long term.

5.3.4 The importance of including the effects of herd immunity in models

The above sections have highlighted that the impact of introducing a vaccination programme among young children is complicated, leading to a reduction in the force of infection and overall number of new infections per unit time in a population (Figure 5.13). For older individuals, these reductions can lead to increases in the proportion of individuals that are susceptible and increases in the number of new infections occurring per unit time. Given the costs associated with the introduction and implementation of a vaccination programme, it is important that these effects are considered when a vaccination programme is designed.

The sizes of these effects are difficult to predict without using a model which incorporates the effect of herd immunity, i.e which allows the force of infection to depend on the prevalence of infectious individuals. A limitation of so-called 'static models' (Panel 2.1), which are sometimes used in health economic evaluations, is that they assume that vaccination only protects those vaccinated and does not affect the force of infection. Several studies have contrasted predictions of the impact of a vaccination programme obtained using a dynamic transmission model against those from static models and have typically found that the latter underestimate the impact.[37–39]

For example, Figure 5.24 compares predictions of the number of cases of meningococcal C disease following the introduction of meningococcal C vaccination in England

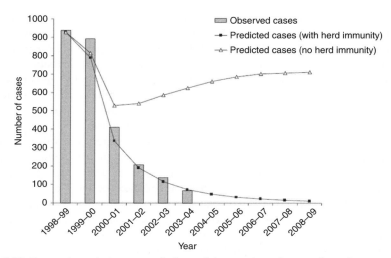

Fig. 5.24 Comparisons between predictions of the number of cases of meningococcal C disease in England and Wales between 1998 and 2008–9 obtained using the model described in Panel 5.5[37] against that predicted using a static model—labelled 'Predicted cases (herd immunity)' and 'Predicted cases (no herd immunity)' respectively. Both models incorporate the actual vaccination coverage. The grey bars reflect the observed numbers of cases. Reproduced with permission from Trotter and Edmunds, 2006.[37]

and Wales using the dynamic transmission model developed by Trotter *et al.*[37, 40] described in Panel 5.5 and a static model, against the observed numbers of cases. In general, in contrast with the dynamic transmission model, the static model over-estimated the number of cases seen following the introduction of vaccination and was unable to reproduce their observed decline.

Likewise, a static model would underestimate the impact of vaccinating children on the the number of new infections occurring per unit time in older age groups, as illustrated by the following calculation.

5.3.4.1 Example: calculating the long-term average annual number of new rubella infections among 20-year-olds following the introduction of childhood vaccination in a high transmission setting using a static model

In section 5.3.3.1, the average annual number of new rubella infections among 20-year-olds in a high transmission setting, in the absence of vaccination, was calculated to be 559 per 100,000.

In the long term following the introduction of vaccination, assuming that 50 per cent of newborns were vaccinated, that vaccination did not affect the force of infection and that vaccination provides lifelong protection, the predicted annual number of new rubella infections among 20-year-olds would have been half of this value, i.e. 0.5×559 per 100,000 = 229.5 per 100,000.

This is much lower than the value which was estimated by taking account of changes in the force of infection, i.e. 770 per 100,000 (section 5.3.3.1).

5.3.5 Extending the logic to other pathogens

Much of our discussion of the effect of declines in the force of infection on the proportion of individuals that are susceptible and the number of new infections in different age groups has focussed on the immunizing infections. These issues are also relevant for infections, such as pertussis, for which immunity resulting from the vaccine or the infection wanes over time.[41, 42]

We note that reductions in the force of infection can also occur through improvements in sanitation for infections transmitted through the faecal–oral route such as hepatitis A or polio. There is evidence to suggest that the force of infection for hepatitis A has declined over time,[43] and therefore many of the issues are relevant for interpreting trends in hepatitis A incidence. We continue the theme of the effect of changes in the force of infection on the incidence of infections in Chapter 9, where we discuss varicella, pneumococcal infections and tuberculosis.

5.4 Summary

This chapter has illustrated that age patterns in the proportion of the population that is susceptible and the number of new infections occurring per unit time depend on R_0, which in turn determines the force of infection and the average age at infection. For ubiquitous immunizing infections, R_0, the average life expectancy and the force of infection (λ) are related through the equations $R_0 = 1 + \lambda L$ and $R_0 = \lambda L$, assuming that the population has an exponential and rectangular age distribution, respectively. These equations are often written as $R_0 = 1 + L/A$ and $R_0 = L/A$, respectively, assuming further that the average age of infection (A) is approximately equal to $1/\lambda$. Methods for estimating the force of infection and describing serological data, taking account of maternal immunity and changes in the force of infection with age, are also discussed. Estimates of age-dependent forces of infection will be used in Chapter 7 to calculate age-dependent contact parameters and R_0.

This chapter has also highlighted that the impact of vaccination programmes introduced among children is not straightforward. Whilst having the beneficial effect of leading to reductions in the numbers of new infections in the overall population, they can also lead to increases in the numbers of infections among older age groups. Such increases result from the reduction in the force of infection which occurs after vaccination is introduced, which leads to increases in the proportion of individuals who reach older age groups still susceptible to infection. These increases have important implications for infections, such as rubella, mumps and measles for which infection at older ages is associated with an increased risk of adverse outcomes.

5.5 Exercises

5.1 The following table shows the percentage of adults who did not have antibodies to rubella in China, Fiji and the UK before the introduction of MMR vaccination among young children.[13, 14, 44] Use the force of infection estimates provided to calculate the average annual numbers of new infections in the age groups provided. In which setting was the burden of CRS likely to have been the greatest, if no women had been vaccinated against rubella?

Age group (years)	% without antibodies		
	China $\lambda = 20\%/\text{year}$	Fiji $\lambda = 4\%/\text{year}$	UK $\lambda = 12\%/\text{year}$
15–19	4.0	43.5	12.8
20–29	4.3	28.8	8.7
30–39	5.4	19.3	7.1

5.2 The following table shows data on the proportion of individuals who did not have antibodies to rubella in Bangladesh during a study published in 2008.[45]

Age group (years)	Number tested	Number negative	% negative	Proportion of the population that is in the given age range (p_a)*
1–5	61	48	78.7	0.1139
6–10	61	29	47.5	0.1135
11–15	63	21	33.3	0.1109
16–20	62	14	22.6	0.1087
21–25	83	15	18.1	0.104
26–30	67	11	16.4	0.0923
31–35	63	12	19.0	0.0775
36–40	60	7	11.7	0.0641
≥41[†]	62	6	9.7	0.2151

* Based on data from [46]

[†] The study provided data on the proportion of individuals that did not have antibodies to rubella in the age group 41–45 years. For the purpose of this exercise, we treat this age group as being representative for all individuals aged over 41 years.

a) Estimate the median age at infection and use this to estimate the average force of infection.

b) Use the values for p_a and the approximate methods discussed in section 5.2.2.1 to estimate:

i. the average proportion of the population that is susceptible;

ii. R_0;

iii. the average force of infection, assuming that it is not age dependent and assuming an average life expectancy of 65 years;

iv. the average age at infection.

c) Use the methods discussed in section 5.2.2.1 to calculate the average annual force of infection experienced by individuals in each age group. What do your estimates suggest about how the force of infection changes with age?

d) Confirm your answer to question (c) using the methods discussed in section 5.2.3.5.2.

5.3 Apply the techniques discussed in section 5.2.3.5.2 to the data in section 5.2.3.2.2 to determine whether the force of mumps infection in the UK during the 1980s was age-dependent.

5.4 Show that for large values for the force of infection (>5 per cent) and realistic values for the life expectancy, Equations 5.10 and 5.11 approximate to $1/\lambda$.

5.5 The following table shows data on the number of individuals who had hookworm ova in their stools in Changshou, China in 1981.[21] What kind of catalytic model might you use to describe the data and why?

Age group (years)	Number tested (N_a)	Number positive (S_a)
0–4	44	6
5–9	179	106
10–14	208	154
15–19	149	120
20–29	149	119
30–39	183	153
40–49	88	79
50–59	90	75
60–69	48	39
70–79	9	7

5.6 (a) Prove the result that, when maternal immunity is lost at a constant rate, the proportion of individuals that are susceptible at a given age a is $\dfrac{\mu(e^{-\mu a} - e^{-\lambda a})}{\lambda - \mu}$.

(b) Use the expression in part a) to prove that the age at which the smallest proportion of individuals are susceptible is given by $a = \dfrac{\ln(\lambda/\mu)}{\lambda - \mu}$.

5.7 Use Equation 5.9 to prove the result that the average age at infection is given by $\dfrac{1}{\lambda + 1/L}$ and $\dfrac{1}{\lambda}\left(\dfrac{1 - (1 + \lambda L)e^{-\lambda L}}{1 - e^{-\lambda L}}\right)$ for a population with an exponential and rectangular age distribution respectively.

5.8 Prove the result that the level of the plateau for the reversible model is given by the equation $\lambda/(\lambda + r_s)$ (Table 5.4). *Hint: write down the differential equations for the rate of change by age in the prevalence of susceptible and infected individuals and use the facts that (i) the proportion infected at any given age equals 1–proportion susceptible at that age and (ii) at any point on the plateau, $\dfrac{ds}{da} = \dfrac{dz}{da} = 0$, i.e. the rate of change in the proportion of susceptible and infected individuals with age is zero.*

5.9 Country X is considering introducing MMR vaccination among infants. The average age at infection for mumps is about 4 years, the life expectancy is 60 years and the population has an exponential age distribution. It expects that, at best, it will only be able to sustain a vaccination coverage of 60 per cent.

a) Assuming, for simplicity, that vaccination occurs at birth, calculate:

  (i) the long-term average age at infection in the population after vaccination is introduced;

  (ii) the long-term average force of infection;

  (iii) the proportion of 15, 25, and 35-year-olds that are likely to be susceptible in the long term;

  (iv) the number of new infections per 100,000 population among 15, 25, and 35-year-olds.

b) Should the government go ahead with the vaccination programme?

c) How would your answer to parts (iii) and (iv) have changed if you had used a static model?

5.10

a) Rearrange equation 5.29 to obtain an expression for the long-term average force of infection after the introduction of vaccination among newborns, λ', in terms of R_0, L and v.

b) Use your answer to part a) to plot values for λ' against the proportion immunized (v) for values of v of between 0 and 1, assuming an average life expectancy (L) of 70 years and values of R_0 of 7 and 12.

c) How might you expect this plot to compare against one assuming that the reduction in the force of infection is directly proportional to the immunization coverage (i.e. a plot of $\lambda(1-v)$ against the proportion immunized) and why?

d) Add a plot of $\lambda(1-v)$ against the proportion immunized (using the same values for R_0 and L that were used in part b) to verify your answer to part c), and to check whether the patterns seen in Figure 5.14 are also predicted for populations with an exponential age distribution.

e) Try to follow steps a)-d) to reproduce Figure 5.14, i.e. using the equation
$R_0 = \dfrac{\lambda' L}{(1-v)(1-e^{-\lambda' L})}$ for a population with a rectangular age distribution instead
of equation 5.29.

References

1 Clarke SK, Heath RB, Sutton RN, Stuart-Harris CH. Serological studies with Asian strain of influenza A. *Lancet* 1958; 1(7025):814–818.

2 Mulder J, Masurel N. Pre-epidemic antibody against 1957 strain of Asiatic influenza in serum of older people living in the Netherlands. *Lancet* 1958; 1(7025):810–814.

3 Black FL. Measles antibodies in the population of New Haven, Connecticut. *J Immunol* 1959; 83(1):74–82.

4 Farrington CP. Modelling forces of infection for measles, mumps and rubella. *Stat Med* 1990; 9(8):953–967.

5 Cutts FT, Abebe A, Messele T *et al.* Sero-epidemiology of rubella in the urban population of Addis Ababa, Ethiopia. *Epidemiol Infect* 2000; 124(3):467–479.

6 Styblo K, Meijer J, Sutherland I. Tuberculosis Surveillance Research Unit Report No. 1: the transmission of tubercle bacilli; its trend in a human population. *Bull Int Union Tuberc* 1969; 42:1–104.

7 Griffiths DA. A catalytic model for infection for measles. *Appl Statist* 1974; 23(3):330–339.

8 Cutts FT, Vynnycky E. Modelling the incidence of Congenital Rubella Syndrome in developing countries. *Int J Epidemiol* 1999; 28(6):1176–1184.

9 Anderson RM, May RM. Infectious diseases of humans. *Dynamics and control.* Oxford: Oxford University Press; 1992.

10 Ades AE. Methods for estimating the incidence of primary infection in pregnancy: a reappraisal of toxoplasmosis and cytomegalovirus data. *Epidemiol Infect* 1992; 108(2):367–375.

11 World Health Organization. Measles vaccines. *Wkly Epidemiol Rec* 2004; 79(14):129–144.

12 de Azevedo Neto RS, Silveira AS, Nokes DJ *et al.* Rubella seroepidemiology in a non-immunized population of São Paulo State, Brazil. *Epidemiol Infect* 1994; 113(1):161–173.

13 Wannian S. Rubella in the People's Republic of China. *Rev Infect Dis* 1985; 7:S72–S73.

14 Macnamara FN, Mitchell R, Miles JA. A study of immunity to rubella in villages in the Fiji islands using the haemagglutination inhibition test. *J Hyg (Lond)* 1973; 71(4):825–831.

15 Ades AE, Nokes DJ. Modeling age- and time-specific incidence from seroprevalence: toxoplasmosis. *Am J Epidemiol* 1993; 137(9):1022–1034.

16 Münch H. *Catalytic models in epidemiology.* Cambridge, MA: Harvard University Press; 1959.

17 Remme J, Mandara MP, Leeuwenberg J. The force of measles infection in Africa. *Int J Epidemiol* 1984; 13(3):332–339.

18 Fine PE, Bruce J, Ponnighaus JM, Nkhosa P, Harawa A, Vynnycky E. Tuberculin sensitivity: conversions and reversions in a rural African population. *Int J Tuberc Lung Dis* 1999; 3(11):962–975.

19 Kitua AY, Smith T, Alonso PL *et al. Plasmodium falciparum* malaria in the first year of life in an area of intense and perennial transmission. *Trop Med Int Health* 1996; 1(4):475–484.

20 Vanamail P, Subramanian S, Das PK *et al.* Estimation of age-specific rates of acquisition and loss of *Wuchereria bancrofti* infection. *Trans R Soc Trop Med Hyg* 1989; 83(5):689–693.

21 Zhang YX. A compound catalytic model with both reversible and two-stage types and its applications in epidemiological study. *Int J Epidemiol* 1987; 16(4):619–621.

22 Whitaker HJ, Farrington CP. Estimation of infectious disease parameters from serological survey data: the impact of regular epidemics. *Stat Med* 2004; 23(15):2429–2443.

23 Fine PE. Herd immunity: history, theory, practice. *Epidemiol Rev* 1993; 15(2):265–302.

24 Gay N, Miller E, Hesketh L *et al.* Mumps surveillance in England and Wales supports introduction of two dose vaccination schedule. *Commun Dis Rep CDR Rev* 1997; 7(2):R21–R26.

25 Panagiotopoulos T, Antoniadou I, Valassi-Adam E. Increase in congenital rubella occurrence after immunisation in Greece: retrospective survey and systematic review. *BMJ* 1999; 319(7223):1462–1467.

26 Panagiotopoulos T, Georgakopoulou T. Epidemiology of rubella and congenital rubella syndrome in Greece, 1994–2003. *Euro Surveill* 2004; 9(4):17–19.

27 Fine PE, Clarkson JA. Measles in England and Wales–II: the impact of the measles vaccination programme on the distribution of immunity in the population. *Int J Epidemiol* 1982; 11(1):15–25.

28 Ramsay M, Gay N, Miller E *et al.* The epidemiology of measles in England and Wales: rationale for the 1994 national vaccination campaign. *Commun Dis Rep CDR Rev* 1994; 4(12):R141–R146.

29 Knox EG. Strategy for rubella vaccination. *Int J Epidemiol* 1980; 9(1):13–23.

30 Anderson RM, May RM. Age-related changes in the rate of disease transmission: implications for the design of vaccination programmes. *J Hyg (Lond)* 1985; 94(3):365–436.

31 Anderson RM, May RM. Vaccination against rubella and measles: quantitative investigations of different policies. *J Hyg (Lond)* 1983; 90(2):259–325.

32 Anderson RM, Grenfell BT. Quantitative investigations of different vaccination policies for the control of congenital rubella syndrome (CRS) in the United Kingdom. *J Hyg (Lond)* 1986; 96(2):305–333.

33 Hethcote HW. Measles and rubella in the United States. *Am J Epidemiol* 1983; 117(1):2–13.

34 Dietz K. The evaluation of rubella vaccination strategies. In Hiorns RW, Cooke D, eds, *The mathematical theory of the dynamics of biological populations*. London: Academic Press; 1981, pp. 81–97.

35 Savage E, Ramsay M, White J *et al*. Mumps outbreaks across England and Wales in 2004: observational study. *BMJ* 2004; 330(7700):1119–1120.

36 Preventing Congenital Rubella Syndrome. *Wkly Epidemiol Rec* 2000; 75(36):290–295.

37 Trotter CL, Edmunds WJ. Reassessing the cost-effectiveness of meningococcal serogroup C conjugate (MCC) vaccines using a transmission dynamic model. *Med Decis Making* 2006; 26(1):38–47.

38 Brisson M, Edmunds WJ. Economic evaluation of vaccination programs: the impact of herd-immunity. *Med Decis Making* 2003; 23(1):76–82.

39 Edmunds WJ, Medley GF, Nokes DJ. Evaluating the cost-effectiveness of vaccination programmes: a dynamic perspective. *Stat Med* 1999; 18(23):3263–3282.

40 Trotter CL, Gay NJ, Edmunds WJ. Dynamic models of meningococcal carriage, disease, and the impact of serogroup C conjugate vaccination. *Am J Epidemiol* 2005; 162(1):89–100.

41 Grenfell BT, Anderson RM. Pertussis in England and Wales: an investigation of transmission dynamics and control by mass vaccination. *Proc R Soc Lond B Biol Sci* 1989; 236(1284):213–252.

42 Crowcroft NS, Pebody RG. Recent developments in pertussis. *Lancet* 2006; 367(9526):1926–1936.

43 Jacobsen KH, Koopman JS. Declining hepatitis A seroprevalence: a global review and analysis. *Epidemiol Infect* 2004; 132(6):1005–1022.

44 Morgan-Capner P, Wright J, Miller CL, Miller E. Surveillance of antibody to measles, mumps, and rubella by age. *BMJ* 1988; 297(6651):770–772.

45 Nessa A, Islam MN, Tabassum S, Munshi SU, Ahmed M, Karim R. Seroprevalence of rubella among urban and rural Bangladeshi women emphasises the need for rubella vaccination of pre-pubertal girls. *Indian J Med Microbiol* 2008; 26(1):94–95.

46 World Population Prospects. *The 2006 Revision and World Urbanization Prospects: The 2005 Revision*. Population Division of the Department of Economic and Social Affairs of the United Nations Secretariat. 2005. Available at http://esa.un.org/unpp.

47 Grenfell BT, Anderson RM. The estimation of age-related rates of infection from case notifications and serological data. *J Hyg (Lond)* 1985; 95(2):419–436.

48 Schenzle D. An age-structured model of pre- and post-vaccination measles transmission. *IMA J Math Appl Med Biol* 1984; 1(2):169–191.

49 Meningococcal. Meningococcal meningitis and septicaemia notifiable. Immunisation against infectious disease. *The Green Book*. London: Department of Health; 2008.

50 Trotter CL, Gay NJ, Edmunds WJ. The natural history of meningococcal carriage and disease. *Epidemiol Infect* 2006; 134(3):556–566.

51 Trotter CL, Andrews NJ, Kaczmarski EB, Miller E, Ramsay ME. Effectiveness of meningococcal serogroup C conjugate vaccine 4 years after introduction. *Lancet* 2004; 364(9431):365–367.

Chapter 6

An introduction to stochastic modelling

6.1 **Overview and objectives**

All the models covered in the book so far have been deterministic, and have aimed to describe what is likely to happen on average in a population. This chapter is intended to introduce the methods for setting up stochastic models, which incorporate chance variation. By the end of this chapter, you should:

◆ Know how to set up stochastic models;

◆ Understand the differences between three key approaches for setting up stochastic models;

◆ Know how stochastic models are used to generate predictions;

◆ Know some of the areas of applications of stochastic models and the insights that stochastic models can provide.

6.2 **A simple problem**

In Chapters 2 and 3, we discussed the methods for setting up models to describe the course of an outbreak, following the introduction of a person with an acute contagious infection such as influenza or measles into a large population, comprising 100,000 individuals. Suppose, instead, that the population had been small, comprising only 10 susceptible individuals, as might be the situation in a hospital ward. What would be the most likely size of the subsequent outbreak?

Figure 6.1 summarizes predictions for this situation from a deterministic model. This predicts that, on average, after the infectious person enters the population, <1 new infectious person will be added to the population each day. Predictions from this model are not very meaningful for three reasons. First and most obviously, it is unrealistic to have fractions of individuals in the population at any time. Second, chance will probably greatly affect the outbreak size. In a real population, we may sometimes see an outbreak occur under similar conditions; at other times, no outbreak will occur. Third, given the small population size, a susceptible individual may contact more than one infectious person and in reality, they would have been infected by only one of the infectious persons. The deterministic model formulated in Chapters 2 and 3 did not account for this possibility.

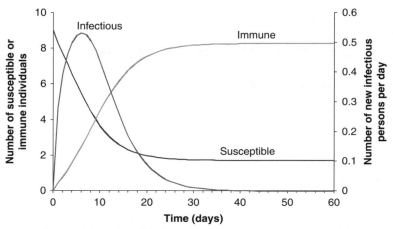

Fig. 6.1 Predictions of the 'number' of susceptible, infectious and immune individuals following the introduction of one infectious person into a population comprising ten susceptible individuals, assuming that $R_0 = 2$ and the pre-infectious and infectious periods are both two days. Obtained using Model 2.1, online.

To better describe transmission in a small population, we need to develop a stochastic model which incorporates the effect of chance on the possible outcome. There are several kinds of stochastic models:

1) **Individual-based models (method 1)**—these track what happens to *each individual* in the population and allow chance to determine whether or not they become infected and infectious at each time step (i.e. an individual-based approach).

2) **Discrete-time compartmental models (method 2)**—these treat the susceptible population as a single compartment, and allow chance to determine the total number of individuals infected by the infectious persons from the previous generation.

3) **Continuous time (or 'time to next event') compartmental models (method 3)**— these treat the susceptible population as a single compartment, and allow chance to determine when the next event (i.e. infection of a person or the recovery of an infectious person) will occur.

We discuss each of these methods in turn.

6.3 **Individual-based models (method 1)**

6.3.1 **The principles of method 1**

This method is intuitive, but is the most computer-intensive of the three methods: keeping track of what happens to every individual in a population requires more equations than does keeping track of changes in the total number of individuals in a compartment.

The 'mathematical' approach for allowing chance to determine whether or not an individual is infected is to draw a number at random for each individual, and to specify the range in which it should lie for the individual to become infected. If the random number falls outside that range, then that individual remains susceptible. This range is based on the risk of infection at that time point.

For example, if the risk of infection is 20 per cent, then in a model which tracks each individual in the population, we could draw a random number between 0 and 1 and specify that it must lie in the range 0–0.2 for that person to become infected, and between 0.2 and 1 for the person to remain susceptible. If the random number drawn was 0.85, for example, then, as 0.85 is larger than 0.2, the person in question does not become infected. If the random number had been 0.12, then because 0.12 is less than 0.2, that person would have become infected in the model.

To calculate the outbreak size in a given population, we would need to draw random numbers for each susceptible person, update the number of susceptible and infectious individuals based on the random number drawn, and repeat this process until there are no further infectious or susceptible individuals and transmission ceases. The following summarizes the succession of steps in the simplest scenario, whereby we take time steps of one serial interval and assume that, once infected, individuals are infectious but become immune by the subsequent time step.

Summary of the steps for method 1

Step 1: Calculate the risk $\lambda_{i,t}$ that the ith susceptible individual (where $i = 1, 2, \ldots N$) becomes infected in the next time interval. We discuss the methods for calculating $\lambda_{i,t}$ in section 6.3.2.

Step 2: Draw a random number between 0 and 1 for each of the susceptible individuals.

Step 3a: If the random number drawn for the ith individual is less than $\lambda_{i,t}$, then that individual becomes infected and hence infectious by time $t+1$; otherwise, that individual remains susceptible.

Step 3b: Any individuals who were infectious at the previous time step are now immune.

Step 4: Count up the number of infectious persons at time $t+1$ (I_{t+1}).

Step 5: If $I_{t+1} = 0$, transmission ceases and the size of the outbreak is given by the sum of the number of infectious persons at time $t=1, 2, 3, 4, \ldots, t$; otherwise return to step 1.

Before we illustrate this process, we discuss the formula for the risk of infection in a small population.

6.3.2 Calculating the risk of infection in each time step—the Reed–Frost equation

In previous chapters, when we assumed that individuals mix randomly and we were dealing with large populations and describing what happens on average in the population, the risk of infection (proportion of susceptible individuals who were infected in each time step, λ_t) was assumed to be proportional to the number of infectious individuals in the population, according to the equation:

$$\lambda_t = \beta I_t \qquad\qquad 6.1$$

where β is the rate at which two specific individuals come into effective contact per unit time (or per time step, if we are considering events occurring at discrete time intervals) and I_t is the number of infectious individuals at time t (section 2.7.1).

In small populations, such as hospital wards, schools, and workplaces, Equation 6.1 overestimates the actual infection risk. For example, in a hospital ward with 10 patients, of whom three are infectious, the risk of infection does not double if six patients are infectious (as would be implied by Equation 6.1), since a susceptible person can contact more than one infectious person and only one of those contacts will lead to infection.

Instead, we use the following equation for λ_t:

$$\lambda_t = 1 - (1 - p)^{I_t} \qquad\qquad 6.2$$

where p is the probability of an effective contact between two specific individuals in each time step. For simplicity, we assume that the infection risk is the same for all individuals and we will therefore use the notation λ_t, rather than $\lambda_{i,t}$. In this equation, p is analogous to β: the distinction between the two is that p is a *probability per time step*, whereas β is a *continuous time rate*. If the time step size is very small, then $p \approx \beta$. This formula is known as the Reed–Frost formula and was developed by Lowell Reed and Wade Hampton Frost during the 1920s.[2, 3] It can be derived by applying the following logic:

1) In order to become infected (and infectious), an individual must come into contact with *at least one* infectious person. The probability of this occurring is equivalent to 1—{the probability that an individual avoids contact with all I_t infectious persons}.

2) The probability that an individual avoids contact with all I_t infectious person is given by the expression $(1 - p)^{I_t}$. This follows from the fact that if, in each time period, $(1-p)$ is the probability that an individual avoids contact with one infectious person, $(1-p) \times (1-p)$ is the probability that an individual avoids contact with two infectious persons, $(1-p) \times (1-p) \times (1-p)$ is the probability that that individual avoids contact with 3 infectious persons, etc.

3) Combining the logic from steps 1 and 2 gives the Reed–Frost formula.

As shown in Figure 6.2, for small numbers of infectious individuals in the population, the Reed–Frost equation and Equation 6.1 give very similar values for λ_t. A mathematical proof showing that the two equations give similar values for λ_t when p is small (as would be the case in a large population) or when the number of infectious individuals is small is provided in the Appendix section A.4.1.

We shall now return to the example discussed in section 6.2 and consider how we apply method 1 to predict the course of an outbreak.

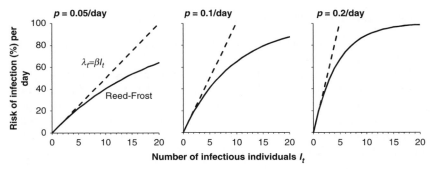

Fig. 6.2 Comparison between predictions of the risk of infection per day for values of the probability of an effective contact between two specific individuals per day (p) ranging between 5 and 20 per cent, assuming either that the risk of infection increased directly with the number of infectious individuals ($\lambda_t = \beta I_t$) or according to the Reed–Frost equation. In these calculations, β is taken to equal p.

Panel 6.1 Extensions to the Reed–Frost equation

The Reed–Frost equation can be extended to describe the risk of infection resulting from contact between different subgroups of a population. For example, if we wish to stratify between infection resulting from contact in the household and in the community, we would need to have two different values for p, e.g. p_h, reflecting the probability of an effective contact between two specific individuals in the household per time step and p_c, reflecting the probability of an effective contact between two specific individuals in the community per time step.

Denoting the numbers of infectious persons in the household and community at time t by $I_{h,t}$ and $I_{c,t}$ respectively, we obtain the following formula for the risk of infection:

$$\lambda_t = 1 - (1 - p_h)^{I_{h,t}} (1 - p_c)^{I_{c,t}} \qquad 6.3$$

If we wanted to include a further stratification to describe contact in the workplace, the equation would be as follows:

$$\lambda_t = 1 - (1 - p_h)^{I_{h,t}} (1 - p_c)^{I_{c,t}} (1 - p_w)^{I_{w,t}} \qquad 6.4$$

where p_w is the probability of an effective contact between two specific individuals in the workplace per time step and $I_{w,t}$ is the number of infectious persons in the workplace at time t. This equation forms the basis of most of the individual-based models in the literature.

Whilst the equation is relatively easy to write down, the actual values for p_h, p_c and p_w are not always readily available. The earliest individual-based models, such as that of Elveback during the 1970s,[15] which described influenza transmission between families, neighbourhoods, schools and pre-school, simply used values

Panel 6.1 Extensions to the Reed–Frost equation *(continued)*

which led to model predictions of the age-specific incidence of illness, secondary attack rates and the epidemic curve which were consistent with observed data. Other, more recent studies[16, 20] have used estimates obtained by fitting statistical models to household-level data. Based on data collected during an influenza season during the 1970s, for example, such studies have suggested that a person with a low level of pre-season antibody had a 16 per cent chance of being infected from the community during the epidemic period, and a 26 per cent chance of being infected by another household member during that person's infectious period.[26]

6.3.3 Example: an illustration of the individual-based approach—method 1

To illustrate method 1, we will use a simple approach, taking time steps of one serial interval so that individuals are infectious one time step after infection, and by the subsequent time step, they are immune. We will consider a population comprising 10 individuals following the introduction of one infectious person with influenza ($R_0 = 2$) and assume that individuals mix randomly, so that the risk of infection is identical for all individuals in the population. We shall refer to this risk between time t and $t+1$ as λ_t.

Adapting Equation 2.7 to account for the fact that we are using time steps of one serial interval, p is related to R_0 and the population size N by the formula:

$$p = R_0 / N$$
$$= 0.2 \text{ per time step} \qquad 6.5$$

We will now work through the steps listed earlier.

Iteration 1

Step 1: Applying the Reed–Frost formula leads to the risk, λ_0, that a susceptible individual becomes infected between time $t = 0$ and $t = 1$ is $1 - (1 - 0.20)^1 = 0.20$.
Steps 2 and 3: After drawing a random number for each of the 10 susceptible individuals, we obtain the following table for the status of individuals at time $t = 1$:

Individual number	Random number	Status at $t = 1$
1	0.764571	Susceptible
2	0.0067925	Infectious
3	0.304373	Susceptible
4	0.462942	Susceptible

5	0.762053	Susceptible
6	0.331372	Susceptible
7	0.61417	Susceptible
8	0.975166	Susceptible
9	0.312151	Susceptible
10	0.850425	Susceptible

In this instance, only one random number, that drawn for individual 2, was less than the risk of infection, $\lambda_0 = 0.20$, and so only individual 2 becomes infected and is infectious by time $t = 1$ (i.e. $I_1 = 1$).

Iteration 2

Step 1: Substituting for $I_1 = 1$ into the Reed–Frost equation gives the risk of infection between time $t = 1$ and $t = 2$ of $\lambda_1 = 1 - (1 - 0.20)^1 = 0.20$.

Steps 2 and 3: These lead to the following table for the number of infectious persons at time $t = 2$:

Individual number	Random number	Status at $t = 2$
1	0.239757	Susceptible
2	–	Immune
3	0.863884	Susceptible
4	0.412843	Susceptible
5	0.737687	Susceptible
6	0.039088	Infectious
7	0.094879	Infectious
8	0.020703	Infectious
9	0.535499	Susceptible
10	0.347521	Susceptible

In this instance, three random numbers were less than (= 0.20), and so the individuals for whom these random numbers were drawn are infected and are infectious by time $t = 2$, and so $I_2 = 3$. Individual 2, who was infectious at the previous time ($t = 1$) is now immune.

Iteration 3

Step 1: Substituting for $I_2 = 3$ into the Reed–Frost formula leads to $\lambda_2 = 1 - (1 - 0.20)^3$ = 0.488.

Steps 2, 3a and 3b: We obtain the following table for the time $t = 3$, with $I_3 = 4$ at Step 4:

Individual number	Random number	Status during $t = 3$
1	0.215361	Infectious
2	–	Immune
3	0.270405	Infectious
4	0.862182	Susceptible
5	0.696761	Susceptible
6	–	Immune
7	–	Immune
8	–	Immune
9	0.098544	Infectious
10	0.012308	Infectious

Iteration 4

Step 1: $\lambda_3 = 1 - (1 - 0.15)^4 = 0.478$.

Steps 2 and 3: Result in the following table at time $t = 4$:

Individual number	Random number	Status during $t = 4$
1	–	Immune
2	–	Immune
3	–	Immune
4	0.751125	Susceptible
5	0.602339	Susceptble
6	–	Immune
7	–	Immune
8	–	Immune
9	–	Immune
10	–	Immune

In this instance, none of the random numbers drawn for the susceptible individuals was less than λ_3, so no-one was infected, and therefore $I_4 = 0$. Thus transmission ceases at time $t = 4$, and so the total size of the outbreak in this simulation is given by $I_1 + I_2 + I_3 = 1 + 3 + 4 = 8$.

The online file Model 6.2 illustrates how this model might be set up in a spreadsheet.

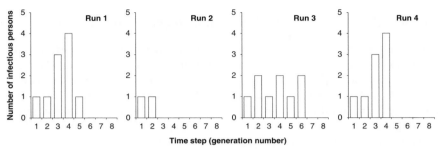

Fig. 6.3 Predictions of the number of infectious persons in each time step from four runs of the steps in section 6.3.1 after the introduction of one infectious person into a population comprising 10 susceptible individuals. Each infectious person has the potential to lead to two infectious persons (i.e. $R_0 = 2$ and so $p = 0.2$ per serial interval). Note that since the time step is 1 serial interval, the number of infectious persons predicted in each time step equals the number of infectious persons in each generation.

6.3.4 Interpreting findings from stochastic models

Because method 1 relies on numbers drawn at random, repeating the steps for method 1 (see section 6.3.1) again will usually lead to a different outbreak size, as shown in Figure 6.3. This illustrates the fact that with a stochastic model, the results from a single simulation are difficult to interpret. The dangers of interpreting results from a single run of a stochastic model are discussed in Panel 6.2.

Instead, the findings from each run are usually pooled together to provide the distribution of the outcome of interest, and the results are summarized in an analogous way to those from any epidemiological study, for example, showing the average outcome and the 95 per cent range in which the outcomes occurred.

Because the outcome of each run depends on chance, the distribution of the outbreak size or other outcome of interest, or the 95 per cent range in which it occurred depends on the number of runs that have been carried out. In general, if the number of runs is small, e.g. 20 or 50, the distribution will be highly variable and difficult to interpret (Figure 6.6). In general, for stochastic modelling studies, the number of runs is typically increased until further increases have no effect on the apparent distribution. For the model discussed in section 6.3.3, for example, the distribution of outbreak sizes is similar for model runs numbering 500 or more (Figure 6.6).

Panel 6.2 Interpreting findings from stochastic models

The difficulty of deriving conclusions from a single run of a stochastic model are illustrated in work by Cooper *et al.*,[1] which analysed the transmission of nosocomial hand-borne pathogens, such as *Staphylococcus aureus* in a general medical–surgical ward between health care workers (HCWs) and patients (see Figure 6.4). On average, the ward was assumed to comprise 3 HCWs and 20 patients, with the average length of stay being 10 days and 1 per cent of patients being already colonized on admission. On average, carers were assumed to wash their hands (decontaminating their hands from the pathogen) 14 times/day and made 5 contacts with a patient per day.

The model was set up using the stochastic modelling method 3 (Section 6.6). At the start of the simulations, all patients and all HCWs were assumed to be uncolonized and uncontaminated respectively. An outbreak in the ward can occur only once an infected or colonized patient enters the ward.

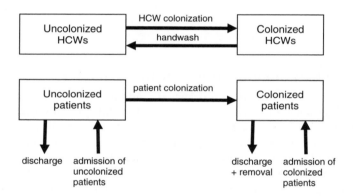

Fig. 6.4 Flow diagram of the model describing transmission of nosocomial pathogens between patients and HCWS in Cooper *et al*. Reproduced with permission from Cooper *et al*, 1999.[1]

The outcomes for three model runs which considered 365-day period, which were based on the same average parameters, but which gave different predictions of the persistence of nosocomial pathogens on a hospital ward are shown in Figure 6.5. Specifically, in run A, colonized patients are present on the ward for a large proportion of the year. In run B, few colonized patients are seen on the ward. In run C, a major outbreak occurs on around day 230. Given the contribution of chance variation to these predictions, conclusions of the persistence of the nosocomial infections would be obtained after running the model many times, and examining the proportion of runs which resulted in a given scenario.

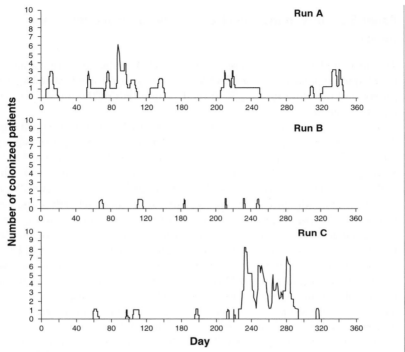

Fig. 6.5 Sample simulation runs from the model by Cooper *et al*. All the input parameters were identical, with $R_0=0.57$. Reproduced with permission from Cooper *et al*, 1999.[1]

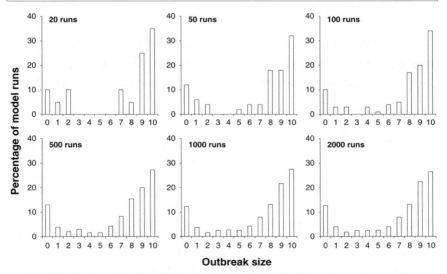

Fig. 6.6 Distribution of outbreak sizes resulting from different numbers of runs of method 1 for the model described in section 6.3.3.

Panel 6.3 How many runs from a stochastic model do we need?

The small models described in section 6.3, which describe small populations and have few input parameters, typically take seconds to run on standard desktop computers, and therefore running such models hundreds or thousands of times is typically straightforward.

However, this can be difficult for large models, such as those developed during the early 2000s to predict the impact of different interventions against pandemic influenza.[16, 18, 20, 21] The models of Germann et al. and Ferguson et al.[18, 21] for example, described the US population and modelled approximately 300 million individuals. They also incorporated detailed movement patterns between homes, workplaces, long-distance travel, contact patterns in schools, churches, and workplaces etc. At the time of writing, intensive computing resources were required to run the models and obtain interpretable results. Each realization of the model of Ferguson et al.[21], for example, ran in 1–2 hours (on 8 CPU Opteron 854-based servers) and the predictions of the impact of the different strategies, which were published in,[21] required 20,000 CPU hours. Some of the outcomes of interest (e.g. the cumulative attack rate and numbers of antiviral doses require for given scenarios varied by less than 0.1 per cent between simulations, and an overall average outcome could be determined just by using 5–20 simulation runs.

The earlier work of Ferguson et al.[20] (published in 2005) on the impact of strategies for containing an influenza pandemic, should it emerge in South East Asia, limited the computational burden by running up to 1,000 simulations for a given control strategy, and stopping when 50 simulation runs in which control had failed had occurred.

6.4 Discrete-time stochastic compartmental models (method 2)—allow chance to determine the number of secondary cases resulting from each generation of cases

6.4.1 Overview of method 2

This method is slightly less laborious than the individual-based approach of method 1. Instead of keeping track of the status of each individual as in method 1, it keeps track of the *total* number of susceptibles and infectious persons at each time step. Random numbers are used to determine the *total number of susceptibles infected by the infectious persons in each generation*, assuming that this number follows some distribution.

The steps for method 2 are identical to those used for method 1, except that we use the *distribution* of the number of individuals likely to be infected to determine how many individuals are infected in the next time step. The steps for simulating an outbreak using time steps of one serial interval are as follows.

Summary of the steps for method 2

Step 1: Calculate the risk of infection in the next time interval using the Reed–Frost formula of $\lambda_t = 1-(1-p)^{I_t}$

Step 2: Calculate the distribution of the number of susceptible individuals that are likely to be infected by the infectious persons present at time t.

Step 3: Sample a random number, n_i, between 0 and 1 from the distribution calculated in step 2 to determine k_i, the number of susceptible individuals who are infected. I_{t+1} is then given by k_i, and S_{t+1} is given by $S_t - k_i$. The subscript in the notation k_i and n_i is used to denote the process of infection. (Note that many packages provide in-built routines for sampling random numbers from a given distribution; the mechanics of doing this are discussed in Panel 6.4).

Step 4: if $I_{t+1} = 0$, transmission ceases and the size of the outbreak is given by the sum of the number of infectious terms at time $t = 1, 2, 3, 4,..,t$; otherwise return to step 1.

Before illustrating these steps, we discuss how we calculate the distribution of the number of susceptible individuals who might be infected.

6.4.2 Calculating the distribution of the number of susceptible individuals infected during a given time step

Suppose we have a simple scenario whereby there are two susceptible individuals; we shall refer to these individuals as John and Nigel. To calculate the distribution of the number of individuals who might be infected in the next time step, we first consider what outcomes can occur and the probability of these outcomes. For simplicity we shall assume that the risk of infection between time t and $t+1$, λ_t, is 0.8.

For this scenario, there are three possible outcomes for the next time step, each depending on the risk of infection λ_t:

A. **Both susceptible persons remain susceptible.** Each individual has a probability of $(1-\lambda_t)$ of remaining susceptible; the probability of both remaining susceptible is $(1-\lambda_t)^2$. For example, if the risk of infection is 0.8, then the probability that John remains susceptible is 0.2; likewise the probability that Nigel remains susceptible is 0.2. The probability that both John and Nigel remain susceptible is the product of these two probabilities, i.e. $0.2 \times 0.2 = 0.04$.

Panel 6.4 Sampling random numbers from a distribution

Many packages provide inbuilt routines for sampling random numbers from distributions. For example, in Excel 2007, this routine is available through the 'Data Analysis' options. We describe one possible mechanism by which they work.

For example, if the distribution of the number of susceptible individuals that could be infected follows the pattern in Figure 6.7a, i.e. the probability that no, one or two individuals are infected is 0.04, 0.32 and 0.64 respectively, then we might specify that, if the random number lies in the ranges 0–0.04, 0.04–0.36 and 0.36–1, then no, 1 or both individuals are infected respectively.

These ranges can be obtained by first calculating the *cumulative probability distribution* of the number of individuals who are infected. Each outcome (0, 1 or 2 individuals becoming infected) is then assigned a centile in this distribution, with its width being equal to the probability of that outcome occuring. The range in which a random number should lie for the given outcome to occur is then equal to the centile of the cumulative probability distribution that is occupied by that outcome. For example, considering Figure 6.7a, the centiles could be 0–0.04, 0.04–0.36 and 0.36–1 for no, 1 or both individuals to be infected respectively. Thus, if our random number is 0.3, then as shown in Figure 6.7b, 0.3 lies in the centile corresponding to 1 susceptible individual being infected.

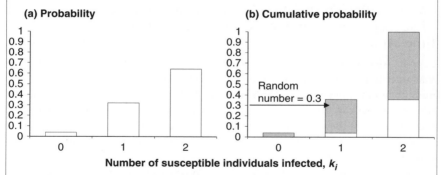

(a) Probability   **(b) Cumulative probability**

Random number = 0.3

Number of susceptible individuals infected, k_i

Fig. 6.7 (a) Distribution of the number of susceptible individuals infected in the next time step, in a population comprising two susceptible individuals, and assuming that the risk of infection equals 0.8 per time step, calculated using Equation 6.6. (b) Cumulative probability distributions corresponding to the probability distributions shown for (a). The grey areas reflect the centiles in which a number drawn at random would have to lie in order to lead to a given number of individuals infected.

B. **Only one of the two susceptible persons becomes infected.** This occurs with a probability of $2\lambda_t(1-\lambda_t) = 2 \times 0.8 \times 0.2 = 0.32$. This probablity can be derived using the following logic:

{Probability that only one of the two susceptible persons is infected}

=

$\left\{\begin{array}{c}\text{probability that a given individual is infected and the other individual}\\\text{remains susceptible}\end{array}\right\}$

×

$\left\{\begin{array}{c}\text{The number of ways of selecting one individual to remain susceptible and}\\\text{the other individual to become infected}\end{array}\right\}$

The probability that John is infected in the next time step equals $\lambda_t = 0.8$; the probability that Nigel remains susceptible equals $1- \lambda_t = 0.2$. The probability that John is infected *and* Nigel remains susceptible equals the product of these two probabilities i.e. $\lambda_t(1- \lambda_t) = 0.8 \times 0.2 = 0.16$.

Since there are two individuals, there are two ways in which we can select a given individual to be infected and the other to remain susceptible. The overall probability that either John or Nigel is infected and the other remains susceptible is therefore given by $2\lambda_t(1- \lambda_t) = 2 \times 0.16 = 0.32$.

C. **Both susceptible persons are infected.** John and Nigel each have a probability of $\lambda_t = 0.8$ of being infected; the probability of both being infected is $\lambda_t^2 = 0.8 \times 0.8 = 0.64$.

The resulting distribution of the number of susceptible individuals infected in the next time step is plotted in Figure 6.7a. Methods used to sample from this distribution to determine the number of individuals that are infected in the next time step are discussed in Panel 6.4.

The equation that is used to calculate the probability that only one of the two susceptible individuals is infected (outcome B) is the standard binomial expression for the probability of 1 success out of S_t trials. We can extend this logic to consider the general situation whereby there are S_t susceptible individuals. As shown in Panel 6.5, the equation for the probability that exactly k_i out of S_t individuals will be infected in the next time step is given by the standard binomial expression for the probability of k_i successes out of S_t trials:

$$P(\text{exactly } k_i \text{ out of the } S_t \text{ susceptible individuals are infected}) = \binom{S_t}{k_i}\lambda_t^k(1-\lambda_t)^{S_t-k_i} \quad 6.6$$

where $\binom{S_t}{k_i}$ is the binomial coefficient, reflecting the number of ways of choosing k_i out of the S_t susceptible individuals to become infected.

6.4.3 An illustration of method 2

Table 6.1 shows the result of one simulation run of method 2 for the population of 10 susceptible individuals considered for method 1, and using the same value for

Panel 6.5 Derivation of the general equation for the probability that exactly k_i out of S_t individuals will be infected in the next time step

If there are S_t susceptible individuals, then there are S_t+1 possible outcomes:

Outcome 1: All S_t susceptible individuals remain susceptible. The probability of this occurring equals $(1-\lambda_t)^{S_t}$.

Outcome 2: One out of the S_t susceptible individuals remains susceptible and the other S_t-1 susceptible individuals are infected.

Outcome 3: Two out of the S_t susceptible individuals remain susceptible and the other S_t-2 susceptible individuals are infected.

…

Outcome k_i+1: Exactly k_i out of the S_t susceptible individuals remain susceptible and the other S_t-k_i susceptible individuals are infected.

…

Outcome S_t+1: All S_t susceptible individuals are infected. The probability of this occurring equals $\lambda_t^{S_t}$.

The probability of outcome k_i can be expressed generally as follows:

$$\left\{\begin{array}{c}\text{probability that a given set of } k_i \text{ individuals are infected and the other}\\ S_t - k_i \text{ individuals remain susceptible}\end{array}\right\}$$

$$\times$$

$$\left\{\begin{array}{c}\text{The number of ways of selecting } k_i \text{ individuals to remain susceptible and}\\ \text{the remaining } S_t - k_i \text{ individuals to become infected}\end{array}\right\}$$

The probability that a given set of k_i individuals is infected equals $\lambda_t^{k_i}$; the probability that a given set of $S_t - k_i$ individuals remain susceptible equals $(1-\lambda_t)^{S_t-k_i}$. The probability of the given set of k_i individuals being infected *and* the given set of S_t-k_i individuals remaining susceptible equals the product of these two probabilities, i.e. $\lambda_t^{k_i}(1-\lambda_t)^{S_t-k_i}$.

The number of ways of choosing k_i out the S_t susceptible individuals to become infected is given by the binomial coefficient $\binom{S_t}{k_i}$, which can also be written as $^{S_t}C_{k_i}$ or $\dfrac{S_t!}{(S_t-k_i)!\,k_i!}$.

The overall probability of k_i out of the S_t susceptible individuals being infected is therefore given by the equation:

$$P(\text{exactly } k_i \text{ out of the } S_t \text{ susceptible individuals are infected}) =$$

$$\binom{S_t}{k_i}\lambda_t^{k_i}(1-\lambda_t)^{S_t-k_i}$$

6.7

This equation is the standard binomial expression for the probability of k_i successes out of S_t trials.

Table 6.1 Summary of the results of one simulation run using method 2 of the effect of the introduction of one infectious person into a totally susceptible population comprising 10 individuals. $I_0 = 1$, $S_0 = 10$. The simulation finishes on the third iteration with an outbreak size of $I_1 + I_2 = 7$ infectious individuals.

	Iteration 1	Iteration 2	Iteration 3
Step 1: Estimate λ_t.	$\lambda_0 = 1 - (1 - 0.2)^1 = 0.2$	$\lambda_1 = 1 - (1 - 0.2)^4 = 0.5904$	$\lambda_2 = 1 - (1 - 0.2)^3 = 0.4880$

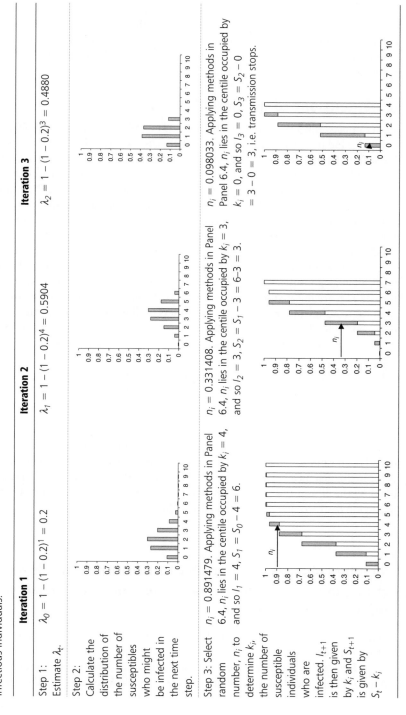

Step 2: Calculate the distribution of the number of susceptibles who might be infected in the next time step.

Step 3: Select random number, n_i to determine k_i, the number of susceptible individuals who are infected. I_{t+1} is then given by k_i and S_{t+1} is given by $S_t - k_i$.

$n_i = 0.891479$. Applying methods in Panel 6.4, n_i lies in the centile occupied by $k_i = 4$, and so $I_1 = 4$, $S_1 = S_0 - 4 = 6$.

$n_i = 0.331408$. Applying methods in Panel 6.4, n_i lies in the centile occupied by $k_i = 3$, and so $I_2 = 3$, $S_2 = S_1 - 3 = 6 - 3 = 3$.

$n_i = 0.098033$. Applying methods in Panel 6.4, n_i lies in the centile occupied by $k_i = 0$, and so $I_3 = 0$, $S_3 = S_2 - 0 = 3 - 0 = 3$, i.e. transmission stops.

p (0.2 per serial interval). This highlights the fact that, as the number of susceptible and infectious individuals changes, the distribution of the number of individuals contacted by each infectious person (and by implication, number of infectious persons predicted in the next generation) changes. Model 6.3 online illustrates how this model might be set up in a spreadsheet.

6.5 Extensions to methods 1 and 2

The examples which we considered for methods 1 and 2 were relatively simple because only one kind of transition was incorporated, namely susceptible individuals becoming infected and infectious. They did not explicitly describe infectious individuals recovering and becoming immune. Also, transitions were assumed to occur after fixed time steps, which were implicitly assumed to be one serial interval. Both methods 1 and 2 can be adapted to deal with other transitions, for example, to allow chance to determine the number of infectious cases who recover and become immune, or to allow the time steps to be of less than one serial interval (e.g. of size δt).

For example, considering method 2, the number of infectious individuals who recover between time t and a small time interval, $t+\delta t$ thereafter can be calculated by using an analogous method to that used to calculate the number of susceptible individuals who are infected in each time interval. A random number in the range 0–1 is sampled from the binomial distribution and is used to determine the number, k_r, of infectious individuals to recover in that time interval. The expression for the probability that k_r out of I_t infectious individuals recover in that time interval is analogous to Equation 6.6:

P(exactly k_r out of the I_t infectious individuals recover) =

$$\binom{I_t}{k_r} r_t^k (1-r_t)^{I_t-k_r} \qquad 6.8$$

where r_t is defined as the risk that an infectious individual recovers between time t and $t+\delta t$. For most practical purposes, small time steps are used in the calculations, and r_t is approximated by the rate at which individuals recover from being infectious, multiplied by the size of the time step δt. The steps for method 2 that are summarized in Section 6.4.1 would now be adapted as follows:

Summary of the steps for method 2, extending it to allow chance to determine the number of infectious individuals who recover in each time step

Step 1a: Calculate the risk of infection in the next time interval using the Reed–Frost formula of $\lambda_t = 1-(1-p)^{I_t}$.

Step 1b: Calculate the average proportion of infectious persons who should recover during the next time interval using the expression $r_t = r\delta t$, where δt is the size of the time interval and r is the rate at which infectious persons recover from being infectious (given by 1/duration of infectiousness—see Section 2.7.2).

Step 2a: Calculate the distribution of the number of susceptible individuals that are likely to be infected by the infectious persons present at time t.

Step 2b: Calculate the distribution of the number of infectious individuals who should recover in the next time step.

Step 3a: Draw a random number n_i in the range 0–1 from the distribution calculated in step 2a to determine k_i, the number of susceptible individuals who are infected (and become infectious) in the next time step (see Panel 6.4 for the mechanics of how this is done).

Step 3b: Draw a random number n_r in the range 0–1 from the distribution calculated in step 2b to determine k_r, the number of infectious individuals who recover in the next time step (see Panel 6.4 for the mechanics of how this is done).

Step 4: $I_{t+\delta t}$ is then given by $I_t + k_i - k_r$ and $S_{t+\delta t}$ is given by $S_t - k_i$.

Step 5: if $I_{t+\delta t}=0$, transmission ceases; otherwise return to step 1.

6.6 **Continuous time ('time to next event') compartmental models (method 3)**

Both methods 1 and 2 assume that all transitions occur after the same fixed time step δt, and are known as *discrete time* stochastic models. They are analogous to deterministic difference equations. A third method uses chance to determine when the next event occurs (i.e. the size of δt) and, if more than one kind of transition is considered, for example, susceptibles becoming infected or infectious individuals recovering, the type of transition which occurs. Because the size of the time step is variable, the models based on this approach are referred to as *continuous time* or *time to next event* models, and can be considered to be stochastic implementations of differential equations. Figure 6.8 provides an example of predictions obtained using this method.

This method can be implemented in a spreadsheet (see Model 6.4, online) although this is practical only for describing the transmission of an infection in small populations.

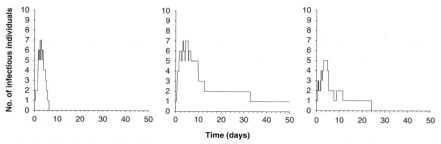

Fig. 6.8 Examples of different predictions of the prevalence of infectious individuals with influenza, following the introduction of one infectious person into a totally susceptible population comprising 10 individuals, obtained by using method 3. See Model 6.4, online.

In practice, it is usually implemented using a programming language. The key steps in the calculations are as follows.

Summary of the steps for method 3

Step 1: Calculate the rate (M_t) at which individuals can change their current status (i.e. become infected, recover from being infectious, die etc.).

M_t is known as a *hazard rate*, as it gives the hazard or chance of an event occurring over a small time interval. Mathematically, the chance of any event leading to a change of status in a small interval of time δt is approximately given by $M_t \delta t$. The approximation can be made as precise as we choose by selecting a small enough value for δt.

In the following model, only two kinds of transitions are described explicitly, namely susceptible individuals being infected and becoming infectious, and infectious individuals recovering and becoming immune.

$$\boxed{\text{Susceptible}} \longrightarrow \boxed{\text{Infectious}} \longrightarrow \boxed{\text{Immune}}$$

It would be written using the following differential equations:

$$\frac{dS}{dt} = -\beta S(t)I(t)$$

$$\frac{dI}{dt} = \beta S(t)I(t) - rI(t)$$

$$\frac{dR}{dt} = rI(t)$$

where β is the rate at which two specific individuals come into effective contact per unit time, and r is the rate at which infectious individuals recover. In this example, the total rate at which individuals could change their current status is given by the sum of the rates at which individuals become infected and infectious, and infectious persons recover to become immune:

$$M_t = \beta\, S(t)\, I(t) + rI(t) \qquad 6.9$$

Step 2: Draw a random number, n_1, between 0 and 1 and calculate the time after which the next transition occurs, given by:

$$T = -\ln(n_1)/M_t \qquad 6.10$$

This expression for T follows from the fact that when events occur at random at a constant rate, the time until the event occurs follows the exponential distribution (see Section 2.7.2). Given that the hazard rate is M_t, it can be shown that the probability p_T that there has been no event by time T is given by the following:

$$p_T = e^{-M_t T} \qquad 6.11$$

Reference[4] and the references cited in that work provide further details. Replacing p_T with the random number n_1, and rearranging the resulting equation leads to Equation 6.10.

Step 3: Calculate the probability that each type of transition (e.g. susceptible –> infected or infectious –> immune) will occur. Use this to calculate the range in which a number drawn at random must lie for a given transition to occur.

In the above example, the probability that one susceptible individual becomes infected (and then infectious) during the next time step is given by $\beta S(t)I(t)/M_t$; the probability that one infectious individual recovers during the next time step is $r(t)I(t)/M_t$.

Thus, if the random number drawn is in the interval $(0,\beta S(t)I(t)/M_t)$ then one susceptible individual is infected (and becomes infectious); otherwise one infectious person recovers and becomes immune.

Step 4: Draw a random number n_2 to determine the transition event which occurs next.

Step 5: Use the result from step 4 to update the number of susceptible, infectious and immune individuals present in the population and return to step 1.

An illustration of method 3 is provided in Appendix section A.4.2. Readers may wish to refer to Keeling and Rohani[4] for a technical discussion of different methods for implementing these steps.

6.7 Which approach is best?

Each of the methods described above for setting up stochastic models has its advantages and disadvantages. For example, the individual-based approach of method 1 is more computationally demanding than is the approach of method 2. Method 3 is also computationally demanding if the population size is large or if there are many events, but it is attractive because it allows the size of the time step to vary and comes close to describing events occurring continuously. On the other hand, as is the case with difference equations, we can approximate events occurring in continuous time using methods 1 and 2 simply by using a sufficiently small time step. Consequently, the approach used when developing a stochastic model typically depends on the size of the problem and the available computing resources.

6.8 Insights and applications of stochastic models

6.8.1 Inferring reproduction numbers from distributions of outbreak sizes

The model runs which are illustrated in Figure 6.3 highlight an importance distinction between deterministic models and stochastic models. As discussed in Chapter 4, for a deterministic model, when an infectious person is introduced into a totally susceptible population and the reproduction number of the infection is greater than one, then the model will always predict that an outbreak will occur. Conversely, when the reproduction

Table 6.2 Example of the expected number of individuals observed in different compartments after the introduction of 1 infectious individual into a population consisting of 10 susceptible individuals, as predicted using method 3, assuming that $p = 0.1$/day and the recovery rate is 0.5/day. For these parameters, $R_0 = 2$. See Appendix section A.4.2 for further details of the calculations.

Time	Susceptibles	Infectious	Immune	M_t	Random number (n_1)	T	Probability that the next event is:		Random number (n_2)	Next event
							Infection event	Recovery event		
0.000	10	1	0	1.5	0.46	0.518	0.667	0.333	0.56	S->I
0.518	9	2	0	2.8	0.81	0.077	0.643	0.357	0.73	I->R
0.595	9	1	1	1.4	0.22	1.079	0.643	0.357	0.05	S->I
1.674	8	2	1	2.6	0.07	1.004	0.615	0.385	0.93	I->R
2.678	8	1	2	1.3	0.85	0.128	0.615	0.385	0.25	S->I
2.806	7	2	2	2.4	0.18	0.725	0.583	0.417	0.32	S->I
3.531	6	3	2	3.3	0.42	0.264	0.545	0.455	0.13	S->I
3.795	5	4	2	4	0.53	0.161	0.500	0.500	0.39	S->I
3.956	4	5	2	4.5	0.06	0.609	0.444	0.556	0.22	S->I
4.564	3	6	2	4.8	0.66	0.087	0.375	0.625	0.61	I->R
4.651	3	5	3	4	0.44	0.205	0.375	0.625	0.39	I->R
4.857	3	4	4	3.2	0.95	0.018	0.375	0.625	0.41	I->R
4.874	3	3	5	2.4	0.32	0.480	0.375	0.625	0.84	I->R
5.355	3	2	6	1.6	0.43	0.525	0.375	0.625	0.73	I->R
5.879	3	1	7	0.8	0.86	0.183	0.375	0.625	0.42	I->R
6.0062	3	0	8	0	0.85	No event	No event	No event	0.62	No event

number is less than one, the model always predicts that transmission of the infection dies out.

In contrast, for a stochastic model, even if the reproduction number is greater than one, then an outbreak is predicted to occur in only some of the model runs. Likewise, in a stochastic model, an outbreak can occur even if the reproduction number is less than one, because of chance variation. The probability of an outbreak, however, depends, among other things, on the size of the reproduction number. This is illustrated in Figure 6.9, which shows the distribution of outbreak sizes predicted by running the model discussed in section 6.3 using different values of R_0. For low values of R_0, for example, large outbreaks occurred in a small proportion of the simulations; for $R_0 = 2$, outbreaks involving seven or more persons were predicted for over 50 per cent of the simulations.

Given the different distributions of outbreak sizes which are associated with different values of the basic reproduction number, methods have been developed to estimate the basic or net reproduction number from observed distributions of outbreak sizes.[6, 7] According to theory which is too complex to reproduce here (see De Serres et al.[6] for further details), the distribution of outbreak sizes in a given population is related to the reproduction number (denoted by R, as it could be the net or basic reproduction number) through the equation:

$$P(Outbreak\,size = k) = \frac{R^{k-1}e^{-Rk}k^{k-2}}{(k-1)!} \quad k = 1,2,3,\ldots$$

6.12

The corresponding distribution is shown in Figure 6.12. Equation 6.12 assumes further that the reproduction number is less than 1.

The theory was first developed to estimate the net reproduction number for infections in populations in which there was little indigenous transmission as a result of a successful vaccination programme. In such populations, the introduction of an infectious person from an area where control has been less successful could lead to an outbreak. Estimates of the net reproduction number and the extent to which it is less than 1, should provide insight into whether there is a need for further interventions or whether transmission will cease on its own.

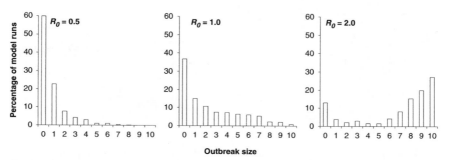

Fig. 6.9 Distribution of outbreak sizes obtained using the model discussed for method 1 in section 6.3 for $R_0 = 0.5$, 1 and 2 (equivalent to $p = 0.05$, 0.1 and 0.2 per serial interval). The distributions are based on 500 model runs.

During the period 1995–8 in the UK, for example (and following a national vaccination campaign), there had been about 14, 4, 2, and 1 outbreaks involving 3–4, 5–9, 10–24 and ≥100 individuals respectively.[6] These outbreaks sizes were compatible with a net reproduction number of between 0.5 and 0.6, which was consistent with estimates obtained using other methods, and suggested that sustained transmission was unlikely.[6]

Data on outbreak sizes for new or emergent infection (e.g. a new strain of influenza) may be analysed in a similar way to estimate the basic reproduction number, which can provide insight into the risk of a major outbreak.[7]

6.8.2 Modelling transmission in small populations and the persistence of infection

One weakness of deterministic models is that, even if fractions of individuals are present in the model population, they predict that transmission of an infection always continues. In contrast, this situation typically does not occur in stochastic models, which tend to deal only with integer numbers of individuals, for which, by definition, transmission will stop once the number of infectious persons drops below 1 (i.e. zero). This makes stochastic models appropriate for addressing questions involving small populations comprising, e.g. 10 or 100 individuals, such as hospital wards or schools, in which chance effects may lead to small numbers of infectious persons and transmission ceasing. It also makes them appropriate for addressing questions relating to the persistence of infections in populations of a given size. Such questions cannot be addressed using deterministic models.

For example, stochastic models were applied to elucidate why, in some populations, the numbers of cases of measles dropped to low levels and no cases were seen for

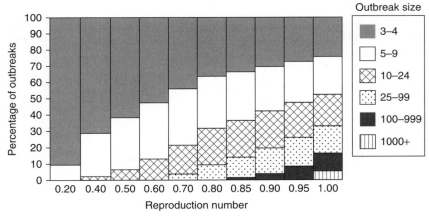

Fig. 6.10 Distribution of the size of outbreaks of disease resulting from an importation. Reproduced with permission from De Serres *et al*, 2000.[6] Given that small outbreaks are less likely to be reported than large outbreaks, this distribution relates only to outbreaks involving three or more persons.

several months in small island populations ('endemic fade out'), until the infection was reintroduced[8–10] (see Figure 4.27). The analyses suggested that the population needed to comprise more than 250,000 individuals for transmission of the infection to persist; subsequent analyses have highlighted that the distribution of the infectious period[5] and the birth rate[11] also strongly influence the critical population size.

Of practical relevance, stochastic models (based on method 3) were applied during the 1990s to explore issues relating to the persistence of polio and calculating the probability that polio had been eradicated if no cases had been observed for different time periods.[12] Less than 1 per cent of infections lead to paralysis and the study suggested that no cases of paralytic polio would have to be observed for three years before one could be 95 per cent certain that the virus was locally extinct.

6.8.3 Individual-based microsimulation models

As the name suggests, these models track the status of every individual in a population generally using combinations of the different methods, with or without some deterministic elements. One of the earliest individual-based microsimulation models was that of Elveback et al.,[15] which was developed during the 1970s to explore the impact of interventions against influenza in a population comprising 1,000 persons, structured into 254 families. Individuals were stratified into five age groups (pre-school, grade school, high school, young adult and older adult), with each of the pre-school children belonging to one of 30 playgroups and mixing between individuals in the neighbourhood and other social groups being defined by given clusters. Models which were developed during the 2000s to explore the impact of interventions against pandemic influenza[16–21] have used a similar approach, although the population sizes considered have been larger and the movement patterns have been more detailed than those in the Elveback model (see Panel 6.3).

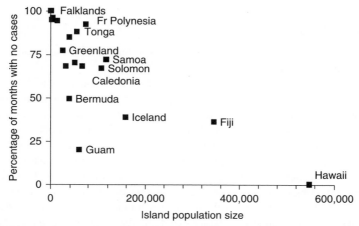

Fig. 6.11 The persistence of measles in island populations spanning up to 15 year periods until 1966. Adapted from Anderson and May, 1992.[13] Data from Black 1966.[14]

The ONCHOSIM model is another example of a microsimulation model which was developed specifically for addressing questions relating to control. This was developed during the late 1980s in collaboration with the Onchocerciasis Control Programme to assess the implications of cessation of larviciding on the transmission dynamics of onchocerciasis in different settings.[22] It describes the infection process of every individual and every parasite in different village populations using combinations of methods 1 and 2 above, taking account of different levels of exposure to the vector, biting densities, lifespan of the fly, parasite etc. Since the development of ONCHOSIM, other large-scale simulation models have also been developed for HIV (SIMULAIDS and STDSIM) and schistosomiasis (SCHISTOSIM).[23–25]

The obvious disadvantage of such highly structured models is that they are difficult to set up and they can be slow to run (see Panel 6.3). A further challenge is that the most detailed models require many input parameters (some of which are not readily available). As the number of input parameters increases, it becomes increasingly more difficult to elucidate the contribution of a given input parameter on the overall outcome, and thus many simulations may need to be run in order to obtain useful predictions. On the other hand, with the development of fast computers, these disadvantages should become less of a problem in future years.

One advantage that these models have over less structured deterministic models is that they can be used to explore the impact of interventions targeted at the household, school or workplace. For example, the influenza models described above have been able to explore the impact of providing antivirals to contacts of influenza cases in the household. A further advantage is that, by attempting to describe reality, they are intuitively easier to understand than are deterministic models, in that they track the status among all individuals in the population, rather than collectively as a group. In addition, by tracking the experience of each individual in a population, they are better than deterministic models at describing the transmission of infections for which the risk of disease or another outcome depends on the person's previous exposure history.

6.9 Summary

In this chapter, we discussed the key methods for setting up stochastic models and the insights and areas of applications of these models.

Stochastic models incorporate the effect of chance on an outcome and can provide estimates of the range in which a possible outcome may occur. Stochastic models are typically set up using one or more of three approaches: (i) tracking what happens to each individual in a population, and allowing chance to determine whether or not each individual becomes infected; (ii) treating the susceptible population as a single compartment, and allowing chance to determine the total number of individuals infected by the infectious persons in the previous generation; (iii) treating the susceptible population as a single compartment, and allowing chance to determine when the next event (i.e. infection of a person or the recovery of an infectious person) will occur.

In general, as a consequence of chance variation inherent in the stochastic approach, model runs are typically collated into a distribution which provides insight into the range of outcomes which might occur and their relative likelihood. The number of runs needs to be balanced against computational burden.

Stochastic models have provided insight into how distributions of outbreak sizes may be used to estimate reproduction numbers. Besides modelling transmission in small populations, stochastic models have been used to address questions relating to persistence of an infection and critical population sizes. The development of fast computers has led to an increasing number of stochastic microsimulation models, which have been used to explore the effect of interventions.

References

1 Cooper BS, Medley GF, Scott GM. Preliminary analysis of the transmission dynamics of nosocomial infections: stochastic and management effects. *J Hosp Infect* 1999; 43(2): 131–147.

2 Abbey H. An examination of the Reed–Frost theory of epidemics. *Hum Biol* 1952; 24: 201–233.

3 Fine PE. A commentary on the mechanical analogue to the Reed–Frost epidemic model. *Am J Epidemiol* 1977; 106(2):87–100.

4 Keeling MJ, Rohani P. *Stochastic dynamics in Modeling infectious diseases in humans and animals.* Princeton, NJ and Oxford: Princeton University Press; 2008, pp. 190–232.

5 Keeling MJ, Grenfell BT. Understanding the persistence of measles: reconciling theory, simulation and observation. *Proc Biol Sci* 2002; 269(1489):335–343.

6 De Serres G, Gay NJ, Farrington CP. Epidemiology of transmissible diseases after elimination. *Am J Epidemiol* 2000; 151(11):1039–1048.

7 Ferguson NM, Fraser C, Donnelly CA, Ghani AC, Anderson RM. Public health. Public health risk from the avian H5N1 influenza epidemic. *Science* 2004; 304(5673):968–969.

8 Bartlett MS. Measles periodicity and community size. *J R Statist Soc* 1957; A120:48–70.

9 Bartlett MS. The critical community size for measles in the United States. *J R Statist Soc* 1960; 123:37–44.

10 Anderson RM, May RM. The invasion, persistence and spread of infectious diseases within animal and plant communities. *Philos Trans R Soc Lond B Biol Sci* 1986; 314(1167): 533–570.

11 Conlan AJ, Grenfell BT. Seasonality and the persistence and invasion of measles. *Proc Biol Sci* 2007; 274(1614):1133–1141.

12 Eichner M, Dietz K. Eradication of poliomyelitis: when can one be sure that polio virus transmission has been terminated? Am J Epidemiol 1996; 143(8):816–822.

13 Anderson RM, May RM. *Infectious diseases of humans. Dynamics and control.* Oxford: Oxford University Press; 1992.

14 Black FL. Measles endemicity in insular populations: critical community size and its evolutionary implication. *J Theor Bio* 1966; 11(2):207–211.

15 Elveback LR, Fox JP, Ackerman E, Langworthy A, Boyd M, Gatewood L. An influenza simulation model for immunization studies. *Am J Epidemiol* 1976; 103(2):152–165.

16 Longini IM, Jr., Halloran ME, Nizam A, Yang Y. Containing pandemic influenza with antiviral agents. *Am J Epidemiol* 2004; 159(7):623–633.

17 Longini IM, Jr., Nizam A, Xu S *et al.* Containing pandemic influenza at the source. *Science* 2005; 309(5737):1083–1087.

18 Germann TC, Kadau K, Longini IM, Jr., Macken CA. Mitigation strategies for pandemic influenza in the United States. *Proc Natl Acad Sci USA* 2006; 103(15):5935–5940.

19 Halloran ME, Ferguson NM, Eubank S *et al.* Modeling targeted layered containment of an influenza pandemic in the United States. *Proc Natl Acad Sci USA* 2008; 105(12):4639–4634.

20 Ferguson NM, Cummings DA, Cauchemez S *et al.* Strategies for containing an emerging influenza pandemic in Southeast Asia. *Nature* 2005; 437(7056):209–214.

21 Ferguson NM, Cummings DA, Fraser C, Cajka JC, Cooley PC, Burke DS. Strategies for mitigating an influenza pandemic. *Nature* 2006; 442(7101):448–452.

22 Plaisier AP, van Oortmarssen GJ, Habbema JD, Remme J, Alley ES. ONCHOSIM: a model and computer simulation program for the transmission and control of onchocerciasis. *Comput Methods Programs Biomed* 1990; 31(1):43–56.

23 Vlas SJ, van Oortmarssen GJ, Gryseels B, Polderman AM, Plaisier AP, Habbema JD. SCHISTOSIM: a microsimulation model for the epidemiology and control of schistosomiasis. *Am J Trop Med Hyg* 1996; 55(5 Suppl):170–175.

24 Korenromp EL, Van VC, Grosskurth H *et al.* Model-based evaluation of single-round mass treatment of sexually transmitted diseases for HIV control in a rural African population. *AIDS* 2000; 14(5):573–593.

25 Robinson NJ, Mulder D, Auvert B, Whitworth J, Hayes R. Type of partnership and heterosexual spread of HIV infection in rural Uganda: results from simulation modelling. *Int J STD AIDS* 1999; 10(11):718–725.

26 Longini IM, Jr., Koopman JS, Haber M, Cotsonis GA. Statistical inference for infectious diseases. Risk-specific household and community transmission parameters. *Am J Epidemiol* 1988; 128(4):845–859.

Chapter 7

How do models deal with contact patterns?

7.1 Overview and objectives

This chapter illustrates the important role that contact patterns between individuals have on the transmission and control of infections. It also describes the methods for incorporating age-dependent contact into models and for predicting the impact of interventions using reproduction numbers.

By the end of this chapter, you should:

- Be aware of some of the evidence for age-dependent mixing;
- Be able to define and set up matrices of 'Who Acquires Infection from Whom' (WAIFW) to describe non-random ('heterogeneous') mixing between individuals;
- Be able to use force of infection estimates to calculate WAIFW matrices;
- Understand the possible effect of non-random mixing patterns between individuals on the transmission dynamics and control of infectious diseases;
- Be able to calculate the basic or net reproduction number taking account of non-random mixing, and use them to predict the impact of interventions.

7.2 Why might mixing patterns be important?

So far in this book, we have assumed that contact between individuals is random, for example, that children are equally likely to contact other children and adults or that individuals in different social-economic groups are equally likely to contact each other. When exploring the impact of control strategies, however, especially those targeting specific subgroups of the population, modelling studies need to consider the effect of non-random contact patterns.

For example, Figure 7.1 shows hypothetical contact patterns in two populations:

1) In population A, children have many more contacts than do adults (seven versus three), and most of the contacts of children are with other children;

2) In population B, children have as many contacts as do adults (four) and mainly contact adults, whereas adults mainly contact other children.

If the same proportion of children in the two populations is vaccinated against a new infection, such as pandemic influenza, in which population would the subsequent overall incidence be the lowest?

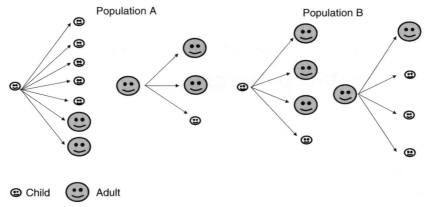

Fig. 7.1 Examples of two hypothetical contact patterns.

One intuitive answer to this question might be population A, given that children in population A have more contacts than do children in population B. On the other hand, more of the contacts of children in population A than in population B are with other children. Thus, adults in population A will benefit less from the reduced incidence among children in their population resulting from the introduction of vaccination, than will adults in population B, in which there is much contact between children and adults. These different factors make it difficult to use intuition alone in order to predict the effect of vaccinating children on the overall incidence.

Answering questions such as these is important for predicting the level of coverage of an intervention that is required to control transmission, and models can be used to do this. Before describing the methods for incorporating assumptions about non-random (heterogeneous) mixing into models, we first review the evidence for age-dependent contact.

7.3 What is the evidence for age-dependent contact for infections transmitted via the respiratory route?

7.3.1 Age dependencies in presumed transmission-linked cases

Figure 7.2a shows data on the ages of pairs of Dutch tuberculosis cases in The Netherlands, during the period 1993–1996,[1] for whom the *M. tuberculosis* strain isolated from their sputum shared an identical DNA fingerprint pattern. It would be reasonable to assume that these pairs of cases consisted of a primary and a secondary case, although it is possible that both cases were infected by another person, who had onset outside the study period.

In general, the ages of the two cases were highly correlated, strongly suggesting that individuals are most likely to transmit infection to others of a similar age (Figure 7.2a). For example, the average age difference between two cases was 13.9 years (standard deviation of 12.2 years) which was statistically significantly smaller than the difference

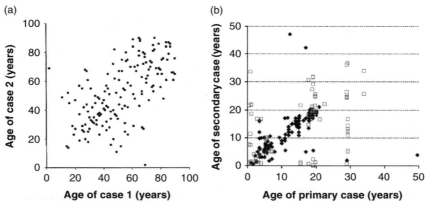

Fig. 7.2 (a) Scatter diagram of the ages of people in pairs of epidemiologically-linked Dutch tuberculosis patients in The Netherlands during the period 1993–1996, as defined using Restriction Fragment Length Polymorphism with the insertion element IS6110 as a probe. Strains whose fingerprint patterns had fewer than 5 IS6110 copies were subtyped further using the PGRS (polymorphic GC-rich sequence probe).[3] Each pair is represented by two dots in the graph, as each person is represented on both the X and Y axes. Reproduced with permission from Borgdorff et al, 1999.[1] (b) Scatter diagram of the age of the presumed primary and secondary cases, as implied by date of onset, of measles (open squares) and meningococcal meningitis (filled diamonds) in England and Wales during the period 1995–1998. Reproduced with permission from Edmunds et al, 2006.[2]

which would be predicted in a random sample of all pairs of cases (25.5 years, 95% CI: 21.5–29.5 years).

Analogous age patterns have also been reported among presumed primary and secondary cases of measles and meningococcal meningitis in the UK[2] (Figure 7.2b).

7.3.2 Time trends in morbidity following the (re)introduction of a pathogen

Figure 7.3 shows that the GP consultation rate during the 1957 (Asian) influenza pandemic was higher and peaked earlier for children than for adults.[4] The high and early peak observed among children probably partly reflects age-dependent contact patterns. For example, once a case appears among children, the infection is transmitted rapidly to other children due to intense mixing at school, before the infection reaches adults. Differences in consultation rates between children and adults may also partly reflect differences in health-seeking behaviour, e.g. parents are more likely to consult physicians when their child is sick than they are when they themselves feel unwell.

In contrast, reviews of measles and rubella outbreaks on remote island populations where these infections were reintroduced after a long absence found that the attack rate among children and adults was generally similar.[5] These populations differ from many populations seen today, given that they often comprised large family sizes, living in crowded conditions and spending much time indoors because of the cold climate.

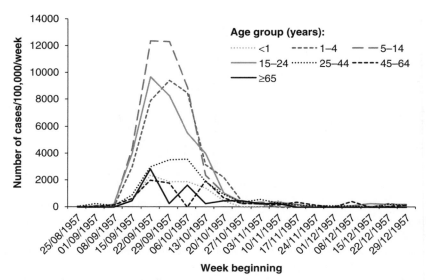

Fig. 7.3 Numbers of cases of influenza reported per 100,000 population per week in different age groups in a GP practice in Wales during the 1957 (Asian) influenza pandemic.[4]

These factors would have contributed to high levels of exposure among adults to infections introduced by children.

7.3.3 Age-dependencies in the force of infection

As we saw in Chapter 5, the force of infection is often higher for children than for adults (Section 5.2.3.5.2). Whilst there are several plausible explanations for this difference, the most plausible (and the one that has received most attention) is that contact between individuals is age-dependent.

7.3.4 Social contact surveys

Few studies have attempted to measure directly the number of contacts that individuals make with individuals in other age groups. Until recently, most of these studies were relatively small or they involved individuals in a narrow age range, such as schoolchildren,[6] university staff or students.[7-9] The largest of the early studies, conducted in Utrecht in 1986, surveyed 1,813 individuals (59 per cent of those initially invited).[9] This study questioned individuals about the number of conversations that they had in a typical week and indicated that contact between individuals was strongly age-dependent, with individuals being most likely to converse with others who were similar in age (Figure 7.4).

The largest study of contact patterns to date was published in 2008.[10] Individuals from eight European countries were asked to complete a diary documenting their physical and non-physical contacts on a single day between May 2005 and September 2006.[10] In total, 7,290 diaries were collected, ranging from 267 diaries in The Netherlands to

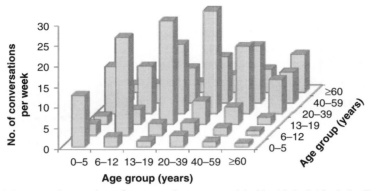

Fig. 7.4 Data on the number of conversations per week held with individuals in different age groups in a random survey of the population of Utrecht, 1986 (data extracted from Wallinga *et al*.).[9]

1,328 diaries in Germany. A physical contact was defined as skin-to-skin contact (e.g. a kiss or a handshake); a non-physical contact was defined as a two-way conversation with two or more words in the physical presence of another person, but with no physical contact. The extent to which such contacts are sufficient to transmit infection is unclear and probably varies between infections.

The contact patterns seen in each of the countries were generally similar, e.g. with individuals being most likely to contact others of a similar age (Figure 7.5). As might be expected, mixing between 30–39-year-olds and young children, and between middle-aged adults and older children (reflecting parents mixing with their children) was also strong, albeit weaker than that between individuals who were of the same age. Similar age patterns were seen even when only physical contacts were considered, although the amount of contact between adults was greatly reduced, presumably reflecting the fact that adults mainly contact each other at work, where contact is usually non-physical.

Differences in the average numbers of contacts made by individuals in different countries (for example, the larger number of individuals contacted by individuals in Italy, as compared with Germany or the UK—Figure 7.5) are difficult to interpret, given differences in the study design between countries. In some countries, responders who had many contacts, such as bus drivers or shop assistants, were asked to provide only an *estimate* of the number of contacts, rather than the actual number.

7.4 How do we incorporate age-dependent mixing into models?

7.4.1 Expressions for the force of infection

As discussed in Sections 2.7.1 and 3.4.1, when we assume that individuals mix randomly, the rate at which susceptible individuals are infected (i.e. the force of infection, $\lambda(t)$) is related to β (the rate at which two specific individuals come into effective

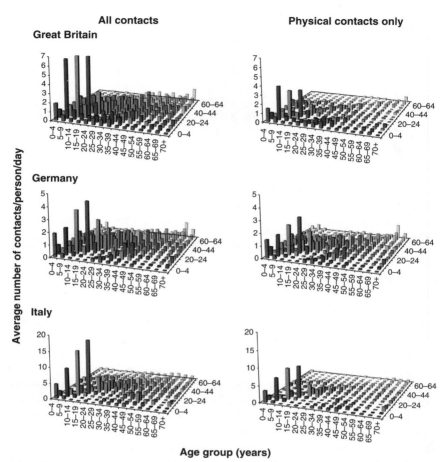

Fig. 7.5 Estimates of the average number of all (i.e. physical and non-physical) reported contacts and only physical contacts per person per day in the UK, Germany and Italy, as found by Mossong et al. (2008).[10] Note that the scales on the vertical axes for these figures differ between settings. The age groups used for both horizontal axes are indentical.

contact per unit time) and the number of infectious individuals at a given time t ($I(t)$) as follows:

$$\lambda(t) = \beta I(t) \qquad\qquad 7.1$$

When we assume that individuals do not mix randomly, individuals in different subgroups of the population will become infected at different rates depending on how they interact with others in their own subgroup and other subgroups.

For example, if we assume that contact patterns differ only between children and adults, the rate at which children will be infected depends on how closely they mix with other children and how closely they interact with adults. We will use subscripts y and o to refer to younger (children) and older (adult) individuals respectively. The overall force of infection among children ($\overline{\lambda_y(t)}$) can then be expressed as the sum of the force of infection attributable to contact with other children ($\lambda_{yy}(t)$) and that attributable to contact with adults (the 'old') ($\lambda_{yo}(t)$), as follows:

$$\overline{\lambda_y(t)} = \lambda_{yy}(t) + \lambda_{yo}(t) \qquad\qquad 7.2$$

We will use the line over the symbol $\lambda_y(t)$ to denote the fact that we are considering the 'overall' force of infection in a subgroup of the population (children in this instance).

Similarly, the force of infection experienced by adults (the 'old') at a given time t ($\overline{\lambda_o(t)}$) is given by the sum of the force of infection attributable to contact with children ($\lambda_{oy}(t)$) and that attributable to contact with adults ($\lambda_{oo}(t)$) as follows:

$$\overline{\lambda_o(t)} = \lambda_{oy}(t) + \lambda_{oo}(t) \qquad\qquad 7.3$$

Each of the components $\lambda_{yy}(t)$, $\lambda_{yo}(t)$, $\lambda_{oy}(t)$ and $\lambda_{oo}(t)$ is difficult to measure directly; however, we can express them by extending the logic in Equation 7.1 (see Panel 7.1):

$$\lambda_{yy}(t) = \beta_{yy} I_y(t) \qquad\qquad 7.4$$

$$\lambda_{yo}(t) = \beta_{yo} I_o(t) \qquad\qquad 7.5$$

$$\lambda_{oy}(t) = \beta_{oy} I_y(t) \qquad\qquad 7.6$$

$$\lambda_{oo}(t) = \beta_{oo} I_o(t) \qquad\qquad 7.7$$

where

$I_y(t)$ and $I_o(t)$ are the number of infectious children and adults at time t;

β_{yy} is the rate at which two specific children come into effective contact per unit time;

β_{yo} is the rate at which a specific (susceptible) child and a specific infectious adult come into effective contact per unit time;

β_{oy} is the rate at which a specific (susceptible) adult and a specific infectious child come into effective contact per unit time;

β_{oo} is the rate at which two specific adults come into effective contact per unit time.

Substituting for $\lambda_{yy}(t) = \beta_{yy} I_y(t)$ and $\lambda_{yo}(t) = \beta_{yo} I_o(t)$ into Equation 7.2, we obtain the following:

$$\overline{\lambda_y(t)} = \beta_{yy} I_y(t) + \beta_{yo} I_o(t) \qquad\qquad 7.8$$

By the same logic, we can obtain an expression for the force of infection among adults:

$$\overline{\lambda_o(t)} = \beta_{oy} I_y(t) + \beta_{oo} I_o(t) \qquad\qquad 7.9$$

Panel 7.2 discusses the notation used in these equations.

Panel 7.1 Derivation of the equations $\lambda_{yy}(t) = \beta_{yy}I_y(t)$ and $\lambda_{yo}(t) = \beta_{yo}I_o(t)$

The expression $\lambda_{yy}(t) = \beta_{yy}I_y(t)$ can be derived by considering two expressions for the number of new infections per unit time among children that are attributable to contact with other children.

The first expression can be obtained by using the argument that, if there are $S_y(t)$ susceptible children, then in total, there are $S_y(t) \times I_y(t)$ possible contacts which the susceptible children could make with the $I_y(t)$ infectious children. Of these, a fraction β_{yy} will be effective contacts, and therefore the total number of new infections among children which are attributable to contact with other children per unit time is given by the equation:

$$\beta_{yy}S_y(t)I_y(t) \qquad\qquad 7.10$$

The total number of new infections among children per unit time which are attributable to contact with other children is also given by the following expression:

$$\lambda_{yy}(t)S_y(t) \qquad\qquad 7.11$$

Equating Equation 7.10 and 7.11, we obtain the following result:

$$\lambda_{yy}(t)S_y(t) = \beta_{yy}S_y(t)I_y(t) \qquad\qquad 7.12$$

Cancelling $S_y(t)$ from both sides of this equation, we obtain the equation $\lambda_{yy}(t) = \beta_{yy}I_y(t)$.

By an analogous argument, we can obtain the equation $\lambda_{yo}(t) = \beta_{yo}I_o(t)$.

Equations 7.8 and 7.9 can be concisely summarized using matrix notation (see Basic maths section B.7.1 for the definition of matrices) as follows:

$$\begin{pmatrix} \overline{\lambda_y(t)} \\ \overline{\lambda_o(t)} \end{pmatrix} = \begin{pmatrix} \beta_{yy} & \beta_{yo} \\ \beta_{oy} & \beta_{oo} \end{pmatrix} \begin{pmatrix} I_y(t) \\ I_o(t) \end{pmatrix} \qquad\qquad 7.13$$

The matrix $\begin{pmatrix} \beta_{yy} & \beta_{yo} \\ \beta_{oy} & \beta_{oo} \end{pmatrix}$ (or its equivalent when contact is stratified into more than two subgroups in the population – see Panel 7.3) is usually referred to as the matrix of 'Who Acquires Infection From Whom'[5] or, most commonly, as the WAIFW matrix (pronounced 'WAYFU', 'WHYFU' or 'WAYFWER'). As we shall see, the advantage of using matrix notation is that it makes it easier to identify certain types of contact patterns, especially when contact is assumed to differ between more than two subgroups in the population. The matrices are often represented graphically in the form shown in Figure 7.5.

7.4.2 How do we calculate the β parameters?

As discussed in Section 2.7.1, the rate at which two specific individuals come into effective contact per unit time (i.e. β) depends on both the frequency of contact with

---

Panel 7.2 Notation for β_{yy}, β_{yo}, β_{oy}, β_{oo}

Note the way in which subscripts are used with this notation—the first component of the subscript reflects the age of the person being infected; the second subscript reflects the age group of the source of infection.

For example, β_{yo} reflects the rate at which a specific young susceptible person and an old infectious person come into effective contact per unit time, and β_{oy} reflects the rate at which a susceptible old person and a young infectious person come into effective contact per unit time.

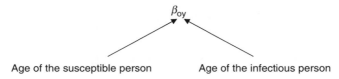

Age of the susceptible person   Age of the infectious person

Thus, in the equation for $\overline{\lambda_y(t)}$ or $\overline{\lambda_o(t)}$, the first subscript for each β parameter matches the subscript used for the force of infection (i.e. 'y' if we are considering the force of infection among children) and the second subscript matches the subscript of the infectious person, as follows:

$$\overline{\lambda_o(t)} = \beta_{oy}I_y(t) + \beta_{oo}I_o(t)$$

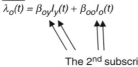

The 2nd subscript of the β parameter matches the subscript of the infectious individuals.

The notation for the subscripts used when writing down reproduction numbers (see section 7.5.1) is analogous.

This notation is used by convention in infectious disease modelling and stems from the convention used in mathematics for writing sets of equations using matrices, whereby the element in the ith row and j^{th} column in a matrix has the subscript for the row first, followed by the subscript for the column.

---

others in a given age group (i.e. the values plotted in Figure 7.5) and the proportion of those contacts which are 'effective', i.e. sufficient to transmit infection if the contact occurs between a susceptible and an infectious person. This proportion differs between infections. For example, the kind of contact which is sufficient to transmit measles infection may be different from that which is required to transmit meningococcal or *M tuberculosis* infection. As we shall see in the next chapter, β parameters for sexually transmitted infections are typically separated out into these components. However, for directly transmitted infections, very few published studies have done this to date.

Panel 7.3 Expressions for the force of infection when contact is assumed to differ between more than two subgroups in the population

If we wanted to assume that the force of infection differs between three age groups in the population (e.g. the young, middle-aged and old), our equations for the force of infection among children, middle-aged individuals and the old would be as follows:

$$\overline{\lambda_y(t)} = \beta_{yy}I_y(t) + \beta_{ym}I_m(t) + \beta_{yo}I_o(t)$$
$$\overline{\lambda_m(t)} = \beta_{my}I_y(t) + \beta_{mm}I_m(t) + \beta_{mo}I_o(t)$$
$$\overline{\lambda_o(t)} = \beta_{oy}I_y(t) + \beta_{om}I_m(t) + \beta_{oo}I_o(t) \qquad 7.14$$

Using matrix notation, the equations would be written as follows:

$$\begin{pmatrix} \overline{\lambda_y(t)} \\ \overline{\lambda_m(t)} \\ \overline{\lambda_o(t)} \end{pmatrix} = \begin{pmatrix} \beta_{yy} & \beta_{ym} & \beta_{yo} \\ \beta_{my} & \beta_{mm} & \beta_{mo} \\ \beta_{oy} & \beta_{om} & \beta_{oo} \end{pmatrix} \begin{pmatrix} I_y(t) \\ I_m(t) \\ I_o(t) \end{pmatrix} \qquad 7.15$$

The notation which might be used if we had n age groups and the force of infection differed between each of these age groups is as follows:

$$\overline{\lambda_i(t)} = \beta_{i1}I_1(t) + \beta_{i2}I_2(t) + \beta_{i3}I_3(t) + \ldots + \beta_{in}I_n(t)$$
$$= \sum_{j=1}^{n} \beta_{ij}I_j(t) \qquad 7.16$$

where $\overline{\lambda_i(t)}$ is the force of infection in the ith age group, β_{ij} is the rate at which susceptible individuals in the ith age group and infectious individuals in the jth age group come into effective contact per unit time, and $I_j(t)$ is the number of infectious individuals in the jth age group. Using matrix notation, Equation 7.16 would be written as follows:

$$\begin{pmatrix} \overline{\lambda_1(t)} \\ \overline{\lambda_2(t)} \\ \overline{\lambda_3(t)} \\ \ldots \\ \overline{\lambda_{n-1}(t)} \\ \overline{\lambda_n(t)} \end{pmatrix} = \begin{pmatrix} \beta_{11} & \beta_{12} & \beta_{13} & \cdots & \beta_{1\,n-1} & \beta_{1n} \\ \beta_{21} & \beta_{22} & \beta_{23} & \cdots & \beta_{2n-1} & \beta_{2n} \\ \beta_{31} & \beta_{32} & \beta_{33} & \cdots & \beta_{3n-1} & \beta_{3\,n} \\ \ldots & \ldots & \ldots & \cdots & \ldots & \ldots \\ \beta_{n-1\,1} & \beta_{n-1\,2} & \beta_{n-1\,3} & \cdots & \beta_{n-1\,n-1} & \beta_{n-1\,n} \\ \beta_{n1} & \beta_{n2} & \beta_{n3} & \cdots & \beta_{n\,n-1} & \beta_{nn} \end{pmatrix} \begin{pmatrix} I_1(t) \\ I_2(t) \\ I_3(t) \\ \ldots \\ I_{n-1}(t) \\ I_n(t) \end{pmatrix}$$

Instead, the β parameters are typically inferred indirectly from epidemiological data, namely either from estimates of the average force of infection in specific age groups, such as those discussed in Chapter 5, if the infection is endemic, or from data on the age-specific numbers of new infections or cases over time, if the infection is new or re-emergent. Note that it is often unclear as to what constitutes a contact; however, a clear definition is not necessary if the β parameters are estimated indirectly. We discuss various approaches used below.

7.4.2.1 Estimating contact parameters for endemic infections, given estimates of the average group-specific force of infection

As shown in chapter 5, for endemic infections, we can estimate the average force of a given infection in specific age groups from cross-sectional data on the age-specific prevalence of previous infection. Using the estimated force of infection, we can then estimate the average number of infectious individuals in specific age groups (see Panel 7.4).

For example, based on age-specific data on the proportion of individuals who had antibodies to rubella, the average annual force of rubella infection for children and adults (aged 0–<15 and ≥15 years respectively) in the UK during the 1980s was 13 per cent and 4 per cent (see Section 5.2.3.5.2) and, on average, there were 18,956 and 2,859 infectious young and old individuals respectively (Panel 7.4). If we substitute these values for the forces of infection and the number of infectious children and adults into Equations 7.8 and 7.9, we obtain the following equations:

$$0.13 = 18,956\beta_{yy} + 2,859\beta_{yo} \qquad 7.17$$

$$0.04 = 18,956\beta_{oy} + 2,859\beta_{oo} \qquad 7.18$$

We can calculate the β parameters using these equations. However, in their current form, we cannot calculate distinct values for all four of the unknown β parameters β_{yy}, β_{yo}, β_{oy}, and β_{oo} since we have two equations with four unknown parameters (note that we can only calculate two unknown parameters from two equations).

To overcome this problem, we can constrain the structure of the WAIFW matrix so that the above equations reduce to *two equations with two unknowns*. Similarly, if we were considering a population stratified into three age groups, we would have three equations relating the force of infection in the three age groups and nine unknown β parameters; we would then need to constrain the WAIFW structure so that we have three equations with three unknown β parameters.

There are several ways of constraining these matrices. One commonly-imposed constraint is that contact is symmetrical, such that the rate at which *a child contacts and transmits infection to an adult equals the rate at which an adult contacts and transmits infection to a child*, i.e. $\beta_{oy} = \beta_{yo}$. Since this constraint reduces our two equations in four unknowns to two equations with three unknowns, we need to apply one more

Panel 7.4 Methods for calculating the numbers of susceptible and infectious individuals in specific age groups

In general, the number of infectious individuals can be approximated using the relationship:

Number of infectious persons ≈ Number of new infectious persons
per unit time × Duration of infectiousness

For acute infections for which all individuals are infectious shortly after infection, the short pre-infectious period means that the numbers of new infectious persons and the numbers of new infections are approximately equal. For a given age group, the latter equals the product of the force of infection and the number of susceptible individuals in that age group (see section 5.2.3.4). Using the above approximation and assuming that D is the duration of infectiousness, we obtain the following for the average number of infectious children and adults (denoted by I_y and I_o respectively):

$$I_y \approx \overline{\lambda}_y S_y D \qquad\qquad 7.19$$

$$I_o \approx \overline{\lambda}_o S_o D \qquad\qquad 7.20$$

Here, $\overline{\lambda}_y$ and $\overline{\lambda}_o$ are the average forces of infection among children and adults respectively, and S_y and S_o are the average numbers of susceptible children and adults. Note that we have dropped the 't' in parentheses from the notation since we are considering the average values for these variables. For immunizing infections, the number of susceptible individuals of age a follows the pattern shown in Figure 7.6a, with the shaded and unshaded areas in this figure reflecting the total number of susceptible children (aged $<a_y$) and adults (aged a_y-L) respectively. These areas can be calculated by integrating (see Basic maths section B.6) expressions for the numbers of susceptible individuals of age a between the ages 0-a_y and a_y-L, as follows:

$$S_y = \int_0^{a_y} N(a)s(a)da \qquad\qquad 7.21$$

$$S_o = \int_{a_y}^{L} N(a)s(a)da \qquad\qquad 7.22$$

Here, $N(a)$ is the total number of individuals of age a, $s(a)$ is the proportion of individuals of age a who are susceptible, and so $N(a)s(a)$ is the total number of susceptible individuals of age a. We provide expressions for $N(a)$ and $s(a)$ below.

For a population of size N with a rectangular age distribution and a life expectancy of L, the number of individuals in a given age group equals the population size multiplied by the proportion of the population that is in that age group. Thus, the number of individuals in a single year age category a ($N(a)$) is N/L, and the numbers of children and adults (denoted by N_y and N_o respectively) are given by

$$N_y = \frac{Na_y}{L} \text{ and } N_o = \frac{N(L-a_y)}{L} \text{ (Figure 7.6b).}$$

If the force of infection differs only between children and adults, $s(a)$ is given by the following (see Panel 5.2):

$$s(a) = \begin{cases} e^{-\bar{\lambda}_y a} & 0 \le a < a_y \qquad\qquad 7.23 \\ e^{-\bar{\lambda}_y a_y} e^{-\bar{\lambda}_o(a-a_y)} & a_y \le a \le L \qquad\qquad 7.24 \end{cases}$$

Using the expression $N(a)=N/L$, together with equations 7.19–7.24 eventually (with some manipulation) leads to the expressions below for the total numbers of children and adults in the population, or the numbers who are susceptible or infectious.

	Total	Susceptible	Infectious
Children	$N_y = \dfrac{Na_y}{L}$	$S_y = \dfrac{N(1-e^{-\bar{\lambda}_y a_y})}{\bar{\lambda}_y L}$	$I_y = \dfrac{N(1-e^{-\bar{\lambda}_y a_y})D}{L}$
Adults	$N_o = \dfrac{N(L-a_y)}{L}$	$S_o = \dfrac{Ne^{-\bar{\lambda}_y a_y}(1-e^{-\bar{\lambda}_o(L-a_y)})}{\bar{\lambda}_o L}$	$I_o = \dfrac{Ne^{-\bar{\lambda}_y a_y}(1-e^{-\bar{\lambda}_o(L-a_y)})D}{L}$

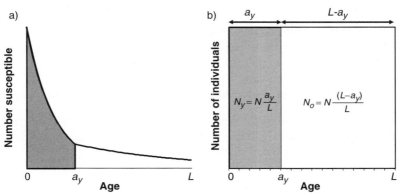

Fig. 7.6 a) Example of how the number of susceptible individuals changes with age. The shaded and unshaded areas correspond to children (aged $<a_y$) and adults (aged a_y-L) respectively. b) Graphical representation of the expressions for the numbers of children and adults in a population with a rectangular age distribution. The number of children (N_y) equals the area of the shaded rectangle, calculated as the (population size)×(proportion of the population that is young). The latter proportion equals a_y/L (width of the shaded rectangle ÷ width of the whole rectangle), and so $N_y=Na_y/L$.

Worked example:
The average force of rubella infection for children and adults (aged <15 and ≥15 years respectively) in the UK during the 1980s was $\bar{\lambda}_y = 13\%$ and $\bar{\lambda}_o = 4\%$ per year respectively (section 5.2.3.5.2).

> **Panel 7.4 Methods for calculating the numbers of susceptible and infectious individuals in specific age groups** *(continued)*
>
> Assuming that the population comprised 55 million individuals (N=55,000,000), a life-expectancy (L) of 75 years, a duration of infectiousness of 11 days (D=11/365 years), and taking a_y to equal 15 years, we obtain the following values for the average numbers of infectious children and adults:
>
> $$I_y = \frac{55,000,000 \times (1 - e^{-0.13 \times 15}) \times 11}{75 \times 365} = 18,965$$
>
> $$I_o = \frac{55,000,000 \times e^{-0.13 \times 15} \times (1 - e^{-0.04(75-15)}) \times 11}{75 \times 365} = 2,859$$

constraint. The following are the possible matrix structures that we could use for the matrix $\begin{pmatrix} \beta_{yy} & \beta_{yo} \\ \beta_{oy} & \beta_{oo} \end{pmatrix}$, where β_1 and β_2 are distinct values:

1) $\begin{pmatrix} \beta_1 & \beta_2 \\ \beta_2 & \beta_2 \end{pmatrix}$ which assumes that an adult is as likely to contact and infect a child as another adult, and as a child is to infect an adult (i.e. $\beta_{oy} = \beta_{oo} = \beta_{yo} = \beta_2$). Contact between children differs from that between adults, and between adults and children.

2) $\begin{pmatrix} \beta_1 & \beta_1 \\ \beta_1 & \beta_2 \end{pmatrix}$. This assumes that a child is as likely to contact and infect another child as an adult (i.e. $\beta_{yy} = \beta_{yo} = \beta_{oy} = \beta_1$), and the contact between adults differs from that between adults and children or between children (i.e. $\beta_{oo} = \beta_2 \neq \beta_{yy}$). According to Figure 7.5, this assumption is unrealistic.

3) $\begin{pmatrix} \beta_1 & k\beta_2 \\ k\beta_2 & \beta_2 \end{pmatrix}$. For this structure, the rate at which an adult contacts and infects a child differs by some assumed factor, k, from the rate at which an adult contacts and infects an adult (i.e. $\beta_{yo} = \beta_{oy} = k\beta_{oo}$). When $k = 1$, this matrix is equivalent to the matrix described in point 1)—see above; $k = 0$ implies that there is no contact between children and adults (which is unrealistic); if $k>1$, adults have more contact with children than they do amongst themselves.

Each of the above matrices is *symmetric*. By convention in a matrix, the line from its top left hand corner to its bottom right-hand corner is the line of symmetry, as indicated by the dashed line below:

$$\begin{pmatrix} \beta_1 & \beta_2 \\ \beta_2 & \beta_1 \end{pmatrix}$$

Using mathematical notation, we would say that a matrix is symmetric if $\beta_{ij} = \beta_{ji}$ for all values of $i \neq j$.

The following are examples of *asymmetric* matrices: $\begin{pmatrix} \beta_1 & \beta_2 \\ \beta_1 & \beta_2 \end{pmatrix}$, $\begin{pmatrix} \beta_1 & \beta_1 \\ \beta_2 & \beta_2 \end{pmatrix}$ and $\begin{pmatrix} 0 & \beta_2 \\ \beta_1 & 0 \end{pmatrix}$

Asymmetric matrices are considered to be unrealistic for many infections as they assume that, for example, the rate at which *a child contacts and infects an adult* differs from the rate at which *an adult contacts and infects a child*. On the other hand, asymmetric matrices may be appropriate for describing transmission of infections via the faecal–oral route, for sexually transmitted infections (assuming that the two groups in the model are heterosexual males and females, see Chapter 8) or for vector-borne infections (where the two groups reflect humans and the vector).

7.4.2.1.1 Examples of calculations of β parameters Returning to our rubella example on page 187, if we assume that the WAIFW matrix has the following structure $\begin{pmatrix} \beta_1 & \beta_2 \\ \beta_2 & \beta_2 \end{pmatrix}$ then we would need to solve the equations:

$$0.13 = 18{,}956\beta_1 + 2{,}859\beta_2 \qquad\qquad 7.25$$

$$0.04 = 18{,}956\beta_2 + 2{,}859\beta_2 \qquad\qquad 7.26$$

Equation 7.26 is equivalent to the following:

$$0.04 = 21{,}815\beta_2 \qquad\qquad 7.27$$

We can calculate β_2 directly from Equation 7.27, which gives $\beta_2 = 0.04/21{,}815 = 1.83\times10^{-6}$ per year. After dividing this equation by 365 to obtain β_2 in units of per day, we obtain $\beta_2 = 5.02 \times 10^{-9}$ per day.

By substituting the value that we have obtained for β_2 into Equation 7.25, and rearranging the resulting equation, we obtain $\beta_1 = (0.13-2{,}859\beta_2)/18{,}956 = 6.58 \times 10^{-6}$ per year or 1.80×10^{-8} per day.

Our WAIFW matrix, with the β parameters in units of per day, is as follows: $\begin{pmatrix} 1.80\times10^{-8} & 5.02\times10^{-9} \\ 5.02\times10^{-9} & 5.02\times10^{-9} \end{pmatrix}$. Alternatively, if we had assumed the following matrix structure: $\begin{pmatrix} \beta_1 & 0.5\beta_2 \\ 0.5\beta_2 & \beta_2 \end{pmatrix}$, we would have obtained the following WAIFW matrix:

$\begin{pmatrix} 1.81\times10^{-8} & 4.44\times10^{-9} \\ 4.44\times10^{-9} & 8.88\times10^{-9} \end{pmatrix}$ (see Exercise 7.3).

As shown in Figure 7.7, for both matrices (denoted by R1 and R2 respectively), the rate at which an effective contact is made between two specific children is very high; the main difference between the two matrices is that the amount of contact between adults is higher for matrix R2 than for matrix R1.

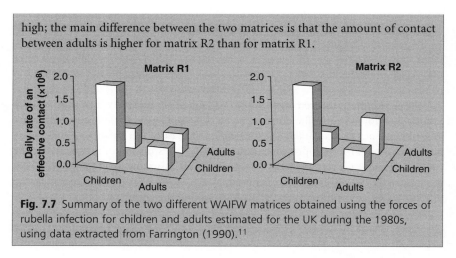

Fig. 7.7 Summary of the two different WAIFW matrices obtained using the forces of rubella infection for children and adults estimated for the UK during the 1980s, using data extracted from Farrington (1990).[11]

Note that in some instances, solving equations such as Equations 7.25 and 7.26 results in negative values for the β parameters, which is unrealistic. In such situations it would be appropriate either to discard the matrix structure altogether, or to follow alternative approaches, such as those discussed in Kanaan and Farrington.[12]

In general, mixing patterns, such as those reflected by matrix R2, are said to be 'with-like' or 'assortative' if there is much contact between individuals in the same group and little contact between individuals in different groups. As illustrated in Figure 7.5, mixing patterns between different age groups appear to be strongly with-like.

Conversely, mixing patterns are said to be 'with-unlike' if there is little contact between individuals in the same group but much contact between individuals in different groups (Figure 7.8). In general, with-unlike mixing patterns are appropriate for describing heterosexual sexual contact by gender, whereby males preferentially mix with females and vice versa (Chapter 8).

The matrices discussed above are simple in that contact was assumed to differ only between children and adults. Modelling studies may refine these assumptions further by, for example, assuming that contact differs between infants, children at pre-school, primary school, secondary school, adults of working age, and the elderly. These might incorporate detailed assumptions about contact between middle age parents and their children, or between the elderly and their grandchildren etc (see [13–16]). We shall discuss

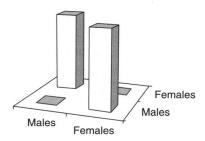

Fig. 7.8 Example of a mixing pattern which is with-unlike.

Panel 7.5 Extending the logic to deal with different kinds of non-random mixing

Much of the emphasis in this chapter has been on describing the methods for dealing with age-dependent mixing. However, these methods can be extended to deal with other kinds of mixing patterns, e.g. considering mixing between individuals in different socio-economic groups, or individuals in different locations. For example, to describe mixing between individuals in urban and rural areas, we might use a matrix such as the following:

$$\begin{array}{cc} & \begin{array}{cc} urban & rural \end{array} \\ \begin{array}{c} urban \\ rural \end{array} & \left(\begin{array}{cc} \beta_{uu} & \beta_{ur} \\ \beta_{ru} & \beta_{rr} \end{array} \right) \end{array}$$

where
β_{rr} is the rate at which two specific individuals in rural areas come into effective contact per unit time;
β_{uu} is the rate at which two specific individuals in urban areas come into effective contact per unit time;
β_{ur} reflects the rate at which a specific (susceptible) person in an urban area comes into effective contact with a specific (infectious) person from a rural area;
β_{ru} reflects the rate at which a specific (susceptible) person in a rural area comes into effective contact with a specific (infectious) person from an urban area.
β_{ur} might be some fraction, k, of the contact between individuals in rural areas e.g. $\beta_{ur} = k \beta_{rr}$, where $k<1$. Again, we can impose constraints on the structure as appropriate, for example that $\beta_{ur} = \beta_{ru}$.

Models developed in recent years of the transmission of pandemic influenza have used detailed versions of the above matrix to describe contact patterns between different cities to describe the spatial spread of infection.[25–27] Likewise, models of the spread of foot and mouth disease have used detailed extensions of the above matrix to describe transmission between different farms, with the probability of contact depending on the distance between farms.[28]

how we might choose between different matrices in section 7.4.3. Panel 7.5 describes how the logic can be extended to deal with other kinds of heterogeneity in contact.

In some instances, the matrix structure could be better selected by using data for infections transmitted via a similar route. For example, since mumps and rubella are transmitted by a similar route, it would be reasonable to choose a matrix structure which is compatible with the age-specific force of infection estimated for both infections.

To date, only a few studies have attempted to estimate WAIFW matrices for respiratory infections which are compatible with data on two infections.[17, 18] A complication of this approach is that due to random variation in the data, it can be difficult to obtain a single matrix structure which matches the data for two infections. Bayesian approaches

Panel 7.6 Estimating β parameters using contact and serological data

A study by Wallinga et al.[9] is, to our knowledge, the first reported study which has attempted to calculate β parameters for a respiratory infection by separating β into components reflecting the frequency of contact between individuals in different age groups, and the probability of transmission given contact. Given the innovative nature of this study and the fact that other studies are conducting similar analyses using the data described in Mossong et al.[10] (see Figure 7.5), we outline the methods used by Wallinga et al below.

The study used the following data:

1. Distributions of the number of conversations per week between individuals in different age groups from the survey of conversational contacts conducted in The Netherlands in 1986 (Figure 7.4). These are reproduced in detail in Figure 7.9.

2. Data on the age-specific proportion of the respondents from this survey who had antibodies to mumps, as indicated by Enzyme-Linked Immunosorbent Assay. These data reflected past infection with the mumps virus, since routine measles–mumps–rubella vaccine had not yet been introduced at the time of the study.

Wallinga et al first corrected the distributions of the numbers of contacts made between individuals in different age groups for reciprocity to ensure that the numbers of conversations made by individuals in, e.g. age group i with individuals in

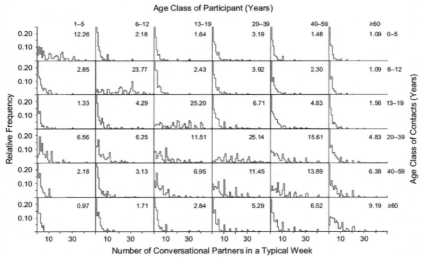

Fig. 7.9 Relative frequencies of numbers of different conversational partners encountered during a typical week in 1986, as estimated from self-reported data, Utrecht, The Netherlands. Data are stratified by the age classes of the participants (horizontal) and their contacts (vertical). The numbers above each histogram indicate the mean value. Reproduced with permission from Wallinga et al, 2006.[9]

age group j equalled the numbers of contacts that individuals in age group j made with individuals in age group i. For example, the number of conversations reported by adolescents with young adults was less than that reported by young adults with adolescents (18,899,430 vs 32,590,670 per week respectively). Such discrepancies frequently occur in contact surveys. For example, in sexual behaviour surveys, women tend to report fewer partnerships with men than do men with women, for many reasons. As discussed by Wallinga *et al*, the inconsistencies in the Dutch study may reflect under-reporting by adolescents of the number of contacts that they make with young adults. It could also reflect participation bias, if, for example, young adults who contact adolescents were more likely to respond than were those who do not have such contacts.

By analogy with expression 2.11, the β parameter reflecting the rate at which two specific individuals in age groups i and j come into effective contact was assumed to be related to the size of age group (w_j) and the average number of contacts made per week between age groups i and j (m_{ij}), as follows:

$$\beta_{ij} =$$

(Average number of contacts made between individuals in
age groups i and j each week, m_{ij})

$$\times$$

(Probability of transmission given contact, q)

$$\div$$

(Number of individuals in age group i, N_i),

i.e.

$$\beta_{ij} = \frac{q m_{ij}}{N_i}$$

7.28

The authors then used these β parameters in expressions which are analogous to Equations 7.8 and 7.9 for the force of infection in a given age group, λ_i, which were then used in expressions for the cumulative exposure to infection to mumps in different age groups. The latter expressions were then fitted to the age-specific proportion of individuals who had antibodies to mumps to obtain the unknown parameter q. This was found to be 0.16, suggesting that the probability of mumps transmission given conversational-type contact was about 16 per cent.

for dealing with this situation have been pioneered by Farrington *et al.* are discussed in [12, 17]. These involve identifying parameter values in the matrices which are said to be 'close', according to some criterion.

A paper by Kanaan and Farrington[12] provides a helpful review of the kinds of structures for WAIFW matrices that typically have been used in modelling studies, some of which are summarized in Table 7.1. At the time of writing, only one published study had attempted to use observed social contact data to calculate the β parameters[9] in the manner described in Panel 7.6, although similar analyses are currently underway using data on contact patterns in European countries.[10]

Table 7.1 Examples of some common matrix structures reviewed by Kanaan and Farrington.[12] The parameters β_1, β_2, β_3, β_4, β_5 reflect distinct values for the β parameters, and contact is assumed to differ between the age groups 0–<3, 3–<8, 8–<13, 13–<20, 20+ years.

Matrix	Structure	Assumptions
A	Age grp (yrs): 0–<3, 3–<8, 8–<13, 13–<20, 20+ Row 0–<3: β_1, β_1, β_3, β_4, β_5 Row 3–<8: β_1, β_2, β_3, β_4, β_5 Row 8–<13: β_3, β_3, β_3, β_4, β_5 Row 13–<20: β_4, β_4, β_4, β_4, β_5 Row 20+: β_5, β_5, β_5, β_5, β_5	Children of pre-school age are assumed to be as likely to contact others of pre-school age as they are to contact children aged 3–<8 years. The rate at which children aged 3–<8 years come into effective contact with others in the same age group is different from that at which individuals in any other two age groups come into effective contact with each other. Individuals aged 8–<13, 13–<20 and 20+ years are assumed to be as likely to contact individuals who are younger than themselves as they are to contact individuals who are in the same age group. The rate at which this contact occurs differs between the age groups 8–<13, 13–<20 and 20+ years.
B	Age grp (yrs): 0–<3, 3–<8, 8–<13, 13–<20, 20+ Row 0–<3: β_1, β_1, β_3, β_4, β_5 Row 3–<8: β_1, β_2, β_2, β_4, β_5 Row 8–<13: β_1, β_2, β_3, β_4, β_5 Row 13–<20: β_4, β_4, β_4, β_4, β_5 Row 20+: β_5, β_5, β_5, β_5, β_5	This is similar to matrix A, except that: (a) Children of pre-school age are assumed to be as likely to mix with children aged 3–<8 and 8–<13 years as they are to mix with other children of pre-school age. (b) Children aged 3–<8 years are as likely to contact others of the same age as they are to contact children aged 8–<13 years. (c) The rate at which children aged 8–<13 years come into effective contact with others in the same age group is different from the rate at which individuals in any other two age groups come into effective contact with each other.

C

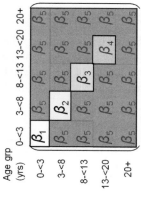

Age grp (yrs): 0–<3 3–<8 8–<13 13–<20 20+

All individuals are assumed to contact individuals in a different age group at some background rate (β_5).

The rate at which individuals in the same age group come into effective contact is assumed to differ for all age groups, excepting those aged over 20 years, who are assumed to be as likely to contact others of the same age as they are to contact individuals in other age groups.

D

Age grp (yrs): 0–<3 3–<8 8–<13 13–<20 20+

This is similar to matrix C, except that:

(a) Children of pre-school age are assumed to be as likely to contact 20+ year olds as they are to contact others of pre-school age;

(b) Contact among children aged 3–<8 years with others in the same age group is assumed to be as likely as that between children aged 8–<13 years and others of the same age group.

7.4.2.2 Estimating contact parameters for infections which are new or which have been recently introduced into a population

The method described in section 7.4.2.1 cannot be used to obtain β parameters for an infection which has recently been introduced into a population and which is therefore not endemic. For such infections we might have data similar to those presented in Figure 7.3, i.e. the number of new infections or cases seen each day or each week.

For such infections, we can estimate the β parameters by first setting up a model which describes the transmission of the infection in different age groups over time, expressing the force of infection in terms of the age-specific β parameters and then fitting model predictions to the data available. Considering the data in Figure 7.3, for example, we could set up a model which calculates the weekly numbers of reported cases of influenza in several different age groups for a given assumption about contact between individuals, and fit these model predictions to the weekly numbers of reported influenza cases to obtain the unknown β parameters (see Model 7.1, online).

For such analyses, we normally need to impose fewer constraints on our matrix structure than in the situation in which we are estimating unknown parameters for an endemic infection. For example, for the scenario discussed in section 7.4.2.1, we needed to impose sufficient constraints on our matrix so that we had only two equations with two unknown parameters. When fitting a transmission model to data, on the other hand, we need to constrain the number of unknown parameters so that it is less than (or equal to) the number of datapoints.

The data in Figure 7.3, for example, provide the numbers of cases reported for each of the 7 age groups each week over a 19 week period i.e. $7 \times 19 = 133$ data points. In principle, if we were to stratify our WAIFW matrix into seven age groups, with $7 \times 7 = 49$ unknown β parameters, we could estimate all 49 of the unknown β parameters by fitting model predictions of the numbers of reported cases to the observed data. In practice, however, it would be sensible to impose some constraints (e.g. that contact is symmetric) on the β parameters to ensure that the values obtained are biologically plausible.

7.4.3 Which WAIFW matrix structure(s) should we use?

It is generally possible to calculate several different WAIFW matrices for given values of a force of infection, which are compatible with the observed data. For example, both of the following WAIFW matrices (with β parameters in units of per day) can be obtained using the forces of rubella infection estimated for children and adults in the UK (see section 7.4.2.1.1):

$$\begin{pmatrix} 1.80 \times 10^{-8} & 5.02 \times 10^{-9} \\ 5.02 \times 10^{-9} & 5.02 \times 10^{-9} \end{pmatrix} \quad \begin{pmatrix} 1.81 \times 10^{-8} & 4.44 \times 10^{-9} \\ 4.44 \times 10^{-9} & 8.88 \times 10^{-9} \end{pmatrix}$$

$$\text{Matrix R1} \qquad\qquad\qquad \text{Matrix R2}$$

Which matrix should we use, if we wish to estimate the impact of different interventions using a model?

If we had estimated these matrices by fitting model predictions of the numbers of reported cases to observed data, i.e. using some goodness of fit statistic which measures how well model predictions using each matrix fits the data, it would be reasonable to use the matrix which provides the best fit to the data. On the other hand, the choice is slightly more complicated than this for the matrices calculated using the approach described for endemic infections (section 7.4.2.1), since all of the matrices were calculated so that they lead to predictions of the same force of infection and therefore all fit the data equally well.

In practice, as illustrated in Panel 7.7, modelling studies typically use many different plausible matrix structures when exploring the impact of interventions, given that underlying contact patterns in a population are usually poorly understood and β parameters in some age groups are difficult to estimate. For common endemic infections, such as measles, rubella, mumps etc, it is sometimes difficult to estimate the β parameters for teenagers and adults. For example, the high proportion of teenagers and adults who have been infected with these infections (see Section 5.2.3.5.2) means that the estimated force of infection in these age groups will be based on small numbers of new infections and hence is unreliable. Therefore estimates of the numbers of infectious individuals and the β parameters in these age groups can be unreliable.

Exploring the effect of several different matrix structures is particularly important when using model predictions to guide policy decisions, given that different matrices tend to lead to different predictions. For example, considering the matrices R1 and R2 that we calculated in section 7.4.2.1.1 using identical data, we see that vaccination with an effective coverage of 72 per cent of newborns is predicted to be sufficient to control rubella transmission if individuals are assumed to contact each other according to matrix R1 (Figure 7.11). However, it is insufficient if we assume that individuals mix according to matrix R2 (Model 7.2, online).

Why do these matrices lead to different predictions?

The explanation lies with the fact that the rate at which two specific adults come into effective contact (β_{oo}) is much higher for matrix R2 than for matrix R1. As we saw in Section 5.3.3, vaccination of newborns leads to an increase in the average age at infection and hence to an increase in the amount of transmission involving adults. This fact, together with the higher value for β_{oo} for matrix R2 than for matrix R1, means that if the population mixes according to matrix R2, the amount of transmission among adults will be greater, following the introduction of vaccination than if individuals mix according to matrix R1. As a result, the vaccination coverage required to control transmission in populations mixing according to matrix R2 needs to be greater than for those mixing according to matrix R1. In fact, as we shall see later, the effective coverage among newborns would need to exceed 78 per cent in order to control transmission if individuals are assumed to contact each other according to matrix R2.

The amount of mixing between different age groups, e.g. between children and adults, also strongly influences the impact of a control strategy. In general, the smaller the amount of contact between different age groups (i.e. the greater the with-like mixing), the smaller the impact in the overall population of control targeted at a specific age group (see Panel 7.7). Thus, in principle, if vaccination or antivirals are provided to schoolchildren during an influenza pandemic, for example, the greatest reduction in the overall incidence is likely to occur in settings in which there is substantial contact between children and other age groups.

We can formalize these arguments by calculating the (basic) reproduction number and the number of secondary infectious persons among children or adults that result from each child or adult, which, in turn, depend on the underlying contact patterns.

Panel 7.7 Analyses of the impact of varicella vaccination in Canada—an example of the sensitivity of model predictions to the assumed mixing patterns

The study of Brisson et al.[15] used an age-structured model to examine the potential impact of several different strategies of varicella (chickenpox) vaccination in Canada, e.g. routine vaccination of 1-year-olds, with or without routine vaccination of 11-year-olds at different stages of the programme. Chickenpox is caused by the varicella zoster virus; following infection, the virus remains latent in an individual and can reactivate many years later to cause varicella zoster ('shingles'). There were several concerns regarding the varicella vaccination programme:

◆ By reducing the prevalence of infectious persons, vaccination reduces the opportunity for individuals to get exposed, and could lead to increases in the numbers of new infections among adults, who have an increased risk of complications following infection.

◆ It might lead to an increased occurrence of so-called 'breakthrough varicella', which is defined as a mild form of varicella, which occurs among vaccine failures following infection.

◆ Individuals whose infection status has not been boosted by exposure to varicella in adult life may face an increased risk of zoster. Thus the reduction in the circulation of varicella because of the vaccination programme could lead to an increase in the numbers of new cases of zoster.

◆ The vaccine used was made from live attenuated virus and could establish latency. The introduction of the vaccination programme could result in increased morbidity, as a result of reactivation of the latent infection among vaccinees.

The study used the five matrix structures shown in Table 7.2.

As shown in Figure 7.10, the impact of vaccinating infants depended strongly on the assumed structure of the WAIFW matrix, and the greatest reduction in the numbers of new varicella cases was predicted for the assumption that contact between individuals was proportional (Figure 7.10a). This can be explained by the fact that for this assumption, there is substantial contact between individuals in different age groups, and therefore any reduction in the numbers of infectious persons which occurs in any one age group greatly benefits individuals in other age groups.

The age distribution of cases was predicted to change following the introduction of vaccination for all of the assumptions about contact (Figure 7.10e), with an increase in the average age of the cases, as reflected in an increase in the proportion of cases who were aged 25 or more years. The smallest increase was predicted for the assumption that mixing between individuals is with-like (assortative). This follows from the fact that for this assumption, there is little contact between children and adults, and therefore any reduction in the prevalence of infectious children, occurring because of the vaccination programme, has a relatively small impact on the numbers of new infections among adults, at least until the vaccinees themselves become adults.

Table 7.2 Summary of the WAIFW matrices assumed in the analyses of Brisson et al.[15] The β parameters are in units of per 100 days. Note the different vertical axis scale of these figures. The age groups used for the horizontal axes are identical

Matrix name (assigned by authors)	Structure	Assumptions
Base matrix	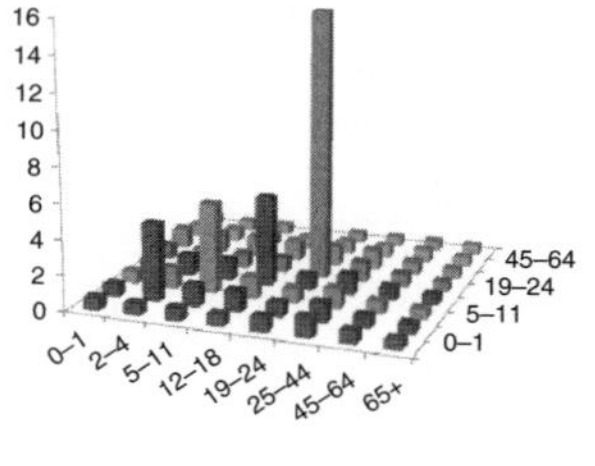	High rates of contact between individuals of pre-school, primary, high school and university age with other in the same age group, with that between 19–24 year olds being the highest. Infants contact 25–44-year-olds at a slightly higher rate than other age groups, reflecting contact between parents and children. Adults are as likely to contact children as they are to contact other adults. Children contact other children, who are not of the same age, at a rate which differs from that between any other age groups.
Matrix 1	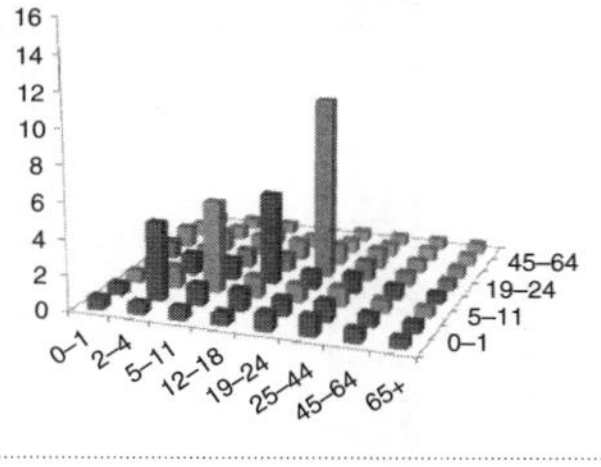	Identical to the base matrix, except that it assumed that 19–24-year-olds contacted each other at a rate which was 2/3 of that assumed in the base matrix.
Matrix 2	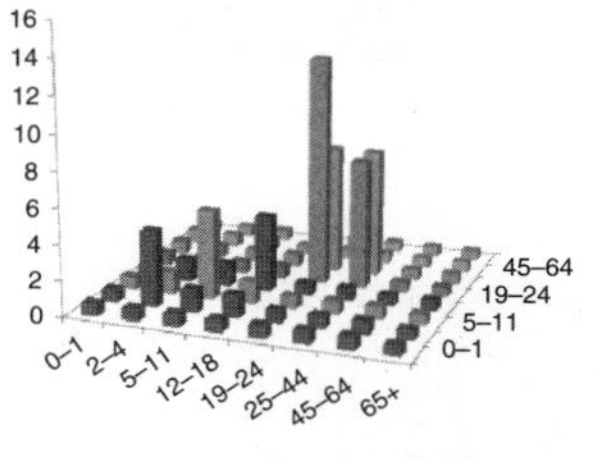	Identical to the base matrix, except that the rate at which an individual aged 25–44 years and those aged 0–1, 2–4, 5–11 and 25–44 years came into effective contact is assumed to be identical, but lower than that for the base matrix. There is a large amount of contact between 19–24 and 25–44-year-olds, which might occur, e.g. as a result of work.
Proportional	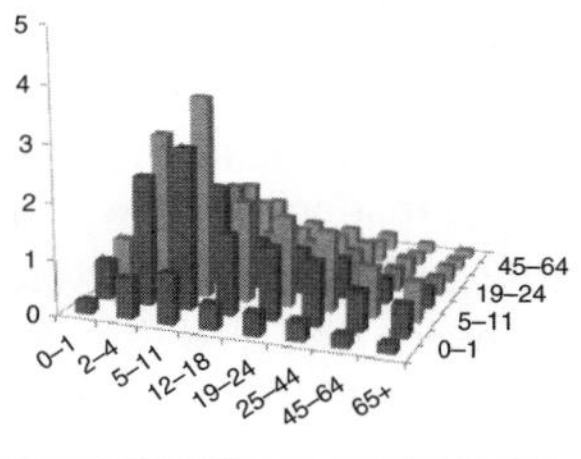	The matrix has the following structure: $$\begin{pmatrix} \beta_1\beta_1 & \beta_1\beta_2 & \beta_1\beta_3 & \cdots & \beta_1\beta_7 & \beta_1\beta_8 \\ \beta_2\beta_1 & \beta_2\beta_2 & \beta_2\beta_3 & \cdots & \beta_2\beta_7 & \beta_2\beta_8 \\ \beta_3\beta_1 & \beta_3\beta_2 & \beta_3\beta_3 & \cdots & \beta_3\beta_7 & \beta_3\beta_8 \\ \cdots & \cdots & \cdots & \cdots & \cdots & \cdots \\ \beta_7\beta_1 & \beta_7\beta_2 & \beta_7\beta_3 & \cdots & \beta_7\beta_7 & \beta_7\beta_8 \\ \beta_8\beta_1 & \beta_8\beta_2 & \beta_7\beta_4 & \cdots & \beta_7\beta_8 & \beta_8\beta_8 \end{pmatrix}$$

Panel 7.7 Analyses of the impact of varicella vaccination in Canada—an example of the sensitivity of model predictions to the assumed mixing patterns (*continued*)

Matrix name (assigned by authors)	Structure	Assumptions
Assortative (with-like)	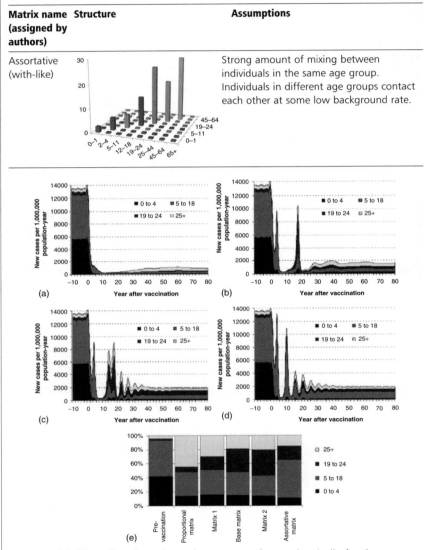	Strong amount of mixing between individuals in the same age group. Individuals in different age groups contact each other at some low background rate.

Fig. 7.10 (a)–(d) Predicted numbers of new cases of natural varicella for the assumptions that mixing is (a) proportional; (b) based on matrix 1; (c) based on matrix 2; (d) assortative (see Table 7.2), assuming that 90 per cent of infants are vaccinated and that vaccination protects for an average of 32 years, with 93 per cent of individuals protected after vaccination (see [15] for further details); (e) shows the age distribution of cases at equilibrium for this scenario. The shaded areas reflect the morbidity in different age groups. Reproduced with permission from Brisson *et al.*[15]

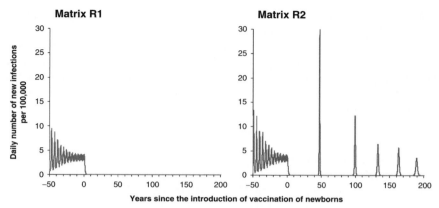

Fig. 7.11 Predictions of the daily number of new rubella infections per 100,000 following the introduction of 72 per cent effective vaccination coverage among newborns in year 0, assuming that individuals contact each other according to WAIFW matrices R1 and R2 (see Section 7.4.2.1.1). The predictions are obtained using the age-structured model discussed in Panel 5.4, after adapting it to allow for age-dependent contact (Model 7.2, online).

7.5 **How do we calculate R_0 if mixing is assumed to be non-random?**

By now, we are familiar with the verbal definition of the basic reproduction number as the 'average number of secondary infectious persons resulting from a single infectious person following his/her introduction into a totally susceptible population'. R_0 also has so-called 'threshold properties', namely if it is greater or less than one, then the incidence increases and decreases respectively if an infectious person enters a totally susceptible population.

When we assume that individuals do not mix randomly, the numbers of secondary infectious persons which result from each infectious person depends on the subgroup to which they belong. According to the mixing pattern described by matrix R1, for example, on average, each adult and child leads to different numbers of infectious persons, and each adult will generate a different number of infectious persons among adults than among children.

As was first described by Heesterbeek *et al*,[19, 29] the basic reproduction number in this situation is some average of all these individual numbers of secondary infectious persons. To calculate this average, we first need to set up something which is known as the 'Next Generation Matrix'(abbreviated to 'NGM'), which summarizes the numbers of secondary infectious persons which result from each child or adult in the population.

7.5.1 **Writing down the Next Generation Matrix**

As we saw in Sections 2.7.1 and 4.2.2.1, when we assume that individuals mix randomly, R_0 is given by the following expression:

$$R_0 = \beta N D \qquad\qquad 7.29$$

where β is the rate at which two specific individuals come into effective contact per unit time, N is the total population size, and D is the duration of infectiousness.

We can adapt this expression to write down the number of infectious persons in a given subgroup which result from individuals in another subgroup. For example, for our population in which children and adults have different numbers of contacts, the number of infectious *children* resulting from the introduction of one infectious child into a totally susceptible population is given by:

$$R_{yy} = \beta_{yy} N_y D \qquad\qquad 7.30$$

where N_y is the total number of children in the population.

Similarly, the number of infectious *adults* resulting from the introduction of one infectious child into a totally susceptible population is given by:

$$R_{oy} = \beta_{oy} N_o D \qquad\qquad 7.31$$

where N_o is the total number of adults in the population.

The expressions for the number of secondary infectious children resulting from each infectious adult (R_{yo}) and the number of secondary infectious adults resulting from each adult infectious (R_{oo}) are analogous:

$$R_{yo} = \beta_{yo} N_y D \qquad\qquad 7.32$$

$$R_{oo} = \beta_{oo} N_o D \qquad\qquad 7.33$$

These numbers are typically written using matrix notation:

$$\begin{pmatrix} R_{yy} & R_{yo} \\ R_{oy} & R_{oo} \end{pmatrix} = \begin{pmatrix} \beta_{yy} N_y D & \beta_{yo} N_y D \\ \beta_{oy} N_o D & \beta_{oo} N_o D \end{pmatrix} \qquad\qquad 7.34$$

This matrix is known as the 'Next Generation Matrix'. Note how the subscripts are used – the subscripts for R_{yy}, R_{yo}, R_{oy} and R_{oo} match those for the β parameters (see Panel 7.2).

7.5.1.1 Example: calculation of the Next Generation Matrix

In section 7.4.2.1.1, we calculated the following WAIFW matrix:

$\begin{pmatrix} 1.80 \times 10^{-8} & 5.02 \times 10^{-9} \\ 5.02 \times 10^{-9} & 5.02 \times 10^{-9} \end{pmatrix}$, in which the β parameters are in units of per day, using

estimates of the force of rubella infection from the UK.

Assuming that the population has a rectangular age distribution, comprising 55 million individuals with a life expectancy of 75 years and a_y (the maximum age of children) equal to 15 years, we can use the equationss $N_y = \dfrac{N a_y}{L}$ and $N_o = \dfrac{N(L - a_y)}{L}$

(see Panel 7.4) to calculate the numbers of children (N_y) and adults (N_o) in the population to be approximately 11 million ($\approx \dfrac{55 \times 10^6 \times 15}{75}$) and 44 million

($\approx \dfrac{55 \times 10^6 \times (75 - 15)}{75}$) respectively.

Substituting for $N_y = 11 \times 10^6$, $\beta_{yy} = 1.80 \times 10^{-8}$ per day, $\beta_{yo} = 5.02 \times 10^{-9}$ per day and a duration of infectiousness (D) of 11 days into Equations 7.30 and 7.32, leads to the following values for R_{yy} and R_{yo}:

$$R_{yy} = 1.80 \times 10^{-8} \times 11 \times 10^6 \times 11 = 2.18$$

$$R_{yo} = 5.02 \times 10^{-9} \times 11 \times 10^6 \times 11 = 0.61$$

Similarly, substituting for $N_o = 44 \times 10^6$, $\beta_{oy} = \beta_{oo} = 5.02 \times 10^{-9}$ per day, and a duration of infectiousness of 11 days into Equations 7.31 and 7.33 leads to the following values for R_{oy} and R_{oo}:

$$R_{oy} = R_{oo} = 5.02 \times 10^{-9} \times 44 \times 10^6 \times 11 = 2.43$$

The corresponding Next Generation Matrix is as follows:

$$
\begin{array}{cc}
 & \begin{array}{cc} y & o \end{array} \\
\begin{array}{c} y \\ o \end{array} & \left(\begin{array}{cc} 2.18 & 0.61 \\ 2.43 & 2.43 \end{array} \right) \\
total & \begin{array}{cc} 4.61 & 3.04 \end{array}
\end{array}
$$

Overall, according to this matrix, each infectious child effectively contacts 4.61 individuals, of whom 2.18 are children and 2.43 are adults. Similarly, each adult effectively contacts 3.04 individuals, of whom 0.61 are children and 2.43 are adults. The average number of secondary infectious persons resulting from one child and one adult is 3.85 (=(4.61+3.04)/2) individuals.

Similar calculations for matrix R2 lead to the following Next Generation Matrix:

$$
\begin{array}{cc}
 & \begin{array}{cc} y & o \end{array} \\
\begin{array}{c} y \\ o \end{array} & \left(\begin{array}{cc} 2.19 & 0.54 \\ 2.15 & 4.30 \end{array} \right) \\
total & \begin{array}{cc} 4.34 & 4.84 \end{array}
\end{array}
$$

As illustrated graphically in Figure 7.12, the main difference between matrix R1 and R2 is that the number of secondary infectious persons among adults resulting from each adult is almost twofold greater for matrix R2 than for matrix R1.

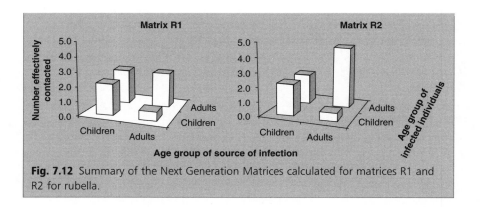

Fig. 7.12 Summary of the Next Generation Matrices calculated for matrices R1 and R2 for rubella.

7.5.2 **Calculating R_0**

How might we calculate R_0 from the Next Generation Matrix? One simple approach might be to take an average of the number of secondary infectious persons which result from each infectious child and the number of secondary infectious persons which result from each infectious adult.

To identify whether this average equals R_0, we could simulate the introduction of infectious persons into a totally susceptible population for a given Next Generation Matrix and check whether the number of infectious persons in each generation increases if the average is greater or less than one.

Before doing this using the matrices calculated in section 7.5.1.1, we shall first do this using the Next Generation Matrices below (matrix A and B), for which the average numbers of individuals effectively contacted by each infectious person are slightly above one (1.7) or below one (0.95). To keep things simple, we shall use a time step of one serial interval.

$$
\begin{array}{cc}
 & y \quad o \\
\begin{array}{c} y \\ o \end{array} & \left(\begin{array}{cc} 0.1 & 0.1 \\ 3 & 0.2 \end{array} \right)
\end{array}
\qquad
\begin{array}{cc}
 & y \quad o \\
\begin{array}{c} y \\ o \end{array} & \left(\begin{array}{cc} 1.6 & 0.1 \\ 0.1 & 0.1 \end{array} \right)
\end{array}
$$

$$total\ \ 3.1\ \ 0.3 \qquad\qquad total\ \ 1.7\ \ 0.2$$

$$average = (3.1 + 0.3)/2 = 1.7 \quad average = (1.7 + 0.2)/2 = 0.95$$

$$\text{Matrix A} \qquad\qquad\qquad \text{Matrix B}$$

Based on these averages, we might expect the number of infectious persons in each generation to increase once infectious persons enter a totally susceptible population if the Next Generation Matrix is given by matrix A, and to decrease if it is given by matrix B. In fact, as shown in Figure 7.13 (Panel 7.8 and Model 7.3 (online)), the opposite occurs: the number of infectious persons in each generation *decreases* if individuals are assumed to contact each other according to matrix A and *increases* for matrix B, irrespective of the numbers of infectious individuals introduced at the start. This suggests that the mean of the numbers of infectious persons generated by one child and one adult does not equal R_0.

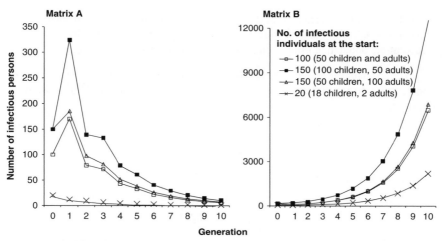

Fig. 7.13 Predictions of the numbers of infectious individuals in each generation following the introduction of different numbers of infectious persons into a totally susceptible population in which the Next Generation Matrix is either matrix A or B. See Model 7.3, online.

Panel 7.8 Worked calculation of the number of individuals predicted in each generation following the introduction of infectious persons into a totally susceptible population using a given Next Generation Matrix

Suppose that 50 infectious children and adults are introduced into a totally susceptible population in which individuals contact each other according to matrix A. The number of infectious children and adults in the first generation (denoted by $I_{y,1}$ and $I_{o,1}$ respectively) can be calculated using the following matrix equation:

$$\begin{pmatrix} I_{y,1} \\ I_{o,1} \end{pmatrix} = \begin{pmatrix} 0.1 & 0.1 \\ 3 & 0.2 \end{pmatrix} \begin{pmatrix} 50 \\ 50 \end{pmatrix}$$

which can be written out and evaluated as follows:

$$I_{y,1} = 0.1 \times 50 + 0.1 \times 50 = 10$$
$$I_{o,1} = 3 \times 50 + 0.2 \times 50 = 160$$

i.e. there should be 10 infectious children and 160 infectious adults in the first generation, giving a total of 10+160=170 infectious individuals.

Panel 7.8 Worked calculation of the number of individuals predicted in each generation following the introduction of infectious persons into a totally susceptible population using a given Next Generation Matrix (continued)

We can adapt the above expressions to obtain the expressions for the numbers of infectious persons in the $k+1^{\text{th}}$ generation in terms of those in the kth generation as follows:

$$I_{y,k+1} = 0.1 I_{y,k} + 0.1 I_{o,k}$$ 7.35

$$I_{o,k+1} = 3 I_{y,k} + 0.2 I_{o,k}$$ 7.36

or, using matrix notation:

$$\begin{pmatrix} I_{y,k+1} \\ I_{o,k+1} \end{pmatrix} = \begin{pmatrix} 0.1 & 0.1 \\ 3 & 0.2 \end{pmatrix} \begin{pmatrix} I_{y,k} \\ I_{o,k} \end{pmatrix}$$

We will now use these equations to calculate the numbers of infectious persons in the second and third generations.

Second generation

Substituting the numbers of infectious children and adults that we estimated above for the first generation ($I_{y,1}=10$ and $I_{o,1}=160$) into Equations 7.35 and 7.36 leads to the following equations for the numbers of infectious children and adults in the second generation:

$$I_{y,2} = 0.1 I_{y,1} + 0.1 I_{o,1} = 0.1 \times 10 + 0.1 \times 160 = 17$$

$$I_{o,2} = 3 I_{y,1} + 0.2 I_{o,1} = 3 \times 10 + 0.2 \times 160 = 62$$

Total number of infectious individuals in the second generation = $I_{y,2}+I_{o,2}$ = 17+62 = 79

Third generation

Substituting for $I_{y,2}=17$ and $I_{o,2}=62$ into Equations 7.35 and 7.36 leads to the following equations for the numbers of infectious children and adults in the third generation:

$$I_{y,3} = 0.1 I_{y,2} + 0.1 I_{o,2} = 0.1 \times 17 + 0.1 \times 62 = 7.9$$

$$I_{o,3} = 3 I_{y,2} + 0.2 I_{o,2} = 3 \times 17 + 0.2 \times 62 = 63.4$$

Total number of infectious individuals in the third generation = $I_{y,3}+I_{o,3}$ = 7.9+63.4 = 71.3

Why is the average of all the numbers in a given Next Generation Matrix inconsistent with the trend in the number of infectious persons in each generation following the introduction of infectious persons into a totally susceptible population?

The reason lies with the fact that the average does not account for the proportion of infectious persons in each generation who are children and adults, as it implicitly assumes that there is an equal proportion of infectious children and adults in each generation. In practice, when we introduce infectious persons into a totally susceptible population, the age distribution of the infectious persons in each generation depends on the Next Generation Matrix. If, for example we introduce 50 infectious children and adults into a population for which the Next Generation Matrix is the same as matrix A, then in the next generation we will have 10 children and 160 adults (Panel 7.8). In the subsequent generation, there should be 17 and 62 infectious children and adults, and the total number of infectious persons will be smaller than that in the previous generation. In fact, as we shall see later, the age distribution converges to some value which is peculiar to each matrix.

Following the approach pioneered by Heesterbeck *et al*,[19, 29] we can gain insight into how we might calculate R_0 by studying how the numbers of infectious persons in Figure 7.13 changes with each generation.

If we just divide the number of infectious persons in a given generation by the number of infectious persons in the preceding generation, we see that for matrix A, for which the number of infectious persons in each generation *decreases* following the introduction of infectious persons into a totally susceptible population (see Figure 7.13), this ratio varies initially, but ultimately converges to a value of about 0.7 (Figure 7.14). For matrix B, for which the number of infectious persons in each generation *increases* following the introduction of infectious persons into the totally susceptible population (Figure 7.13), this ratio converges to a value of about 1.6 (Figure 7.14).

Interestingly, the value to which this ratio converges is independent of the number or ages of infectious individuals which are introduced into the population at the start. In fact, every Next Generation Matrix has some value to which this ratio converges and this value is unique to and a fundamental property of each matrix. The formal mathematical term for this value is the 'characteristic value' of the matrix, or most commonly, the 'dominant eigenvalue', for reasons discussed in section 7.5.3. A further interesting feature of these simulations is that the distribution of children and adults

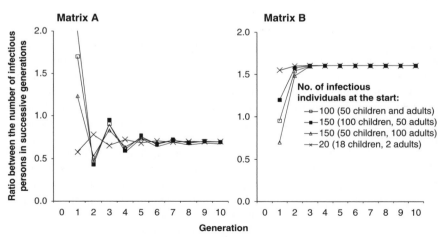

Fig. 7.14 Ratio between the number of infectious persons in a given generation and that in the preceding generation, following the introduction of infectious individuals into a totally susceptible population for which the Next Generation Matrix is either matrix A or matrix B (see Model 7.3, online).

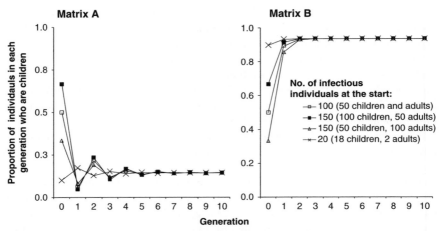

Fig. 7.15 Predicted proportion of individuals in each generation who are children following the introduction of infectious persons into a totally susceptible population, assuming that individuals contact each other according to matrices A and B. See Model 7.3, online.

in each generation also converges to some value, e.g. with about 14 per cent and 86 per cent being children and adults respectively for the simulation relating to matrix A (Figure 7.15). This age distribution is again unique to each matrix, and in mathematical terms, it is referred to as the characteristic vector of the matrix or, most commonly, as the 'dominant eigenvector' of the matrix. Eigenvalues and eigen-vectors are discussed in Basic maths section B.7.3.

Using elegant mathematical theory, which is too elaborate to reproduce here, Heesterbeek *et al*,[19, 29] demonstrated that for any Next Generation Matrix and infection, the ratio between the size of successive generations, as calculated following the introduction of infectious persons into a totally susceptible population (with some restrictions—see below) has the properties of the basic reproduction number. Specifically, for the incidence of an infection to increase following the introduction of infectious persons into a totally susceptible population, this ratio must exceed one. Likewise, for the incidence to decrease, this ratio must be less than one. Finally, and most importantly, we can use it to calculate the herd immunity threshold in the same way as we would calculate it when we assume that individuals mix randomly, using the relationship $1-1/R_0$ (section 1.3).

For example, the basic reproduction number for our rubella matrices R1 and R2 discussed in sections 7.4.2.1.1 and 7.5.1.1 equals 3.53 and 4.75 respectively (Figure 7.16), in turn, implying that at least 72 per cent (= $100 \times (1-1/3.53)$ and 79 per cent (= $100 \times (1-1/4.75)$ respectively of the population should be effectively vaccinated in order to control transmission. These levels of effective vaccination coverage are consistent with the values implied in Figure 7.11 (see Model 7.2, online).

To have all the properties of R_0, the ratio between the number of infectious persons in successive generation must be calculated assuming that the susceptible population is not depleted.[19] This may seem counter-intuitive since, in a real population, the

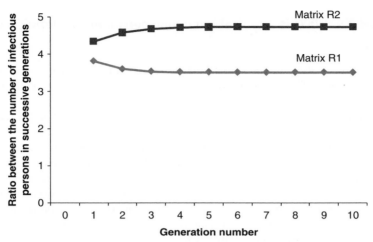

Fig. 7.16 Ratio between the number of infectious persons in a given generation and that in the preceding generation, following the introduction of infectious individuals, into a totally susceptible population for which the Next Generation Matrix is either rubella matrix R1 or R2 (see Section 7.5.1.1 for their definitions and Model 7.3, online).

susceptible population would get depleted, as susceptible individuals contact infectious individuals, become infected and subsequently immune. However, this assumption is made simply for the purposes of identifying the underlying characteristic value of the next generation matrix, which equals R_0.

Since R_0 is calculated as the ratio between the number of infectious persons in successive generations, the term 'basic reproduction number' is also often referred to as the 'basic reproduction ratio'.[19] Whilst the ratio has a clear mathematical definition, its biological interpretation requires further thought. The biological definition that Diekmann and Heesterbeek developed is 'The average number of secondary infectious persons resulting from a *typical* infectious person following his/her introduction into a totally susceptible population.'[19]

This definition is identical to the definition of R_0 that is usually used when we assume that individuals mixed randomly, except that it specifically refers to a 'typical' infectious person. This reference to a typical infectious person is sometimes omitted in definitions of R_0 for randomly mixing populations. We discuss the definition of a typical infectious person in Panel 7.9.

7.5.3 The mechanics of calculating R_0 when we assume that individuals do not mix randomly

There are at least three methods for calculating R_0 from the Next Generation Matrix.

1. Simulation approach

The approach described above can be used to calculate R_0 for any Next Generation Matrix: we simulate the introduction of infectious individuals into a population in which the number of secondary infectious persons generated by individuals in different

---

Panel 7.9 What is a typical infectious person in the definition of R_0?

Heesterbeek *et al*[19, 29] define a typical infectious person in their definition of R_0 as some fictitious individual who partly belongs to each of the subgroups in the population.

We can get insight into what proportion of this hypothetical person belongs to different subgroups by studying how the age distribution of infectious persons changes from one generation to the next, when we introduce infectious persons into a totally susceptible population, with individuals contacting each other according to some Next Generation Matrix. As shown in Figure 7.15 for matrices A and B, the proportions of individuals in each generation who are children or adults converge to some distribution, e.g. with 15 and 85 per cent of individuals in each generation being children and adults for matrix A, with the corresponding proportions being 94 and 6 per cent for matrix B.

We also see that once this age distribution has converged, the ratio between the number of infectious persons in a given generation and that in the preceding generation has also converged. According to Heesterbeek *et al*, the typical infectious person for this matrix is someone who has this age distribution (i.e. 15 per cent young and 85 per cent old for matrix A), since if we were to introduce this 'individual' into a totally susceptible population, the number of secondary infectious persons that 'it' would generate equals R_0.

---

subgroups is determined by that Next Generation Matrix and there is an unlimited supply of susceptible individuals. R_0 can then be calculated as G_{k+1}/G_k, where G_k is the number of infectious persons in generation k, once sufficient numbers of generations have occurred for this ratio to have stabilized.

The advantage of this approach is that it is relatively easy to set up in a spreadsheet (see Model 7.3, online) and, unlike the approaches described below, it always leads to the correct value for the basic reproduction number (i.e. the dominant eigenvalue of the Next Generation Matrix—see Basic maths section B.7.4).

2. 'Mathematical' approaches

R_0 can also be calculated by using the following two mathematical approaches:

(a) *Simultaneous equations approach*: find the values for R_0 and x for which the following equations (or their equivalent when the contact parameters are stratified into more than two subgroups—see below) hold:

$$R_{yy}x + R_{yo}(1 - x) = R_0 x \qquad 7.37$$

$$R_{oy}x + R_{oo}(1 - x) = R_0(1 - x) \qquad 7.38$$

Using Matrix notation, these equations can also be written as follows:

$$\begin{pmatrix} R_{yy} & R_{yo} \\ R_{oy} & R_{oo} \end{pmatrix} \begin{pmatrix} x \\ 1 - x \end{pmatrix} = R_0 \begin{pmatrix} x \\ 1 - x \end{pmatrix} \qquad 7.39$$

This approach is equivalent to the simulation approach (see Appendix section A.5.1.1); Model 7.4 (online) illustrates how we can estimate R_0 from these equations in practice.

(b) *Matrix determinant approach*: find the maximum value for R_0 which satisfies the following equation (or its equivalent when the population is stratified into more than two subgroups—see below).

$$(R_{yy} - R_0)(R_{oo} - R_0) - R_{oy}R_{yo} = 0 \qquad\qquad 7.40$$

This equation can be obtained by rearranging Equations 7.37 and 7.38 (see Appendix A5.1.2). Mathematically-interested readers may recognize this equation as being that of the 'determinant' of the matrix $\begin{pmatrix} R_{yy} - R_0 & R_{yo} \\ R_{oy} & R_{oo} - R_0 \end{pmatrix}$ and that R_0

is the 'eigenvalue' of the Next Generation Matrix $\begin{pmatrix} R_{yy} & R_{yo} \\ R_{oy} & R_{oo} \end{pmatrix}$ (see Basic maths

sections B.7.2 and B.7.3 for further details about matrix determinants and eigenvalues). We therefore refer to this approach for calculating R_0 as the 'matrix determinant' approach.

The methods for extending these approaches to deal with populations stratified into more than two subgroups are provided in Panel 7.10.

Many statistical or mathematical software packages, such as Stata, Mathematica, Maple, and Matlab have inbuilt functions for calculating the determinant or the eigenvalues for a matrix. At time of writing, Excel does not have a function for calculating eigenvalues, although its function (mdeterm()) for calculating the determinant of a matrix can be adapted for this purpose (see Model 7.4, online).

As shown in the following example, two values for 'R_0' can sometimes be found which satisfy Equation 7.40 and therefore Equations 7.37 and 7.38 for a given Next Generation Matrix. As demonstrated by Heesterbeek et al,[19, 29] the value which should be taken for R_0 should be the largest value which satisfies Equation 7.40. This explains why R_0 is known mathematically as the 'dominant' (i.e. largest) eigenvalue of the Next Generation Matrix. A mathematical explanation for why R_0 is taken as the largest eigenvalue is provided in the Basic maths section B.7.3.

7.5.3.1 Example: application of the matrix determinant approach for calculating R_0

For the rubella matrix R1 $\begin{pmatrix} 2.18 & 0.61 \\ 2.43 & 2.43 \end{pmatrix}$, substituting for $R_{yy} = 2.18$, $R_{yo} = 0.61$, $R_{oy} =$

2.43 and $R_{oo} = 2.43$ into Equation 7.40, we obtain the following equation:

$$(R_0 - 2.18)(R_0 - 2.43) - 2.43 \times 0.61 = 0$$

or equivalently:

$$R_0^2 - 4.61R_0 + 3.82 = 0$$

Using the result that the solution to an equation of the form $ax^2 + bx + c$ is given

by $\dfrac{-b \pm \sqrt{b^2 - 4ac}}{2a}$, leads to the result that:

$$R_0 = \frac{4.61 \pm \sqrt{(-4.61)^2 - 4 \times 1 \times 3.82}}{2}$$

$$= 1.08 \quad or \quad 3.53$$

Panel 7.10 Extending the methods for calculating R_0 to populations stratified into more than two subgroups

The approaches described above for calculating R_0 can be extended relatively easily to deal with populations comprising more than two subgroups. For example, if the population comprised three subgroups, a fraction x, y and $1-x-y$ of the typical infectious person could be considered to belong to the first, second and third subgroups. For a Next Generation Matrix such as $\begin{pmatrix} 1 & 5 & 4 \\ 2 & 3 & 6 \\ 3 & 7 & 8 \end{pmatrix}$, the basic reproduction number can be calculated relatively easily by using the simulation approach in a spreadsheet.

Alternatively, it can be obtained by using one of the following mathematical approaches:

1. Solving the following matrix equation:

$$\begin{pmatrix} 1 & 5 & 4 \\ 2 & 3 & 6 \\ 3 & 7 & 8 \end{pmatrix} \begin{pmatrix} x \\ y \\ 1-x-y \end{pmatrix} = R_0 \begin{pmatrix} x \\ y \\ 1-x-y \end{pmatrix}$$

which could also be written as:

$$x + 5y + 4(1 - x - y) = R_0 x$$
$$2x + 3y + 6(1 - x - y) = R_0 y$$
$$3x + 7y + 8(1 - x - y) = R_0(1 - x - y)$$

2. Identifying the value for R_0 for which the determinant of the following matrix is zero (see Basic maths section B.7.2 for the definition of a determinant):

$$\begin{pmatrix} 1 - R_0 & 5 & 4 \\ 2 & 3 - R_0 & 6 \\ 3 & 7 & 8 - R_0 \end{pmatrix}$$

For both of the mathematical approaches, R_0 is the largest value which satisfies these equations.

One 'hand-waving'explanation for why R_0 is the maximum value which satisfies Equations 7.39 or 7.40 is that it leads to the greater value for the proportion of the population which needs to be immune in order to control transmission (through the equation $H = 1-1/R_0$), and it must therefore be sufficiently high to control transmission even in the highest risk group. Another hand-waving explanation is that every biological system is associated with several characteristic values, depending on the number of subgroups in the population. Since each pathogen will tend to be transmitted to as many individuals as possible, this will occur according to the largest characteristic value associated with the system.

7.5.4 Methods for calculating the net reproduction number

We can adapt the above logic to estimate the net reproduction number for a population in which some individuals are immune as a result of natural infection or vaccination. In this instance, we would write down the Next Generation Matrix in the same way that we would write it to calculate R_0, except that the population size in each age group (or subgroup) would need to be replaced by the number of susceptible individuals. Considering a population in which contact differs between children and adults, for example, our Next Generation Matrix would be written as follows:

$$\begin{pmatrix} R_{yy} & R_{yo} \\ R_{oy} & R_{oo} \end{pmatrix} = \begin{pmatrix} \beta_{yy}S_yD & \beta_{yo}S_yD \\ \beta_{oy}S_oD & \beta_{oo}S_oD \end{pmatrix} \qquad 7.41$$

where S_y and S_o are the number of susceptible young and old individuals in the population.

Similarly, to estimate the short-term impact of an intervention targeted at a specific age group, we could calculate the reproduction number following the introduction of the intervention using the next generation matrix, calculated using the number of susceptible individuals in each age group as a result of the intervention (see Exercise 7.5).

Estimating the impact of an intervention using the net reproduction number calculated with this approach is typically quicker than developing detailed transmission models, and in any case, it is helpful for checking that predictions from such models are plausible. As illustrated below, estimates of the net reproduction number that are calculated using the above methods are currently used in England to monitor the potential for a measles epidemic to occur and to guide vaccination policy.

7.5.4.1 Example: using estimates of the net reproduction number to infer the potential for a measles epidemic to occur in England

By 1991, notifications of measles cases in England were lower than they had ever been before (see Figure 5.12a). This followed largely from the introduction of routine MMR vaccination in 1988, accompanied by a catch-up campaign targetting pre-school age children. Measles vaccination had been introduced in England in 1968, although the coverage was low (~50%) until 1980. Small increases in the numbers of notifications had been seen during the first half of 1994 in England, with 39 per cent of notifications occuring among children aged >10 years. A measles epidemic with about 5,000 cases in western Scotland had occurred during the period 1993–1994, and there were concerns that a measles epidemic in England was also imminent.[20]

A study by Gay *et al.*,[21] published in 1995, used age-specific measles serological data which had been collected annually (see, for example, Figure 5.18) to predict the potential for a measles epidemic to occur, by calculating the net reproduction number for different assumptions about mixing between individuals. The study used the following two WAIFW matrices, both of which are similar to matrix B in Table 7.1.

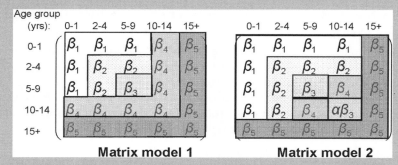

The β parameters for these matrices were calculated using estimates of the force of infection from before the introduction of measles vaccination in England in 1968 (see Table 7.3), which were obtained by fitting catalytic models to data on

Table 7.3 Estimates of the force of measles infection in England, calculated using case notifications for the period 1956–65 (Nigel Gay, personal correspondence) and the average number of susceptible individuals before the introduction of measles vaccination The average numbers of susceptible individuals are calculated assuming that each single-year age group comprised 650,000 individuals and that maternal immunity lasts for three months on average.

Age group (years)	0–1	2–4	5–9	10–14	15–74
Average force of infection (%/year) before the introduction of vaccination in 1968	7.7	23.7	51.7	25.5	9.9
Average number susceptible (prevaccination)	1,062,861	1,216,541	493,355	59,269	59,182
Average number susceptible during the period 1994/5*	730,557	317,850	529,750	353,600	204,922

* Estimates for cohorts born during the period 1973/4–1984/5 are based on serological data collected during the period 1986/7–1991, assuming that force of infection after 1991 was negligible following the introduction of MMR vaccination in 1988; 16.3 per cent of individuals born during or after 1985/7 are assumed to be susceptible; 0.05 per cent of individuals born before 1973/5 are assumed to be susceptible. Estimates for 0–1-year-olds are based on the assumption that individuals were vaccinated at age 15 months.[21]

notifications from the period 1956–65.[14] Because of the uncertainty in the force of infection estimates for individuals aged 10 or more years, resulting from the high prevalence of immunity in this age group, the β parameters for these age groups could not be reliably calculated. The authors therefore used a range of values for the β parameter reflecting contact between 10–14-year-olds, assuming that it differed by a factor α (which varied between 1 and 2) from that between individuals aged 5–9 years.

Using the resulting estimates of the β parameters (see Exercise 7.4), the authors then calculated the net reproduction number for the period 1989–1997 based on different scenarios for the proportion of individuals who were susceptible in each age group. For example, using the estimates of the number of individuals who were susceptible to measles infection in 1994–5 in Table 7.3, leads to the following Next Generation Matrix for WAIFW model 2 (α=1.5) and estimates of the net reproduction number of about 1 by 1994/5.

$$
\begin{array}{c c}
\text{Age group} & \\
\text{(yrs):} &
\begin{array}{c c c c c}
0-1 & 2-4 & 5-9 & 10-14 & 15+
\end{array} \\
\begin{array}{r}
0-1 \\
2-4 \\
5-9 \\
10-14 \\
15+
\end{array} &
\left(
\begin{array}{c c c c c}
0.087 & 0.087 & 0.087 & 0.087 & 0.112 \\
0.038 & 0.129 & 0.129 & 0.129 & 0.049 \\
0.063 & 0.215 & 0.796 & 0.218 & 0.081 \\
0.042 & 0.143 & 0.145 & 0.797 & 0.054 \\
0.031 & 0.031 & 0.031 & 0.031 & 0.031
\end{array}
\right)
\end{array}
$$

As shown in Figure 7.17, for all mixing assumptions considered by the authors, the net reproduction number was estimated to be very close to 1 during the period 1992–7 and therefore a measles epidemic, with over 100,000 cases predicted,[22] appeared likely. Based on these results, which were supported by findings from other dynamic models developed at that time,[14] the UK government conducted a mass measles–rubella vaccination campaign in November 1994, targeting 95 per cent of the 7 million children aged 5–16 years.[23]

Since these first analyses, the potential for measles epidemics continues to be evaluated in England using similar methods.[24]

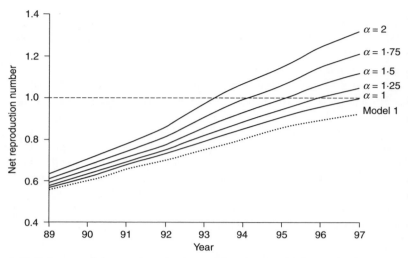

Fig. 7.17 Estimates of the net reproduction number for measles for England, 1989–97.[21] See the footnote to Table 7.3 for assumptions about the proportion susceptible. Reproduced with permission from Gay et al, 1995.[21]

7.6 **Summary**

This chapter has highlighted the fact that contact patterns strongly determine the impact of interventions against infections, but that they are poorly understood. Consequently, modelling studies need to explore the effects of several assumptions about contact if they are intended to guide policy decisions.

The approach used to calculate the contact parameters depend on the data available and can be summarized as follows.

Steps in calculating the matrix of 'Who Acquires Infection From Whom'

Endemic infections

a) Calculate the forces of infection in specific age groups before the introduction of any intervention.

b) Use estimates of the force of infection to calculate the numbers of susceptible individuals in different age groups.

c) Use estimates of the force of infection and the numbers of susceptible individuals to calculate the number of infectious individuals.

d) Decide on the structure of the WAIFW matrix.

e) Use estimates of the forces of infection and the numbers of infectious individuals to calculate the β parameters for the chosen WAIFW matrix.

New or re-emergent infections

a) Set up a transmission model in which the force of infection is expressed in terms of the β parameters of the chosen WAIFW matrix.

b) Fit predictions of the incidence (or the statistic reflected in the data) over time in specific age groups to the available data.

In general, the greater the amount of mixing that is with-like, the smaller the impact in the overall population of an intervention which is targeted at a specific age group. Conversely, the greater the amount of mixing that is with-unlike in different age groups, the greater the impact in the overall population of an intervention targeted at a specific age group.

The level of control that is required to control transmission depends on the basic reproduction number, which can be calculated from the Next Generation Matrix for the given mixing assumption. This involves simulating the introduction of infectious persons into a totally susceptible population, in which there is an unlimited number of susceptible individuals, and taking the ratio between the number of infectious persons in successive generations once sufficient generations have occurred. R_0 can also be calculated using other 'mathematical approaches'. These methods can be adapted to estimate the net reproduction number and are repeatedly being used to predict the potential for a measles epidemic to occur in England.

7.7 **Exercises**

7.1 Adapt the logic in section 7.4.1 and Panel 7.1 to obtain the following equation for the force of infection among old individuals $\overline{\lambda_o(t)} = \beta_{oy}I_y(t) + \beta_{oo}I_o(t)$.

7.2 Suppose that a population has 20 and 50 infectious children and adults respectively, and the WAIFW matrix, in which each β parameter reflects the daily rate at which two specific children/adults come into effective contact per day, is as follows:

$$
\begin{array}{cc}
& \begin{array}{cc} \text{young} & \text{old} \end{array} \\
\begin{array}{c} \text{young} \\ \text{old} \end{array} & \left(\begin{array}{cc} 2\times10^{-4} & 8\times10^{-4} \\ 3\times10^{-4} & 7\times10^{-5} \end{array} \right)
\end{array}
$$

Calculate the force of infection among:

    (a) children which is attributable to contact with:

        (i)   other children;

        (ii) adults;

        (iii) both children and adults.

    (b) adults which is attributable to contact with:

        (i)   children;

        (ii) other adults;

        (iii) both children and adults.

7.3 Calculate the values for β_1 and β_2 assuming that mixing between children and

adults is described using WAIFW matrix $\begin{pmatrix} \beta_1 & 0.5\beta_2 \\ 0.5\beta_2 & \beta_2 \end{pmatrix}$, and using the estimates of

the force of rubella infection for children and adults and the numbers of infectious individuals presented in section 7.4.2.1.

7.4 Table 7.3 shows estimates of the force of measles infection before the introduction of measles vaccination in England, and the number of susceptible individuals (Nigel Gay, personal correspondence).

a) Assuming that the duration of infectiousness was 7 days, use these estimates to calculate the average number of infectious individuals in each age group before the introduction of vaccination.

b) Use these estimates of the average numbers of infectious individuals to calculate:

   (i)   the β parameters for matrix model 2 (see Section 7.5.4.1) assuming that $\alpha = 1$;

   (ii) R_0, assuming that there were 50,000 individuals in each single year age group;

   (iii) the herd immunity threshold.

Vary the size of α for model 2, without changing the size of β.

c) How does the size of α influence assumptions about mixing between individuals and the herd immunity threshold?

d) Use the values for the number of susceptible individuals in Table 7.3 for the period 1994/5 to explore how α affects estimates of R_n and whether this is consistent with the values presented in Figure 7.17.

7.5 The following WAIFW matrix which describes contact between those aged <15 and ≥15 years, was obtained by fitting model predictions of the daily numbers of reported cases of influenza to the data shown in Figure 7.3 (see Model 7.1, online), in which the β parameters are in units of per day:

Age group
(years)   <15   ≥15
$\begin{array}{c} <15 \\ \geq 15 \end{array} \begin{pmatrix} 3.38 \times 10^{-4} & 3.57 \times 10^{-5} \\ 3.57 \times 10^{-5} & 7.14 \times 10^{-5} \end{pmatrix}$

a) Assuming that there were 2,639 children and 5,361 adults in the population, and that the infectious period is two days, write down the Next Generation Matrix and calculate R_0.

b) Assuming that there are sufficient vaccination doses for only 2500 individuals for use before the start of a pandemic, use estimates of the net reproduction number to decide whether it would be best to provide the vaccines to

(i) children only;

(ii) adults only;

(iii) the same proportion of children and adults;

(iv) equal numbers of children and adults.

References

1 Borgdorff MW, Nagelkerke NJ, van SD, Broekmans JF. Transmission of tuberculosis between people of different ages in The Netherlands: an analysis using DNA fingerprinting. *Int J Tuberc Lung Dis* 1999; 3(3):202–206.

2 Edmunds WJ, Kafatos G, Wallinga J, Mossong JR. Mixing patterns and the spread of close-contact infectious diseases. *Emerg Themes Epidemiol* 2006; 3:10.:10.

3 van Soolingen D, Borgdorff MW, de Haas PE et al. Molecular epidemiology of tuberculosis in the Netherlands: a nationwide study from 1993 through 1997. *J Infect Dis* 1999; 180(3):726–736.

4 Ministry of Health. The influenza pandemic in England and Wales 1957–58. 100. 1960. London, Her Majesty's Stationery Office. Reports on Public Health and Medical Subjects.

5 Anderson RM, May RM. Infectious Diseases of Humans. Dynamics and control. Oxford: Oxford University Press; 1992.

6 Mikolajczyk RT, Akmatov MK, Rastin S, Kretzschmar M. Social contacts of school children and the transmission of respiratory-spread pathogens. *Epidemiol Infect* 2008; 136(6):813–822.

7 Beutels P, Shkedy Z, Aerts M, van DP. Social mixing patterns for transmission models of close contact infections: exploring self-evaluation and diary-based data collection through a web-based interface. *Epidemiol Infect* 2006; 134(6):1158–1166.

8 Edmunds WJ, O'Callaghan CJ, Nokes DJ. Who mixes with whom? A method to determine the contact patterns of adults that may lead to the spread of airborne infections. *Proc Biol Sci* 1997; 264(1384):949–957.

9 Wallinga J, Teunis P, Kretzschmar M. Using data on social contacts to estimate age-specific transmission parameters for respiratory-spread infectious agents. *Am J Epidemiol* 2006; 164(10):936–944.

10 Mossong J, Hens N, Jit M et al. Social Contacts and Mixing Patterns Relevant to the Spread of Infectious Diseases. *PLoS Medicine* 2008; 5(3).

11 Farrington CP. Modelling forces of infection for measles, mumps and rubella. *Stat Med* 1990; 9(8):953–967.

12 Kanaan MN, Farrington CP. Matrix models for childhood infections: a Bayesian approach with applications to rubella and mumps. *Epidemiol Infect* 2005; 133(6):1009–1021.

13 Anderson RM, May RM. Age-related changes in the rate of disease transmission: implications for the design of vaccination programmes. *J Hyg (Lond)* 1985; 94(3):365–436.

14 Babad HR, Nokes DJ, Gay NJ, Miller E, Morgan-Capner P, Anderson RM. Predicting the impact of measles vaccination in England and Wales: model validation and analysis of policy options. *Epidemiol Infect* 1995; 114(2):319–344.

15 Brisson M, Edmunds WJ, Gay NJ, Law B, De SG. Modelling the impact of immunization on the epidemiology of varicella zoster virus. *Epidemiol Infect* 2000; 125(3):651–669.

16 Trotter CL, Gay NJ, Edmunds WJ. Dynamic models of meningococcal carriage, disease, and the impact of serogroup C conjugate vaccination. *Am J Epidemiol* 2005; 162(1):89–100.

17 Farrington CP, Kanaan MN, Gay NJ. Estimation of the basic reproduction number for infectious diseases from age-stratified serological survey. *Appl Statist* 2001; 50(3):1–33.

18 Farrington CP, Whitaker HJ. Contact surface models for infectious diseases: estimation from serologic survey data. *Journal of the American Statistical Association* 2005; 100(470):370–379.

19 Diekmann O, Heesterbeek JA, Metz JA. On the definition and the computation of the basic reproduction ratio R_0 in models for infectious diseases in heterogeneous populations. *J Math Biol* 1990; 28(4):365–382.

20 Ramsay M, Gay N, Miller E et al. The epidemiology of measles in England and Wales: rationale for the 1994 national vaccination campaign. *Commun Dis Rep CDR Rev* 1994; 4(12):R141–R146.

21 Gay NJ, Hesketh LM, Morgan-Capner P, Miller E. Interpretation of serological surveillance data for measles using mathematical models: implications for vaccine strategy. *Epidemiol Infect* 1995; 115(1):139–156.

22 Gay N, Ramsay M, Cohen B et al. The epidemiology of measles in England and Wales since the 1994 vaccination campaign. *Commun Dis Rep CDR Rev* 1997; 7(2):R17–R21.

23 Miller E. The new measles campaign. *BMJ* 1994; 309(6962):1102–1103.

24 Vyse AJ, Gay NJ, White JM et al. Evolution of surveillance of measles, mumps, and rubella in England and Wales: providing the platform for evidence-based vaccination policy. *Epidemiol Rev* 2002; 24(2):125–136.

25 Ferguson NM, Cummings DA, Cauchemez S et al. Strategies for containing an emerging influenza pandemic in Southeast Asia. *Nature* 2005; 437(7056):209–214.

26 Germann TC, Kadau K, Longini IM, Jr., Macken CA. Mitigation strategies for pandemic influenza in the United States. *Proc Natl Acad Sci U S A* 2006; 103(15):5935–5940.

27 Cooper BS, Pitman RJ, Edmunds WJ, Gay NJ. Delaying the international spread of pandemic influenza. *PLoS Med* 2006; 3(6):e212.

28 Keeling MJ, Woolhouse ME, May RM, Davies G, Grenfell BT. Modelling vaccination strategies against foot-and-mouth disease. *Nature* 2003; 421(6919):136–142.

29 Heesterbeek JAP. R_0 PhD thesis, University of Leiden 1992.

Chapter 8

Sexually transmitted infections

8.1 Overview and objectives

This chapter introduces you to models of sexually transmitted infections (STIs). By the end of this chapter, you should:

- Understand the important characteristics of sexually transmitted infections and how they differ from the infections modelled so far;
- Use simple deterministic compartmental models to explore the transmission dynamics of short-duration curable STIs such as gonorrhoea to:
  - Explore the importance of heterogeneity in sexual activity for STI invasion and endemic prevalence (insights from the 'Hethcote–Yorke' models)
  - Appreciate the importance of mixing patterns on R_0, the rate of STI spread, the equilibrium STI prevalence and the utility of 'Q', a summary measure of mixing
  - Explore the importance of heterogeneity in sexual activity and mixing patterns for STI control
  - Appreciate the similarity between a heterosexual STI model and a host-vector infection model
- Use a simple deterministic compartmental model to explore the transmission dynamics of HIV/AIDS;
- Explore the effect of partnership concurrency on R_0 and the rate of STI spread;
- Appreciate the insights gained by network modelling of STI transmission and control.

8.2 Characteristics of sexually transmitted infections

There are some important differences between STIs and the infections modelled so far. In contrast to the directly transmitted respiratory infections modelled in earlier chapters, when modelling infections that require intimate contact such as STIs,[1] the rate at which new infections are generated does not depend on the population density.[2] Close crowding of individuals does not necessarily lead to increases in the rate at which individuals make sexual contact whereas it is likely to increase the rate at which individuals make contacts which are sufficient to transmit respiratory infections (Figure 2.6b). Also, the population at risk of an STI is a subset of the community. For a purely sexually transmitted infection, transmission will only occur between sexually active individuals and so these groups will need to be identified. However, data on sexual behaviours are often difficult to collect and subject to significant bias and therefore need to be interpreted carefully.[3] There is often great heterogeneity in the sexual activity of individuals within and between different populations which will be important for predicting the spread and control of STIs.[4]

The natural history of infection differs markedly between different STIs.[1] STIs are also more likely to be asymptomatic in women than in men, which has implications for identifying control strategies. Some short-duration curable STIs, such as gonorrhoea, chancroid and chlamydia infection, do not induce a significant level of immunity in the host, while long-duration syphilis infection results in latent disease and may induce immunity.[1] Before widespread treatment with antibiotics, syphilis infection in adults was a significant cause of death. A more important cause of death nowadays worldwide is the relatively new STI, human immunodeficiency virus (HIV), which kills in the absence of effective treatment and has become pandemic.[1, 5] Some STIs enhance the probability of the transmission of other STIs.[6–9] Most work in this area has focused on the transmission-enhancing effects on HIV of these other STIs, particularly those that cause genital ulcers such as chancroid, syphilis and HSV-2 infection. Such STIs are referred to as *cofactor* STIs.

These characteristics need to be considered when deciding how to set up models of STI transmission. Figure 8.1 gives examples of the natural history of key STIs that have

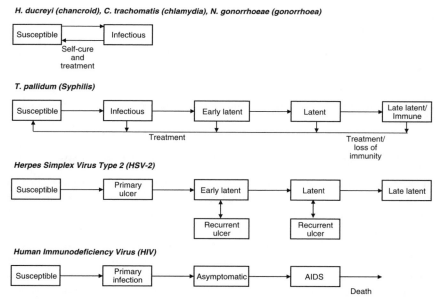

Fig. 8.1 Examples of the natural history of key STIs assumed in modelling studies.[10] Based on White *et al*, 2004.

been assumed in modelling studies. Although model representations are typically based on extensive literature review, some arbitrariness remains in the categorization of STI stages (particularly 'early latent', 'latent' and 'late latent').

An important period in the modelling of STIs occurred during the 1970s and 1980s with the work of Cooke and Yorke, who were the first to develop a mathematical model of gonorrhoea transmission that incorporated many of the characteristics described above.[11] In this paper and in a subsequent monograph,[2] they used deterministic compartmental models of the transmission dynamics of gonorrhoea, together with data on the dramatic increase in the reported number of gonorrhoea cases between 1950 and 1980 in the US (Figure 8.2), to explore the transmission dynamics of gonorrhoea and evaluate possible control strategies.[2]

There was great concern about how best to control this rapid increase. This rise had been attributed to increases in sexual risk behaviour and the introduction of hormonal contraception, replacing condom use, but was probably also partly due to improved surveillance. The elegant and well parameterized modelling studies by Hethcote and

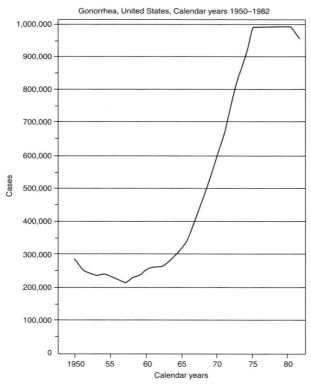

Fig. 8.2 Reported cases of gonorrhoea in the US from 1950 to 1982. Cited in Hethcote and Yorke, 1984.[2] Original source: Statistical Services Section, Division of Venereal Disease Control, Centers for Disease Control, USA.

colleagues provided important insights into the transmission and control of gonorrhoea in the US and were used to inform US STI control policy.

We begin by describing some of Hethcote and Yorke's models, the insights these models provided, and illustrate how extensions to these models have led to an improved understanding of the transmission and control of STIs.

8.3 What prevalence of gonorrhoea infection might we expect? Insights from the Hethcote–Yorke model

Based on the data in Figure 8.2 and an estimate of the size of the sexually active population in the US, it was estimated that the prevalence of individuals infected with *N. gonorrhoea*, the bacteria that causes gonorrhoea, in the sexually active population was around 2 per cent.

Let us start our exploration of the transmission dynamics of gonorrhoea by seeing if we can reproduce this estimated prevalence using a transmission model. To do this, we shall (as Hethcote and Yorke did) first consider the simplest model possible, describing a population that consists of individuals that are not differentiated by gender, age, sexual behaviour or any other characteristic except whether or not they are infected. We assume all infected individuals are infectious (Figure 8.3).

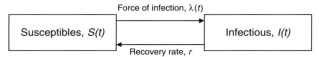

Fig. 8.3 A simple model of STI transmission dynamics (Model 8.1, online).

The equations for our simple model of STI transmission in Figure 8.3 are:

$$\frac{dS(t)}{dt} = -\lambda(t)\,S(t) + rI(t) \qquad\qquad 8.1$$

$$\frac{dI(t)}{dt} = +\lambda(t)\,S(t) - rI(t) \qquad\qquad 8.2$$

Where $S(t)$ and $I(t)$ are the numbers of susceptible and infectious individuals at time t, respectively, $\lambda(t)$ is the force of infection at time t, and r is the recovery rate per year, assumed equal to $1/D$ where D is the duration of infection in years. The population size, N, equals the sum of the number of susceptible and infectious individuals. We assume the population is closed and therefore N does not change over time, ie $N = S(t) + I(t)$.

Let us also assume random mixing and assume that each individual changes sexual partners at a constant rate per year, c, and the probability of transmission of the STI during a sexual partnership between STI discordant partners is β_p.

In earlier chapters where we modelled infections transmitted via the respiratory route, we described two formulations for the force of infection expression assuming *density* or *frequency dependence* (Panel 2.5).

$$\lambda(t) = \beta I(t) \quad \textit{density dependence (pseudo mass action)} \qquad 8.3$$

$$\lambda(t) = c_e \frac{I(t)}{N(t)} \quad \textit{frequency dependence (true mass action)} \qquad 8.4$$

where β was defined differently as the rate at which two specific individuals come into effective contact per unit time and c_e was the average number of individuals effectively contacted by each person per unit time.

Assuming *density dependence* means we assumed the force of infection increases with increased population size while assuming *frequency dependence* means we assumed the force of infection does not change with population size. For STIs and other infections that require intimate contact between individuals, increasing the number of individuals in a room (for example) will not increase the rate at which individuals change sexual partners, and therefore the *frequency dependence* assumption is the most appropriate.

Furthermore, the two implicit components of the transmission parameter ('β' in early chapters)—the contact rate and the transmission probability per contact—are usually separated into two separate parameters when modelling STIs. This is primarily because, for STIs, it is believed the contact rate can be measured more easily than for respiratory infections by, for example, asking the question '*How many sexual partners have you had in the last 12 months?*'.

STI transmission can be modelled at the *per-act* or the *per-partnership* level. Modelling at the per-act level, the correct contact rate parameter is the coital frequency per unit time and the correct transmission probability parameter is the transmission probability per sex-act β_a. Modelling at the per-partnership level, the correct contact rate parameter is the partner change rate, c, and the correct transmission probability parameter is the transmission probability per partnership β_p. In this chapter we model STIs at the per-partnership level as this is most common, but all the models can be reformulated at the per-act level. The relationship between β_a and β_p is discussed in more detail in Panel 8.1.

If we assume random mixing, the equation for the force of infection $\lambda(t)$ is defined as the product of the partner change rate, c, the transmission probability per partnership, β_p, and the prevalence of infection at time t, $\frac{I(t)}{N}$

$$\lambda(t) = c \beta_p \frac{I(t)}{N} \qquad 8.5$$

Using Equation 8.5 and the equations for our simple model of STI transmission (Equations 8.1 and 8.2) we can now make predictions for the spread of gonorrhoea in our population.

However, if we assume plausible parameter values, an average partner change rate, c, of two partners per year, a transmission probability per partnership, β_p, of 0.75, and a duration of infection with some treatment services in the population, D, of two months (0.167 years) we quickly encounter problems because gonorrhoea fails to spread (Figure 8.5).

Panel 8.1 Per-act and per-partnership transmission probabilities

STIs are transmitted during sexual contacts or acts and therefore it is natural to try to model at the level of the sexual act. However, the data on transmission probabilities are commonly available from studies of sexual partnerships. If we have an estimate of the number of acts within a partnership and we assume that the per-act transmission probability does not vary over time (which may not be true), we can easily calculate the per-act transmission probability from the per-partnership probability using a binomial model:[81]

$$\beta_p = 1 - (1 - \beta_a)^n \qquad\qquad 8.6$$

Where β_p is the transmission probability per sexual partnership, β_a is the transmission probability per sexual act, and n is the number of sex acts in the partnership after infection of the index case. This equation is analogous to the Reed–Frost equation discussed in Chapter 6 and can be understood by considering the constituent parts in turn:

$1 - \beta_a$ is the probability of **not getting** infected in 1 sex act

$(1 - \beta_a)^n$ is the probability of **not getting** infected in n sex acts

$1 - (1 - \beta_a)^n$ is the probability of **getting** infected in n sex acts

STIs with high transmission probabilities, such as gonorrhoea and chlamydia infection, will quickly transmit to sexual partners, while STIs with low transmission probabilities such as HIV in the asymptomatic stage and in the absence of other cofactors for transmission will take much longer to transmit to sexual partners. The relationship between β_p and β_a is shown for a range of transmission probabilities in Figure 8.4.

This has important implications for the impact of condom use in preventing infection.[82, 83] For highly infectious STIs such as gonorrhoea, chlamydia and HIV during the primary stage of infection, inconsistent condom use has little effect in preventing transmission. For less infectious STIs such as HIV during the asymptomatic stage and in the absence of other cofactors for transmission, even inconsistent condom use can still have a significant impact.

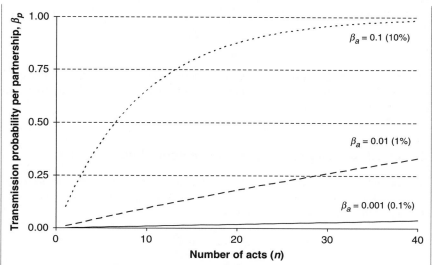

Fig. 8.4 The relationship between the transmission probability per partnership (β_p) and per sex-act (β_a) for n sex acts.

To understand why this occurs we can calculate the R_0 for this infection in this population. The R_0 for this infection in this population is derived in Panel 8.2 and is given by the expression:

$$R_0 = c\beta_p D \qquad\qquad 8.7$$

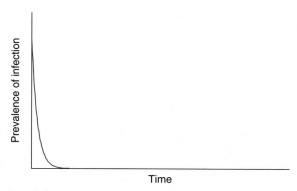

Fig. 8.5 Prediction of the prevalence of infectious individuals over time after the introduction of one infectious case assuming $\beta_p = 0.75$, $D = 0.167$ years, $c = 2$ partners/year. (Model 8.1, online.)

Now we can see why gonorrhoea failed to spread. R_0 was well below one.

$$R_0 = 2 \times 0.75 \times 0.167$$
$$= 0.25$$

Note that the level of sexual activity that is necessary to raise R_0 above one ($c \geq 1 / \beta_p D$) will differ for different STIs because β_p and D vary between STIs (see Boily and Masse 1997 for more examples).[12]

Panel 8.2 Derivation of R_0 for simple gonorrhoea model

We can obtain R_0 for this infection using a similar approach to that used in Section 4.2.2.1. Using Equations 8.2 and 8.5 we can write down an equation for the rate of change of the number of infectious individuals.

$$\frac{dI(t)}{dt} = \lambda(t)S(t) - rI(t)$$
$$= c\beta_p \frac{I(t)}{N} S(t) - rI(t)$$

If the STI is to spread then the rate of change of the number of infectious individuals must be greater than zero, i.e.:

$$c\beta_p \frac{I(t)}{N} S(t) - rI(t) > 0 \tag{8.8}$$

Rearranging, we get:

$$c\beta_p \frac{I(t)}{N} S(t) > rI(t) \tag{8.9}$$

Cancelling $I(t)$ from both sides of the equation and recognizing that when $t=0$, $S(0) \sim N$, we get:

$$c\beta_p > r \tag{8.10}$$

Substituting $1/D$ for r and rearranging we get:

$$c\beta_p D > 1 \tag{8.11}$$

So, for the number of infectious persons to increase following the introduction of an infectious person into a totally susceptible population, the quantity $c\beta_p D$ must be greater than one. During their infectious period of duration D, a single infectious person will have cD sexual partners. Of these, a proportion β_p will be infected and therefore $c\beta_p D$ equals the average number of secondary infectious persons resulting from a single infectious person in a totally susceptible population. As this is the verbal definition of R_0 and $c\beta_p D$ has the correct threshold behaviour, it is reasonable to define $R_0 = c\beta_p D$.

By rearranging Equation 8.7 we can see that if we assume $\beta_p = 0.75$, if gonorrhoea is to invade the population we would need to assume an average partner change rate in the whole sexually active population of eight partners per year, or duration of infection of eight months, or intermediate values for both. These relatively high parameter values are unlikely.

The primary reason we are failing to predict that gonorrhoea will spread in population is not the parameter values we are assuming, but that we are ignoring one of the important characteristics listed above—heterogeneity in human sexual behaviour. Surveys of the sexual behaviour of STI clinics attendees and the general population show that over any period of time most people have relatively low numbers of sexual partners but some have much higher numbers (Figure 8.6). This heterogeneity is very important for the understanding the spread and control of STIs.

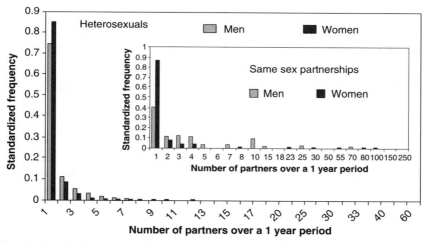

Fig. 8.6 The distribution of reported annual number of partners for heterosexual and homosexual men and women in Britain from the National Survey of Sexual Attitudes and Lifestyles, 2000. The plots show the relative number of partners and excludes individuals who report zero partners. From Schneeberger et al, 2004.[4]

8.4 The importance of heterogeneity in sexual activity for STI transmission dynamics

We can explore the implications of heterogeneity in sexual activity for the spread of a short-duration STI by adapting our model. In line with the findings of Hethcote and Yorke, modelling heterogeneity in sexual activity allows us to predict that gonorrhoea will invade our population while assuming more plausible values for the rate at which individuals change partners than we had to assume using the simple model shown in Figure 8.3. We first describe the key equations and assumptions for the model.

8.4.1 **Incorporating risk heterogeneity in the Hethcote and Yorke model—key assumptions**

We split the population into two groups based on the frequency at which individuals change their partners. More highly sexually active individuals are members of the high-activity group and less active individuals are members of the low-activity group.

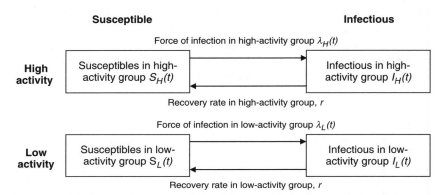

Fig. 8.7 Model of gonorrhoea transmission incorporating heterogeneity in activity (Model 8.2, online).

The equations for rate of change of the number of susceptible and infectious individuals per unit time in this model are very similar to Equation 8.1 and Equation 8.2:

$$\frac{dS_j(t)}{dt} = -\lambda_j(t)S_j(t) + rI_j(t) \tag{8.12}$$

$$\frac{dI_j(t)}{dt} = +\lambda_j(t)S_j(t) - rI_j(t) \tag{8.13}$$

Where $j = {}_H$ for the high-activity group and $j = {}_L$ for the low-activity group

To maintain comparability with our simple model (Figure 8.3) we keep the total number of partnerships formed per year equal in both models but increase the difference (heterogeneity) between the partner change rates in the high and low-activity groups (see Panel 8.3 for details of how to do this). Following Hethcote and Yorke, we assume 2 per cent of the population belong to the high-activity group and 98 per cent belong to the low-activity group. Therefore if we assume the partner change rate in the low-activity group, c_L, is 1.4 partners per year, then, to keep the mean rate of partner change at two partners per year the partner change rate in the high-activity group, c_H, has to be 31.4 partners per year.

Initially we assume *proportionate mixing*, i.e. partners are chosen with a probability that is proportional to the number of partnerships that they generate,[13] and also

---

Panel 8.3 Maintaining overall partner change rate

The equation for the mean rate of partner change is:

$$c_{mean} = c_H \frac{N_H}{N} + c_L \frac{N_L}{N}$$

8.14

To keep the total number of partnerships formed per year equal in both models but increase the difference in the rate of partner change between the high and low-activity groups we rearrange Equation 8.14 to give:

$$c_H = \frac{c_{mean}N - c_L N_L}{N_H}$$

8.15

Equation 8.15 calculates the correct partner change rate for the high-activity group, c_H, if we reduce the partner change rate in the low-activity group, c_L so that the overall mean partner change rate, c_{mean}, remains at two partners per year,

Note: Equation 8.15 can be re-written in terms of the n_H and n_L, the proportions of the population that are in the high and low-activity groups such that $n_H + n_L = 1$:

$$c_H = \frac{c_{mean} - c_L n_L}{n_H}$$

8.16

---

assume that the other parameter values are unchanged, so $\beta_p = 0.75$ and $D = 0.167$ years. Also, for simplicity, we assume that the per-partnership transmission probability is the same in high and low-activity groups (as illustrated in Panel 8.1), although in reality, a high-activity individual is likely to have fewer acts per partnership and therefore β_p may be lower.

The force of infection experienced by a high-activity group member will be higher than for a low-activity group member because of their higher partner change rate (Equation 8.17). However, because we are assuming proportionate mixing, each time a new partner is selected both high and low-activity group members will have the same probability that they select an infected partner, $p(t)$

$$\lambda_j(t) = c_j \beta_p p(t)$$

8.17

Where $j = {}_H$ for the high-activity group and $j = {}_L$ for the low-activity group.

Note that $p(t)$, the probability that a partner selected according to proportionate mixing is infectious, is not the overall prevalence of infectious individuals in the population ($I(t)/N$) as it was for the simple model, but needs to account for the fact that the selected partner can be either a member of the high or low-activity group, and the prevalence of infectious individuals is likely to differ between these two groups.

$$p(t) = g_H \times i_H(t) + g_L \times i_L(t)$$

8.18

where g_H and g_L are the probabilities that a partner selected according to proportionate mixing will be a member of the high or low-activity group, respectively, and $i_H(t)$

and $i_L(t)$ are the prevalence of infectious individuals in the high and low-activity groups, respectively. $i_H(t) = I_H(t)/N_H$ and $i_L(t) = I_L(t)/N_L$ where N_H and N_L are the total number of individuals in the high and low-activity groups, respectively.

Panel 8.4 shows the probability that a partner selected according to proportionate mixing will be a member of the high or the low-activity group, is equal to the proportion of the total number of partnerships generated by each group each year. In our example, this means 31 per cent of partnerships are generated by high-activity group members ($g_H = 0.31$) and 69 per cent are generated by low-activity group members ($g_L = 0.69$).

Panel 8.4 The probability that a partner will be a member of the high or low-activity group assuming proportionate mixing

The probability, g_H, that a partner chosen according to proportionate mixing will be a member of the high-activity group is equal to the number of partnerships generated by high-activity group members per year, $c_H \times N_H$, divided by the total number of partnerships generated in the population each year: $c_H \times N_H + c_L \times N_L$

$$g_H = \frac{c_H \times N_H}{c_H \times N_H + c_L \times N_L} \qquad 8.19$$

By substituting the proportion of the population in these two groups (n_H and n_L) for the sizes of the two groups (N_H and N_L) where $n_H = N_H / N$ and $n_L = N_L / N$, and cancelling the N's, we obtain:

$$g_H = \frac{c_H \times n_H}{c_H \times n_H + c_L \times n_L}$$

$$g_H = \frac{31.4 \times 0.02}{31.4 \times 0.02 + 1.4 \times 0.98} = 0.31 \qquad 8.20$$

Similarly g_L is the probability that partner chosen according to proportionate mixing will be a member of the low-activity group. This can be calculated to be 0.69 using Equation 8.20 and substituting in the values of c_L and n_L in the numerator, or by noting that the probability of selecting either a high or low-activity group member must sum to one, ie, $g_H + g_L = 1$, and therefore $g_L = 1 - g_H = 1 - 0.31 = 0.69$.

8.4.2 Calculating R_0 in a population with heterogeneity in sexual activity

To estimate whether gonorrhoea will invade the population we first need to calculate the number of secondary infections generated in a totally susceptible population by an infected high-activity, R_H, or low-activity, R_L, group member:

$$R_H = c_H \beta_p D$$
$$= 31.4 \times 0.75 \times 0.167$$
$$= 3.93 \qquad\qquad 8.21$$

$$R_L = c_L \beta_p D$$
$$= 1.4 \times 0.75 \times 0.167$$
$$= 0.18 \qquad\qquad 8.22$$

Therefore, at invasion, around 22 times more infections will be caused by each infected high-activity group member than by each infected low-activity group member.

However, we cannot tell from these values whether gonorrhoea will invade because R_H is above one, and R_L is below one.

To find out if gonorrhoea will invade our single-gender model with heterogeneity in activity and proportionate mixing we need to calculate R_0. As described in Chapter 7, we can calculate R_0 using several approaches and these are shown in Panel 8.5 and Appendix A.6.

Method (a) in Panel 8.5 shows that R_0 is the weighted average of the number of secondary infections from high-activity and low-activity members, where the weights, g_H (0.31) and g_L (0.69), are the probabilities that a partner selected according to proportionate mixing will be a member of the high or low-activity group respectively.

$$R_0 = g_H R_H + g_L R_L$$
$$= 0.31 \times 3.93 + 0.69 \times 0.18$$
$$= 1.36 \qquad\qquad 8.23$$

Importantly, this means that by introducing heterogeneity in sexual activity into our model, while we have kept the mean rate of partner change per year constant, we have been able to predict that gonorrhoea will invade the population (Figure 8.8).

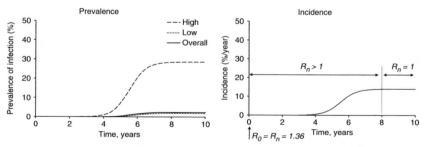

Fig. 8.8 Predicted prevalence and overall incidence of gonorrhoea in a model with heterogeneity in sexual activity. The right-hand figure also shows the relationship between the basic (R_0) and net (R_n) reproduction numbers. $\beta_p = 0.75$, $D = 0.167$ years, $c_L = 1.4$ partners/year, $c_H = 31.4$ partners/year. Two per cent of the population belong to the high-activity group. (Model 8.2, online.)

Panel 8.5 Calculating R_0 in a population with heterogeneity in sexual activity and proportionate mixing

We can use any of the methods described in Chapter 7 to calculate the R_0 for an STI in a population with heterogeneity in sexual activity. In this panel we show how to calculate R_0 for a two-group model with heterogeneity in sexual activity and proportionate mixing by (a) solving the simultaneous equations of the average number of secondary infections caused by a single infection in a typical infectee and (b) based on the mean and variance of the partnership distribution. In Appendix A.6 we show how to calculate R_0 using a matrix determinant approach or by calculating the dominant eigenvalue of the next generation matrix by simulation.

(a) Calculate R_0 by solving the simultaneous equations of the average number of secondary infections caused by a single infection in a typical infectee.

The basic reproduction number of gonorrhoea in this population is the average number of secondary infections caused by a single infection in a *typical infectee* introduced into a susceptible population. The typical infectee is some theoretical average of a high and low-activity individual. If we let x be the probability the typical infectee is a member of the high-activity group, and $1-x$ be the probability the typical infectee is a member of the low-activity group, R_0 is the maximum value that satisfies the following matrix equation.

$$\begin{pmatrix} R_{HH} & R_{HL} \\ R_{LH} & R_{LL} \end{pmatrix} \begin{pmatrix} x \\ 1-x \end{pmatrix} = R_0 \begin{pmatrix} x \\ 1-x \end{pmatrix} \qquad 8.24$$

Where R_{HH} is the number of secondary infections in high-activity members generated by an infected high-activity member, R_{LH} is the number of secondary infections in low-activity members generated by an infected high-activity member, R_{HL} is the number of secondary infections in high-activity members generated by an infected low-activity member, and R_{LL} is the number of secondary infections in low-activity members generated by an infected low-activity member.

Using Equations 8.21 and 8.22 we know that in a completely susceptible population, a high-activity member generates R_H (3.93) infections and a low-activity member generates R_L (0.18) infections. As we assume proportional mixing, using Equation 8.20 we also know that 31 per cent (g_H) of these infections will be transmitted to high-activity members and 69 per cent (g_L) will be transmitted to low-activity members, so we can write:

$$\begin{pmatrix} R_H g_H & R_L g_H \\ R_H g_L & R_L g_L \end{pmatrix} \begin{pmatrix} x \\ 1-x \end{pmatrix} = R_0 \begin{pmatrix} x \\ 1-x \end{pmatrix} \qquad 8.25$$

The two implicit equations can be solved for R_0, eliminating the unknown term, x:

$$R_H g_H x + R_L g_H (1-x) = R_0 x \qquad 8.26$$

$$R_H g_L x + R_L g_L (1-x) = R_0 (1-x) \qquad 8.27$$

Rearranging Equation 8.26 we get:

$$x = \frac{-R_L g_H}{g_H (R_H - R_L) - R_0} \qquad 8.28$$

Substituting Equation 8.28 into Equation 8.27 we get the rather untidy equation:

$$R_H g_L \frac{-R_L g_H}{g_H (R_H - R_L) - R_0} + R_L g_L \left(1 - \frac{-R_L g_H}{g_H (R_H - R_L) - R_0} \right)$$

$$= R_0 \left(1 - \frac{-R_L g_H}{g_H (R_H - R_L) - R_0} \right) \qquad 8.29$$

Multiplying all terms by $g_H(R_H - R_L) - R_0$ and expanding we get:

$$-R_H g_L R_L g_H + R_H g_L R_L g_H - R_L g_L R_L g_H - R_L g_L R_0 + R_L g_L R_L g_H$$

$$= R_H g_H R_0 - R_L g_H R_0 - R_0^2 + R_L g_H R_0 \qquad 8.30$$

Most of these terms cancel and after a little rearrangement this reduces to:

$$-R_H g_H - R_L g_L = -R_0 \qquad 8.31$$

And one further rearrangement yields:

$$R_0 = g_H R_H + g_L R_L \qquad 8.32$$

From Panel 8.4 we know $g_H = 0.31$ and $g_L = 0.69$, so:

$$R_0 = 0.31 \times 3.93 + 0.69 \times 0.18$$

$$= 1.36$$

(b) Calculate R_0 based on the mean and variance of the partnership distribution

Alternatively we can use an approximation based on the mean and variance of the partnership distribution to calculate R_0.[33] In this method R_0 is calculated using the *effective partner change rate*, $\hat{c}$, where $\hat{c}$ is the 'epidemiologically relevant' average number of sexual partners and can be much larger than the simple mean if the variance in the number of partners is high.

In a population with heterogeneity in activity, $\hat{c}$ can be approximated by the sum of the arithmetic mean, c, and the variance, σ^2, divided by the arithmetic mean.[33]

$$\hat{c} = c + \sigma^2 / c \qquad 8.33$$

As 2 per cent of our population have a partner change rate of 31.4 partners per year and 98 per cent of our population have a partner change rate of 1.4 partners per year, the variance is 17.6 (calculated here using the Excel 'VARP' function).

Panel 8.5 Calculating R_0 in a population with heterogeneity in sexual activity and proportionate mixing (continued)

As the mean partner change rate is two partners per year, the *effective partner change* rate is:

$$\hat{c} = 2 + 17.6 \ / \ 2$$
$$= 10.8$$

Substituting $\hat{c}$ into Equation 8.7 we get:

$$R_0 = \hat{c}\beta_p D$$
$$= 10.8 \times 0.75 \times 0.167$$
$$= 1.36 \qquad\qquad 8.34$$

Figure 8.8 also shows that introducing heterogeneity in sexual activity has also enabled us to predict a low overall infection prevalence of 2.3 per cent that is in line with the 2 per cent prevalence estimated by Hethcote and Yorke for the sexually active US population in the 1980s. This was achieved using parameter values for the overall sexual behaviour of the population that are much more plausible than those used in the model that did not incorporate heterogeneity in sexual activity. Other heterogeneities also make it more likely infections will persist.[14] To explore this further see Garnett and Anderson.[15]

Figure 8.9 shows more generally what happens if we increase the difference between the partner change rates in the high and low-activity groups. Once heterogeneity increases above a critical level, R_0 rises above one and gonorrhoea can invade. In our example this occurs when the partner change rate is around 1.5 per year in the low-activity group and therefore around 26 per year in the high-activity group.

Figure 8.9 also shows that if we continue to increase heterogeneity in sexual activity then gonorrhoea prevalence in the overall population first increases and then decreases. In our example, the overall prevalence peaks at around 0.8 and 61 partners per year in the low and high-activity groups respectively, after which further increases in heterogeneity leads to a reduction in the overall prevalence.

This is because the impact of increasing heterogeneity on reducing the partner change rate in the low-activity group starts to exceed the impact of increasing heterogeneity on increasing the prevalence of infection in the high-activity group.

In the extreme case in which the partner change rate in the low-activity group becomes zero, gonorrhoea becomes extinct in the low-activity group.

Heterogeneity in sexual activity is also important in explaining why the infection can be maintained at a low and relatively stable prevalence in the population as a whole. In the absence of immunity, contact with already-infected individuals (called *pre-emptive saturation*[84]), is the only mechanism to prevent the prevalence of infection rising to 100 per cent (see Panel 8.6). However, in a population without heterogeneity in sexual activity and low infection prevalence, the proportion of potentially effective contacts that would be 'wasted' on infected individuals would be very low, and therefore it is an implausible mechanism for limiting transmission. However, as we have

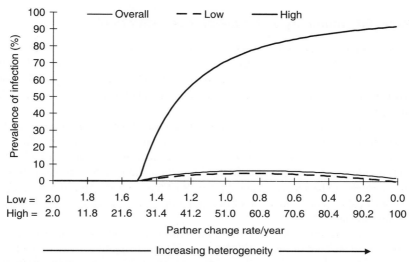

Fig. 8.9 The effect of increasing heterogeneity in sexual activity in a population on equilibrium STI prevalence. The mean rate of partner change remains constant at two partners per year. $\beta_p = 0.75$, $D = 0.167$ years. Two per cent of the population belong to the high-activity group. (Model 8.2, online.)

seen, heterogeneity in sexual activity means that prevalence is very much higher in the high-activity group than in the overall population (Figure 8.9) and therefore in the high-activity group the effects of saturation are much stronger. In our example the prevalence is around 30 per cent in the high-activity group and therefore nearly one in three contacts between infectious individuals and high-activity group members will be 'wasted' on already-infected individuals. As such, *pre-emptive saturation* becomes a much more plausible mechanism to limit transmission.

More generally, what happens after the infection invades a population depends not only on the value of R_0 but also on whether infection is followed by re-susceptibility, immunity or death. For infections such as gonorrhoea that do not invoke an effective immune response in the host, infection prevalence rises steadily to its equilibrium level (Figure 8.8). As this happens the net reproduction number, R_n, falls from its initial value of R_0 (1.36 here) to 1 when equilibrium prevalence is reached (Figure 8.8). Whereas, if infection leads to immunity or death the prevalence of infected and infectious individuals can rise and then fall—see Section 4.2 for an example of this effect due to immunity and Section 8.8 for an example of this effect due to death from HIV/ AIDS.

8.4.3 Proportion of infections due to the high-activity group

As we have seen, although they make up only 2 per cent of the population, the high-activity group generates 31 per cent of the partnerships in the population, suggesting they may generate 31 per cent of new infections, but they actually generate much more

Panel 8.6 Immunity and 'pre-emptive saturation'

An STI can invade a population if the R_0 of the STI in the population is above one, but after introduction the prevalence of infection cannot increase indefinitely as it is bounded by 100 per cent. Therefore some mechanism must be responsible for reducing the number of secondary infections generated by infectious cases from the R_0 value.

For infections such as measles, mumps, rubella and others that induce immunity in the host, transmission is limited primarily by the increasing proportion of contacts that are between infected and immune individuals. These 'wasted' contacts do not cause new infections in the population and therefore do not increase the prevalence. The left-hand side of Figure 8.10 shows an example in which, for a hypothetical infection, three out of four potentially effective contacts are 'wasted' on immune individuals.

Most short-duration STIs do not induce immunity in the host. In fact, short-duration STIs could not persist if they induced sterilizing immunity in the host because they rely on repeatedly re-infecting the same high-risk individuals. Inducing immunity in the host would greatly limit their reproductive success.

So, what limits the rise in prevalence of these STIs? This process was named 'pre-emptive saturation' by Yorke *et al.*[84] It acts in the same way as immunity, and arises because the contacts of infectious individuals are 'wasted' not on immune individuals, but on individuals who are already infected (Figure 8.10 right).

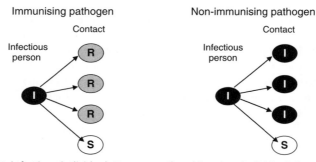

Fig. 8.10 I, infectious individual; R, recovered and immune individual; S, susceptible individual.

This suggests that if two infections are identical in every way (duration of infectiousness, transmission probability per contact, etc.) except that infection with one pathogen results in recovery and re-susceptibility in the host (Figure 8.10 right), and infection with the other pathogen results in recovery and induces immunity in the host (Figure 8.10 left), we would expect the prevalence of infected individuals to be higher for the non-immunizing infection. This is because for non-immunizing infections, only infected individuals can limit the number of secondary infections generated by infectious cases.

because they are also more likely to be infected than low-activity individuals. We can calculate the proportion of all new cases that are generated by high-activity group members when gonorrhoea is in equilibrium using an equation derived by Hethcote and Yorke in their monograph (the derivation is not shown here: see Hethcote and Yorke 1984, pp. 30–31):[2]

$$
\begin{aligned}
h_{eq} &= \frac{g_H i_H(\infty)}{g_H i_H(\infty) + g_L i_L(\infty)} \\
&= \frac{0.31 \times 28.4\%}{0.31 \times 28.4\% + 0.69 \times 1.7\%} \\
&= 88\%
\end{aligned}
\qquad 8.35
$$

Where $i_H(\infty)$ and $i_L(\infty)$ are the equilibrium prevalence of gonorrhoea infection in the high and low-activity group, respectively. These values of $i_H(\infty)$ and $i_L(\infty)$ used in Equation 8.35 were obtained from the model (see in Figure 8.8).

So in our example, the high-activity group is only 2 per cent of the population, but it generates 31 per cent of the partnerships and 88 per cent of new infections (Figure 8.11), highlighting that high-activity individuals are a priority population for STI control efforts because they are at high risk of STI infection and also for onward STI transmission.

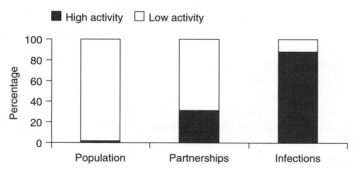

Fig. 8.11 Percentage of population, sexual partnerships and infections generated by the high and low-activity groups in a simple susceptible–infectious–susceptible (SIS) model of the transmission of gonorrhoea assuming proportionate mixing, heterogeneity in sexual behaviour and the parameter values shown in the text.

8.5 **Mixing by sexual activity**

In Chapter 7 we saw that the degree to which the various groups within a population contact each other strongly determines the impact of interventions designed to control respiratory infections. This is also the case for sexually transmitted infections.

8.5.1 Mixing patterns and mixing matrices

Until now we have been assuming *proportionate* mixing by sexual activity, but this is only one possibility. Mixing between population groups can be broadly categorised into three types:

- *Proportionate mixing*, so called because partnerships are formed between population groups based on the proportion of all partnerships generated by these groups. This is also sometimes called *random mixing*, but this can be confused with randomly selecting partners based on the proportion of *individuals* in each group. Therefore describing this type of mixing as *random* is discouraged.

- *With-like mixing*, in which individuals preferentially form partnerships with individuals who have characteristics like their own, for example those with many sexual partners preferentially choose partners who also have many sexual partners. This is often called *assortative mixing*.

- *With-unlike mixing*, in which individuals preferentially form partnerships with individuals who have characteristics unlike their own, for example those with many sexual partners preferentially choose partners with few sexual partners. This is often called *disassortative mixing*.

Mixing can be modelled between subgroups defined by any characteristic of the population that is considered important in explaining the spread or control of the infection, such as age (as you saw in the last chapter), race,[16] or gender, as we show in section 8.6.

Similar to the methods used when we considered respiratory infections, contact patterns can be summarized using *mixing matrices* in which each of the elements g_{jk} in the matrix is the probability that someone in group k forms a partnership with someone in group j. In line with the convention used in the previous chapter, the second subscript, k, refers to the 'choosing' partner and the first subscript, j, refers to the 'chosen' partner. These matrices are similar to the WAIFW matrices described in Chapter 7. They differ because the matrix elements in Chapter 7 represented the rate at which two specific individuals come into effective contact and therefore included the transmission probability per contact, whereas for STIs the transmission probability per contact is typically considered separately.

For proportionate mixing, sexual partners in a given group are selected randomly in proportion to the number of partnerships that the group generates. For this assumption the probability that someone in the high-activity group forms a partnership with someone in the high-activity group, g_{HH}, is the same as the probability that someone in the low-activity group forms a partnership with someone in the high-activity group, g_{HL}, i.e. $g_{HH} = g_{HL} = g_H$. In our example, g_H equals 0.31 (see Panel 8.4). Similarly, the probability that someone in the low-activity group forms a partnership with someone in the low-activity group, g_{LL}, is the same as the probability that someone in the high-activity group forms a partnership with someone in the low-activity group, g_{LH}, i.e. $g_{LH} = g_{LL} = g_L$. Here g_L equals 0.69 (Panel 8.4).

Therefore the proportionate mixing matrix for the partner change rates and group sizes we have assumed is:

$$
\begin{array}{c}
\text{\footnotesize Partner } \; k \\
\begin{array}{cc} H & \quad L \end{array} \\
\text{\footnotesize Partner } \; j \;\;
\begin{array}{c} H \\ L \end{array}
\left(
\begin{array}{cc}
g_{HH} & g_{HL} \\
g_{LH} & g_{LL}
\end{array}
\right)
\end{array}
$$

$$
Proportionate \;=\;
\begin{array}{c}
\begin{array}{cc} H & \quad L \end{array} \\
\begin{array}{c} H \\ L \end{array}
\left(
\begin{array}{cc}
0.31 & 0.31 \\
0.69 & 0.69
\end{array}
\right)
\end{array}
\qquad 8.36
$$

Note also that the probabilities in each column of the matrix sum to one because the partner of individual k must be chosen from either the high or low-activity group. Formally, this can be written as:

$$
\sum_j g_{jk} = 1 \qquad\qquad 8.37
$$

The mixing matrices describing purely with-like and purely with-unlike mixing are:

$$
Purely \text{ with-like} \;
\begin{array}{c}
\begin{array}{cc} H & L \end{array} \\
\begin{array}{c} H \\ L \end{array}
\left(
\begin{array}{cc}
1 & 0 \\
0 & 1
\end{array}
\right)
\end{array}
\qquad 8.38
$$

$$
Purely \text{ with-unlike} \;
\begin{array}{c}
\begin{array}{cc} H & L \end{array} \\
\begin{array}{c} H \\ L \end{array}
\left(
\begin{array}{cc}
0 & 1 \\
1 & 0
\end{array}
\right)
\end{array}
\qquad 8.39
$$

8.5.2 A summary measure of mixing—Q

The *degree of mixing* can be summarized using a statistic that has been given the symbol Q by Gupta and colleagues.[17] Q is equal to 0 when all partners are selected proportionately, equal to 1 when all partners are selected purely with-like, and Q is negative when partners are selected purely with-unlike.

Q depends on the elements of the mixing matrix that measure the proportion of partnerships that are formed within groups. These are the elements on the top-left to bottom-right diagonal of the mixing matrix and in our example these are g_{HH} and g_{LL}.

The formula to calculate Q is:

$$
Q = \frac{\left(\displaystyle\sum_{j=k} g_{jk} - 1 \right)}{b-1} \qquad\qquad 8.40
$$

where b is the number of groups. Q is scaled so that it is equal to 0 when all partners are selected proportionately, 1 when all partners are selected purely with-like, and $\dfrac{-1}{b-1}$ when all partners are selected purely with-unlike. So for our two activity-group example, $b = 2$ and therefore $Q = \dfrac{-1}{2-1} = -1$ when partners are selected purely with-unlike. If there were three activity groups, Q would equal $Q = \dfrac{-1}{3-1} = -1/2$ if mixing was purely with-unlike.

Although commonly used, Q has limitations. Q only measures mixing within identical groups, ignoring mixing between similar groups. Q also equally weights mixing within different population groups regardless of the size of these groups. An alternative measure of mixing that may overcome these limitations has recently been proposed by Keeling and colleagues. 'q' weights mixing between similar groups by the size of the group so that mixing within a smaller group would contribute less to the value of q than mixing within a larger group.[18] To date, however, this measure has not been used extensively.

8.5.3 Data on mixing by sexual activity

Data on the mixing between different sexual activity groups are uncommon because data are required on the characteristics of sexual partners. The data shown in Figure 8.12 suggest that, on average, the individuals in these surveys tended to form sexual partnerships with individuals that were more similar to themselves in terms of sexual activity than the proportionate mixing assumption would predict, so Q is just above 0. The data summarized in the top three rows in this figure are based on data from contact tracing studies among US STI clinic patients collected towards the end of the last century. These individuals are likely to be higher risk than other members of the general population and therefore these data do not necessarily generalize to the rest of the US population. However, the data summarized in the bottom row were collected in a survey of the US general population conducted in 1992 and these data also indicate slightly with-like mixing. That mixing by sexual activity is slightly with-like is intuitively plausible, as in general people tend to socialize with people who are similar to themselves.[19]

8.5.4 Modelling mixing by sexual activity

Many methods have been proposed to model mixing between different population groups.[13, 17, 21, 22] The method we use is based on the method proposed by Gupta et al.[17] which allows a range of mixing patterns between activity groups (with-unlike, proportionate, with-like) to be modelled using one model parameter for a two-activity group model.

To start we note that the number of partnerships formed between activity group k with activity group j must equal the number of partnerships formed by activity group j with activity group k. Here we have two activity groups low ($_L$) and high ($_H$), so:

$$g_{HL}c_L N_L = g_{LH}c_H N_H \qquad\qquad 8.41$$

Using Equation 8.37 and Equation 8.41, if we set the g_{HH}, the probability that someone in the high-activity group forms a partnership with someone in the high-activity group, we can write down equations for g_{HL}, g_{LH} and g_{LL} in terms of g_{HH}:

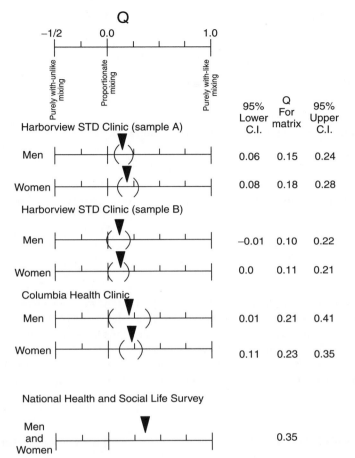

Fig. 8.12 The value of the measure Q for mixing between sexual activity groups in four studies of sexual behaviour in the US, three of which were based on contact tracing in STI clinics, and one (the National Health and Social Life Survey) was based on a survey of the general population. Figure based on Garnett *et al.* 1996.[20] Note in this example Q was calculated on data categorised into three groups, and therefore purely with-unlike mixing was indicated by a Q value of $-1/2$ rather than -1 as in our two-activity group example.

g_{LH}: Using Equation 8.37, $g_{HH} + g_{LH} = 1$, so

$$g_{LH} = 1 - g_{HH} \qquad\qquad 8.42$$

g_{HL}: Rearranging Equation 8.41 for g_{HL} gives:

$$g_{HL} = g_{LH} \frac{c_H N_H}{c_L N_L} \qquad\qquad 8.43$$

Replacing g_{LH} in Equation 8.43 using Equation 8.42, we obtain:

$$g_{HL} = (1 - g_{HH})\frac{c_H N_H}{c_L N_L}$$

$$8.44$$

g_{LL}: From Equation 8.37 we also know:

$$g_{LL} = 1 - g_{HL}$$

$$8.45$$

Substituting g_{LH} in Equation 8.44 into Equation 8.45:

$$g_{LL} = 1 - (1 - g_{HH})\frac{c_H N_H}{c_L N_L}$$

$$8.46$$

These four equations can be summarized as a mixing matrix in terms of g_{HH}:

$$\begin{pmatrix} g_{HH} & g_{HL} \\ g_{LH} & g_{LL} \end{pmatrix} = \begin{pmatrix} g_{HH} & (1 - g_{HH})\dfrac{c_H N_H}{c_L N_L} \\ 1 - g_{HH} & 1 - (1 - g_{HH})\dfrac{c_H N_H}{c_L N_L} \end{pmatrix}$$

$$8.47$$

We can now calculate the values for the elements of the mixing matrix and for Q if the high-activity group selects partners proportionately (i.e. $g_{HH} = 0.31$), purely with-like ($g_{HH} = 1$), or purely with-unlike ($g_{HH} = 0$), and the low-activity group supplies partners to meet these mixing preferences if possible.

To illustrate this, let's assume that the population size is 1000 and therefore there are 20 and 980 individuals in the high and low-activity groups, respectively:

Mixing matrix (using Equation 8.46)	Q value (using Equation 8.40)
Purely with-like mixing by high-activity group	
$\begin{pmatrix} 1 & (1-1)\left(\dfrac{31.4\times20}{1.4\times980}\right) \\ 1-1 & 1-(1-1)\left(\dfrac{31.4\times20}{1.4\times980}\right) \end{pmatrix} = \begin{matrix} \\ H \\ L \end{matrix}\begin{pmatrix} 1 & 0 \\ 0 & 1 \end{pmatrix}$	$Q = (1 + 1 - 1) / (2 - 1)$ $= 1 / 1$ $= 1$
8.48	
Proportionate mixing by high-activity group	
$\begin{pmatrix} 0.31 & (1-0.31)\left(\dfrac{31.4\times20}{1.4\times980}\right) \\ 1-0.31 & 1-(1-0.31)\left(\dfrac{31.4\times20}{1.4\times980}\right) \end{pmatrix} = \begin{matrix} \\ H \\ L \end{matrix}\begin{pmatrix} 0.31 & 0.31 \\ 0.69 & 0.69 \end{pmatrix}$	$Q = (0.31 + 0.69 - 1) / (2 - 1)$ $= 0 / 1$ $= 0$
8.49	

Purely with-unlike mixing by high-activity group

$$\begin{pmatrix} 0 & (1-0)\left(\dfrac{31.4\times20}{1.4\times980}\right) \\ 1-0 & 1-(1-0)\left(\dfrac{31.4\times20}{1.4\times980}\right) \end{pmatrix} = {}^{H}_{L}\begin{pmatrix} {}^{H} & {}^{L} \\ 0 & 0.46 \\ 1 & 0.54 \end{pmatrix}$$

$$Q = (0 + 0.54 - 1) / (2 - 1)$$
$$= -0.46 / 1$$
$$= -0.46$$

8.50

Thus, we can see that for these partner change rates and group sizes, purely with-like, proportionate, or purely with-unlike mixing by high-activity group members is possible (Equation 8.48, Equation 8.49 and Equation 8.50). We can also see that purely with-like or proportionate mixing by the high-activity group members results in purely with-like or proportionate mixing in the population overall, and as expected, Q equals 1 when we model purely with-like mixing and Q equals 0 if we model proportionate mixing.

However, in our example, purely with-unlike mixing by high-activity group members did not result in purely with-unlike mixing by low-activity group members (Equation 8.50). This is because the number of partnerships required by the two activity groups differs. To model purely with-unlike mixing, partner change rates must be altered so that the numbers of partnerships required by both activity groups balance (see Panel 8.7).

In the following section we vary Q between -0.46 and $+1$ so we do not have to alter the partner change rates in the model. This means we can more clearly see the effect of mixing on R_0, and the effect of mixing on the spread of STIs.

8.5.5 Effects of mixing on R_0, rate of STI spread and equilibrium STI prevalence

Let's start by varying Q, while keeping partner change rates and biological parameters (D and β_p) constant, to explore the effect of mixing on R_0. If we vary the proportion of partnerships formed between high-activity group members (g_{HH}) between 0 and 1, Q varies from -0.46 (modelling the most with-unlike mixing pattern without altering partner change rates), through 0 (when mixing is proportionate), to 1 (when mixing is purely with-like).

As Figure 8.13 shows, R_0 increases as the mixing pattern becomes more with-like. This is because increasing with-like mixing means higher-activity individuals tend to contact other higher activity individuals more frequently. As higher-activity individuals are more likely to be infected, increasing with-like mixing leads to an increase in the probability a 'typical-infectee' will be a member of the high-activity group. Higher-activity individuals have higher partner change rates and therefore generate more secondary infections in a completely susceptible population. Therefore the value of R_0 increases.

Panel 8.7 Modelling purely with-unlike mixing by both activity groups

As we saw, in our example, purely with-unlike mixing by high-activity group members did not result in purely with-unlike mixing by low-activity group members (Equation 8.50). This is because the number of partnerships required by the two activity groups differs. The high-activity group requires $c_H N_H = 31.4 \times 20 = 628$ partnerships per year while the low-activity group requires $c_L N_L = 1.4 \times 980 = 1372$ partnerships per year. Therefore even when all of the available partnerships of the high-activity group are formed with low-activity group members, the low-activity group still requires $1372 - 628 = 744$ partnerships. If partner change rates are not altered, these 744 remaining partnerships can only be supplied by other low-activity group members. As such, Q equals -0.46, not -1 as we would expect if purely with-unlike mixing was being modelled (Equation 8.50).

Overall, this means that 46 per cent of the partnerships of low-activity group members are formed with the high-activity group, and 54 per cent of the partnerships of low-activity group members are formed with the low-activity group (Equation 8.50). While this overall mixing pattern is clearly more with-like than was achieved by modelling proportionate mixing by the high-activity group (in which only 31 per cent of the partnerships of low-activity group members were formed with the high-activity group, Equation 8.49), we were not able to model purely with-unlike mixing between the low and high-activity groups as represented by the mixing matrix shown in Equation 8.39.

To model purely with-unlike mixing by both activity groups, the partner change rates must be altered so that the numbers of partnerships required by both activity groups balance. In our example, if we maintain a mean partner change rate of two partners per year, the partner change rate in the high and low-activity groups must change to 50 and 1.02 per year. If this is done both groups require 1000 partnerships per year, ie, $c_H N_H = 50 \times 20 = 1000$ and $c_L N_L = 1.02 \times 980 = 1000$, and each group can supply all the partnerships the other group requires.

Mixing matrix (using Equation 8.47)	Q value (using Equation 8.40)
Purely with-unlike mixing by high-activity group and altered partner change rates	

$$\begin{pmatrix} 0 & (1-0)\left(\dfrac{50\times20}{1.02\times980}\right) \\ 1-0 & 1-(1-0)\left(\dfrac{50\times20}{1.02\times980}\right) \end{pmatrix} = {}_{L}^{H}\begin{pmatrix} H & L \\ 0 & 1 \\ 1 & 0 \end{pmatrix}$$

$$Q = (0 + 0 - 1) / (2 - 1)$$
$$= -1 / 1$$
$$= -1$$

8.51

So if we alter partner change rates we can model purely with-unlike mixing, and the value of Q would equal -1 as expected.

For other methods of modelling mixing between different groups in the population see.[13, 17, 21, 22]

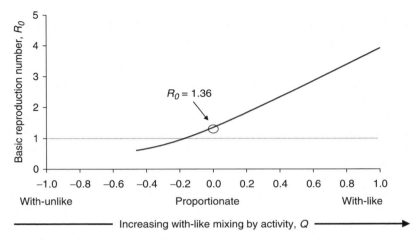

Fig. 8.13 Predictions for the basic reproduction number, R_0, for a curable STI in a single-sex, two-activity group model as the mixing pattern between activity groups varies from 'More with-unlike' ($Q = -0.46$, the most with-unlike mixing possible without altering partner change rates), through proportionate ($Q = 0$), to purely with-like mixing ($Q = 1$). $\beta_p = 0.75$, $D = 0.167$ years, $c_L = 1.4$ partners/year, $c_H = 31.4$ partners/year. Two per cent of the population belong to the high-activity group. An arrow shows the value of R_0 (1.36) assuming proportionate mixing as illustrated in section 8.4. A horizontal line highlights $R_0 = 1$. (Model 8.3, online.)

The derivation of the equation for R_0 that can be used to calculate these R_0 values for any pattern of mixing is shown in Panel 8.8. This derivation is more general than that shown for proportionate mixing in Panel 8.5.

Note that in the limit when $Q = 1$, the two activity groups cease interacting, and we are modelling two independent populations, each with its own R_0 value. The R_0 plotted in Figure 8.13 for $Q = 1$ is the R_0 for high-activity group 3.93. The R_0 value for the lower activity group will be smaller (0.18).

Note also that in this example, the value of R_0 falls below one when mixing becomes moderately with-unlike ($Q < -0.17$) and prevalence will fall ultimately to zero.

8.5.6 Effects of mixing on rate of STI spread and equilibrium STI prevalence (for a given R_0 value)

Increasing with-like mixing tends to lead to the infection invading more rapidly, but rather surprisingly, for a given R_0, it also tends to result in lower equilibrium prevalence (Figure 8.14 and Garnett et al.[23]).

The STI invades more rapidly as with-like mixing increases because infected higher-activity individuals are more likely to transmit infection to other higher-activity individuals, who generate new infections more quickly than lower activity individuals.

The equilibrium STI prevalence is higher in scenarios with less with-like mixing because, for a given R_0, more transmission has to occur in the low-activity group. The lower prevalence in the low-activity group means fewer of these contacts are 'wasted' on

Panel 8.8 Calculating R_0 in a population with heterogeneity in sexual activity and any mixing pattern

We can use any of the methods described in Chapter 7 to calculate the R_0 for an STI in a population with heterogeneity in sexual activity and mixing. Here we use only the simultaneous equations approach.

Here we show the derivation of R_0 for a two-activity group model with any mixing pattern. It is more complicated, but more useful, than the simpler derivations if mixing is assumed to be either proportionate (Panel 8.5) or purely with-unlike (section 8.6.1).

The basic reproduction number of the STI in this population is the average number of secondary infections caused by a single infection in a *typical infectee* introduced into a susceptible population. The typical infectee is some theoretical average of a high and low-activity individual. If we let x be the probability the typical infectee is a member of the high-activity group, and $1-x$ be the probability the typical infectee is a member of the low-activity group, R_0 is the maximum value that satisfies the following matrix equation:

$$\begin{pmatrix} R_{HH} & R_{HL} \\ R_{LH} & R_{LL} \end{pmatrix} \begin{pmatrix} x \\ 1-x \end{pmatrix} = R_0 \begin{pmatrix} x \\ 1-x \end{pmatrix} \qquad 8.52$$

Where R_{HH} is the number of secondary infections in high-activity group members generated by an infected high-activity group member, R_{LH} is the number of secondary infections in low-activity group members generated by an infected high-activity group member, R_{HL} is the number of secondary infections in high-activity group members generated by an infected low-activity group member, and R_{LL} is the number of secondary infections in low-activity group members generated by an infected low-activity group member.

The two implicit equations can be solved for R_0, eliminating the unknown term, x:

$$R_{HH}x + R_{HL}(1-x) = R_0 x \qquad 8.53$$

$$R_{LH}x + R_{LL}(1-x) = R_0(1-x) \qquad 8.54$$

Rearranging Equation 8.53 we get:

$$x = \frac{-R_{HL}}{R_{HH} - R_{HL} - R_0} \qquad 8.55$$

Rearranging Equation 8.54 we get:

$$x = \frac{R_0 - R_{LL}}{R_{LH} - R_{LL} + R_0} \qquad 8.56$$

Eliminating x by setting Equation 8.55 equal to Equation 8.56 and rearranging, we obtain:

$$-R_{HL}(R_{LH} - R_{LL} + R_0) = (R_0 - R_{LL})(R_{HH} - R_{HL} - R_0) \qquad 8.57$$

By rearranging this equation we obtain a quadratic equation in R_0 (ie the R_0 term is squared):

$$R_0^2 + R_0(-R_{HH} - R_{LL}) + (R_{LL}R_{HH} - R_{HL}R_{LH}) = 0 \qquad 8.58$$

This equation can be solved for R_0 using the standard solution for quadratic equation of the form:

$$aR_0^2 + bR_0 + c = 0 \qquad 8.59$$

Which is:

$$R_0 = \frac{-b \pm \sqrt{b^2 - 4 \times a \times c}}{2a} \qquad 8.60$$

By comparing Equation 8.58 with Equation 8.59 we can see that, in this example, $a = 1$, $b = -R_{HH} - R_{LL}$, and $c = R_{LL}R_{HH} - R_{HL}R_{LH}$. (Note b and c represent different quantities elsewhere in this chapter).

So we can write down the formula for R_0 for gonorrhoea in this model population:

$$R_0 = \frac{R_{HH} + R_{LL} + \sqrt{(-R_{HH} - R_{LL})^2 - 4 \times (R_{LL}R_{HH} - R_{HL}R_{LH})}}{2} \qquad 8.61$$

Note, the '$\pm$' symbol has been replaced with a '$+$' because R_0 is the maximum value that satisfies Equation 8.60 and therefore the smaller solution can be ignored.

We can see from this formula that the R_0 will depend on the number of secondary infections that are generated by high and low-activity group members in each of the two activity groups. These numbers will depend on the mixing pattern between the two groups,

Therefore the value of R_0 will depend on the overall number of secondary infections generated by each group, and also the mixing pattern of the population.

infected individuals than if these contacts had been with higher activity individuals. Therefore prevalence rises in the low-activity group until a sufficient proportion of contacts are again 'wasted' on infected individuals to reduce the number of secondary infections from 1.36 (at STI introduction) to 1 (at equilibrium). Therefore, at equilibrium, prevalence is higher in the larger, low-activity group, and therefore the overall equilibrium prevalence is higher.

Note however that in models with heterogeneity, the equilibrium prevalence tends to be lower and the effects of saturation tend to occur earlier than in models without

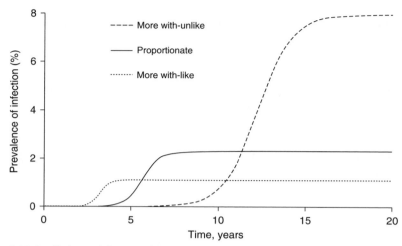

Fig. 8.14 Predictions of the overall prevalence of infectious individuals over time in a curable STI model with more with-unlike ($Q = -0.4$), proportionate ($Q = 0$), or more with-like ($Q = +0.4$) mixing between activity groups. R_0 was set equal to 1.36 in all scenarios by varying the duration of infection ($D = 0.340$, 0.167 and 0.097 years, respectively). $\beta_p = 0.75$, $c_L = 1.4$ partners/year, $c_H = 31.4$ partners/year. Two per cent of the population belong to the high-activity group. (Model 8.3, online.)

heterogeneity. This is clearly true in the example because if homogenous mixing was assumed, an R_0 of 1.36 would result in an equilibrium prevalence of 26 per cent (using $i(\infty) = 1 - 1/R_0$, Equation 1.2). This is much higher than the prevalence in any of the scenarios shown in Figure 8.14 with heterogeneity in risk behaviour.

8.5.7 Effects of mixing on equilibrium STI prevalence (for a given STI natural history and partner change rates)

Figure 8.14 illustrated the effect of changing the mixing pattern if R_0 was held constant by increasing the duration of infection of the STI. It is also interesting to explore what may happen if the mixing pattern changed but the STI natural history and the partner change rates do not change. Plausibly, this could be the intended or unintended consequence of a behaviour change intervention.

Figure 8.15 shows that increasing with-like mixing may not always lead to a reduction in equilibrium prevalence. For lower values of R_0, increasing with-like mixing may actually allow the infection to invade a population and lead to a rise in overall prevalence (Figure 8.15, top). Conversely, for higher values of R_0, increasing with-like mixing will always lead to a fall in overall prevalence because more contacts are 'wasted' on already-infected individuals in the high-activity group (Figure 8.15, middle). For moderate values of R_0, both effects may be seen, so that increasing with-like mixing may lead to an initial rise, but subsequent fall in overall prevalence (Figure 8.15, bottom).

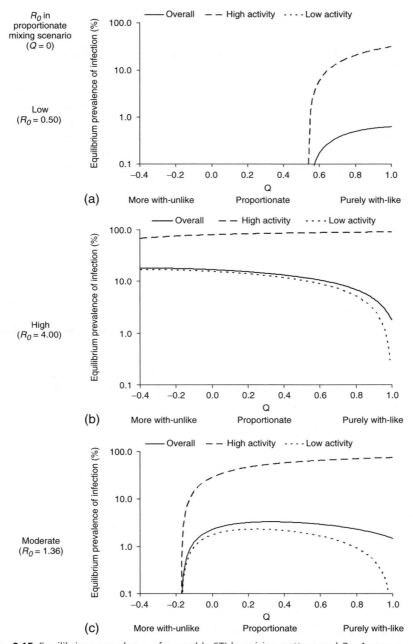

Fig. 8.15 Equilibrium prevalence of a curable STI by mixing pattern and R_0. Assumes partner change rate in high and low-activity groups are 31.4 and 1.4 partners per year, respectively, the high-activity group is 2 per cent of the population, the per-partnership transmission probability is 0.75. In the low, moderate and high R_0 scenarios, the durations of infection are 0.062, 0.167, and 0.493 years, respectively. Note a $\log_{10}$ scale is used on the y axis for clarity. Note that only two lines appear in the low R_0 scenario because the prevalence of infection in the low-activity group remains below 0.1 per cent for all values of Q. (Model 8.4, online.)

8.5.8 Implications of heterogeneity in sexual activity on STI control

Heterogeneity in sexual activity and different mixing patterns between activity groups also has implications for the control of STIs. Figure 8.16 shows how the equilibrium prevalence of gonorrhoea may be affected by a screening programme. Screening is implemented very simply in the model by adding a term to the equations determining the rate of change of the infectious and susceptible individuals in the high and low-activity groups, to simulate a higher rate of recovery. These two rates are then altered so that the number of screenings is kept constant but the screenings are targeted at the high or low activity group, or distributed randomly. Model equations Equation 8.12 and Equation 8.13 become:

$$\frac{dS_j(t)}{dt} = -\lambda_j(t)S_j(t) + rI_j(t) + y_jI_j(t) \qquad\qquad 8.62$$

$$\frac{dI_j(t)}{dt} = +\lambda_j(t)S_j(t) - rI_j(t) - y_jI_j(t) \qquad\qquad 8.63$$

Where y_j is the screening rate of high ($j = _H$) and low ($j = _L$) activity group. For simplicity we assume perfect diagnostic tests and 100 per cent cure if treated.

Figure 8.16 shows how the equilibrium prevalence may change with the annual number of individuals screened and treated for gonorrhoea each year. Three scenarios show the impact of random screening or screening targeted exclusively at high or low-activity group members.

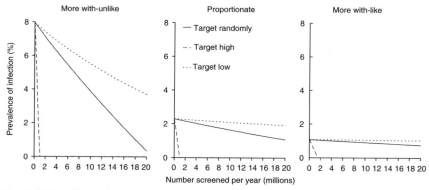

Fig. 8.16 The effect of screening the population on equilibrium curable STI prevalence in the overall population, by mixing pattern and target group. The mixing patterns shown are: more with-unlike ($Q = -0.4$), proportionate ($Q = 0$), more with-like ($Q = +0.4$). Screening is targeted either randomly, or at high or low activity groups. R_0 was set equal to 1.36 in all scenarios by varying the duration of infection ($D = 0.340$, 0.167 and 0.097 years, respectively). Other parameter values are as shown in the heading to Figure 8.14. The assumed population size is 20 million. (Model 8.5, online.)

Looking at each of the panels in Figure 8.16 independently shows that prioritizing higher-risk members of the population is markedly more effective per-person-screened than prioritizing individuals at random or prioritizing members of the low-activity group. For example, if the mixing pattern is proportionate (Figure 8.16, middle), one million screenings per year does not markedly affect prevalence if randomly distributed or targeted at the low-activity group, but eradicates the infection if targeted at the high-activity group.

Looking across all three panels in Figure 8.16 shows that increased with-like mixing tends to make STIs more difficult to control. The same number of screenings has a smaller impact on the equilibrium STI prevalence in populations with more with-like mixing. In our example, 20 million screenings per year randomly distributed would reduce the relative equilibrium prevalence by around a third in the more with-like mixing scenario, by around a half in the proportionate mixing scenario but would almost eradicate the infection in the more with-unlike mixing scenario.

8.6 Mixing on gender (heterosexual mixing model)

In the next model in this chapter, we focus exclusively on high-activity individuals and explore the implications of differences in the natural history of gonorrhoea in males and females. We calculate the number of secondary infections from a single infection in each gender, and the basic reproduction number for gonorrhoea in this population.

Consider the two-gender model shown in Figure 8.17.

In this model we assume exclusively heterosexual activity. Therefore we assume completely with-unlike mixing between the two genders. Note that in a model for a heterosexual population in which individuals are grouped by gender and activity, we are likely to assume moderately with-like mixing by activity and with-unlike mixing by gender. A model that assumes some same-gender sexual activity could be parameterized to model moderately with-like mixing by activity and moderately with-unlike mixing by gender. We also assume the male to female ratio is 1:1 and our population is *closed*, and therefore the numbers of partnerships formed by men and by women are equal.

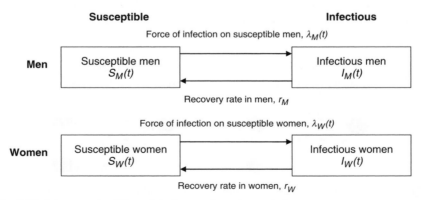

Fig. 8.17 A two-gender SIS model of gonorrhoea transmission.

The equations for rate of change of the number of female susceptible and infectious individuals and the force of infection on females at time t in this model are:

$$\frac{dS_W(t)}{dt} = -\lambda_W(t)S_W(t) + rI_W(t) \qquad 8.64$$

$$\frac{dI_W(t)}{dt} = +\lambda_W(t)S_W(t) - rI_W(t) \qquad 8.65$$

$$\lambda_W(t) = c_W\beta_{WM}i_M(t) \qquad 8.66$$

Where c_W is the average rate at which women change partners, β_{WM} is the per partnership transmission probability from men to women, and $i_M(t)$ is the infection prevalence in males at time t. The equations and parameters for males are obtained by replacing 'W's with 'M's and vice versa.

The left-hand side of Figure 8.18 illustrates heterosexual mixing in which one infectious woman generates four secondary infections in men, and each infection in males generates, on average, 0.5 secondary infections in women (ie four infections → two infections). So overall, one infection in women leads to two tertiary infections in women and therefore we would expect the STI to invade the population.

This looks very similar to host-vector modelling (Figure 8.18 right). Ronald Ross first realized this similarity when he was developing his models for Malaria in 1911.[24] Ross recognized that one gender could be thought of as the 'vector' to the other gender. Indeed, *Hethcote* and colleagues based the equations for their two-gender STI model[25] on the equations and ideas developed by Ross for his host-vector modelling of malaria.

8.6.1 Calculating R_0 for a heterosexually mixing population (host-vector)

As before, to calculate the basic reproduction number for the population as a whole first we need to calculate the number of secondary infections generated by each subgroup in the model. In this case these are men and women:

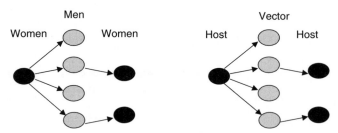

Fig. 8.18 Schematic of STI transmission between men and women (left) and infection transmission between host and vector (right).

The *next generation matrix* of the numbers of secondary infections that would result from a single infection introduced into a susceptible heterosexually mixing two-gender model population is:

$$
\begin{array}{c}
\text{Infectious individual} \\
\text{Man} \quad \text{Woman}
\end{array}
$$

$$
\text{Susceptible Individual} \quad
\begin{array}{c}
\text{Men} \\
\text{Women}
\end{array}
\begin{pmatrix}
0 & R_{MW} \\
R_{WM} & 0
\end{pmatrix}
\qquad 8.67
$$

Where R_{MW} is the number of secondary infections in men due to an infected women and R_{WM} is the number of secondary infections in women due to an infected man. Since, in this purely heterosexual transmission model, there is no direct transmission between males and males or between females and females $R_{MM} = R_{WW} = 0$. Further, R_{WM} and R_{MW} may differ because of variation in sexual behaviour, transmission probability and duration of infection between males and females.

We can use any of the methods described in Chapter 7 to calculate the R_0. Here we calculate R_0 by solving the simultaneous equations of the average number of secondary infections caused by a single infection in a typical infectee. The basic reproduction number of gonorrhoea in this population is the average number of secondary infections caused by a single infection in a *typical infectee* introduced into a susceptible population. The typical infectee is some theoretical average of men and women. If we let x be the probability the typical infectee is a man, and $1–x$ be the probability the typical infectee is a woman, R_0 is the maximum value that satisfies the following matrix equation:

$$
\begin{pmatrix}
0 & R_{MW} \\
R_{WM} & 0
\end{pmatrix}
\begin{pmatrix}
x \\
1-x
\end{pmatrix}
= R_0
\begin{pmatrix}
x \\
1-x
\end{pmatrix}
\qquad 8.68
$$

The two implicit equations can be solved for R_0, eliminating the unknown term, 'x'

$$
R_{MW}(1-x) = R_0 x \qquad 8.69
$$

$$
R_{WM}x = R_0(1-x) \qquad 8.70
$$

Rearranging Equation 8.69 for $(1–x)$ and substituting $(1–x)$ into Equation 8.70 yields

$$
R_{WM}x = \frac{R_0 R_0 x}{R_{MW}}
$$

Cancelling the remaining x terms and rearranging gives the equation for R_0 for a two-gender heterosexually mixing model of as SIS infection like gonorrhoea:

$$
R_0 = \sqrt{R_{WM}R_{MW}} \qquad 8.71
$$

This is a particular case of a more general result for the R_0 of an infection in a host-vector model such that the basic reproduction number is equal to the geometric mean of the number of secondary infections from each of the groups (26). Here we have two groups, males and females, so the geometric mean is the square root of the product of R_{WM} and R_{MW}.

The equations for R_{WM} and R_{MW} are:

$$R_{WM} = c_M \beta_{WM} D_M \qquad\qquad 8.72$$

$$R_{MW} = c_W \beta_{MW} D_W \qquad\qquad 8.73$$

Where c_W and c_M are the annual partner change rates in women and men, respectively, β_{MW} and β_{WM} are the transmission probabilities per partnership from women to men and men to women, respectively, and D_W and D_M is the duration of infection in women and men, respectively.

As we are modelling the highly active group, we assume the partner change rates among females and males, c_W and c_M, are both 31.4 partners per year. To model (crudely) the lower proportion of infections that are symptomatic in women than men[1] and therefore the likely lower treatment seeking rates among women than men, we assume the average duration of infectiousness with some treatment in the population is longer for females than for males (D_W = 3 months and D_M = 1 month). Finally, we assume the male to female transmission probability per partnership is higher than the female to male transmission probability per partnership (β_{WM}=0.9 and β_{MW}=0.6) as is commonly observed for STI transmission.[1]

Using these parameter values:

$$R_{WM} = c_M \beta_{WM} D_M = 31.4 \times 0.9 \times \frac{1}{12} = 2.4 \qquad\qquad 8.74$$

$$R_{MW} = c_W \beta_{MW} D_W = 31.4 \times 0.6 \times \frac{3}{12} = 4.7 \qquad\qquad 8.75$$

Using these values and Equation 8.71 we can calculate the basic reproduction number for this STI in this high-activity population.

$$\begin{aligned} R_0 &= \sqrt{R_{WM} R_{MW}} \\ &= \sqrt{2.4 \times 4.7} \\ &= 3.3 \end{aligned} \qquad\qquad 8.76$$

Thus, our simple model has highlighted the potential importance of gender differences in the natural history and transmission probability of STIs. Although the probability of gonorrhoea transmission from female to males is lower than from males to females, our model predicted that females may generate more secondary infectious than males because of the longer average duration of infection in females than in males.

8.7 **Summary of predictions using simple curable STI models**

The early deterministic compartmental modelling work of gonorrhoea by Cooke, Hethcote and Yorke highlighted some of the important characteristics of sexually transmitted infectious that are important for their transmission and control. They showed that heterogeneity in human sexual activity was critical in explaining the invasion of short-duration non-immunizing bacterial STIs and their relatively low but stable equilibrium prevalence. They coined the term *pre-emptive saturation* for the process that limits transmission for non-immunizing infections in which contacts of infectious individuals are 'wasted' (from the pathogen's perspective) on already-infected individuals. Using only slightly more complicated models than those detailed above, Hethcote and Yorke showed the importance of asymptomatic individuals in the spread of infection, and that strategies that best identified either higher-activity individuals or asymptomatics, or ideally both, would be most effective at controlling infection. Their modelling helped inform US STI control policy in the 1980s.

So far in this chapter we have also explored the likely impact of mixing by sexual activity on the transmission and control of STIs. In general with-like (also called 'assortative') mixing facilitates the invasion of an infection, because fewer contacts are 'wasted' on low activity individuals, but it limits the overall spread of infection because it tends to protect lower-activity individuals as it reduces contact between activity groups. More with-like mixing also tends to make infections more difficult to eradicate because it creates a core of high-activity individuals who continually infect and re-infect each other.

We will now adapt our model for a short duration bacterial STI to represent HIV/AIDS, make an estimate of R_0 for HIV and use this model to make projections for the trend in HIV prevalence, HIV incidence, mortality and sexual behaviour over time.

8.8 **Simple transmission models of human immunodeficiency virus/AIDS**

AIDS is the disease caused by the retrovirus human immunodeficiency virus (HIV).[5] HIV primarily targets CD4 cells and without treatment this leads to the collapse of the host immune system and ultimately death. The clinical syndrome was called Acquired Immune Deficiency Syndrome (AIDS) in 1982 and four years later the causative virus was named HIV-1.[5] HIV has been the focus of a large number of modelling studies since its discovery, some of which are described below. Many of the insights gained from modelling the transmission of short-duration curable STIs also apply to HIV, but there are also important differences between HIV/AIDS and the STIs considered so far that we will need to address.

Most importantly there is currently no cure for HIV so that in the absence of treatment, once the AIDS stage of HIV infection is reached, death quickly follows. Also, in the absence of other 'cofactors' for HIV transmission, HIV is typically much less infectious[27–29] than short-duration bacterial STIs, potentially lowering its R_0 compared to short-duration bacterial STIs. However, HIV is infectious for far longer than the short-duration STIs,[30–32] increasing its R_0 relative to short-duration bacterial STIs. Depending on the research question, we may also need to consider that the infectiousness of HIV-infected individuals varies markedly with time since infection.[29]

8.8.1 Simple transmission model of HIV/AIDS

Let's start by adapting the simple two-activity group SIS model for gonorrhoea we used in section 8.4 by removing the possibility of cure, adding AIDS compartments, and an AIDS-related mortality rate, μ (Figure 8.19).

As we are modelling the long-term dynamics of a persistent infection that leads to death we also need to model the rate of recruitment into sexually active age groups, 'a' otherwise we will run out of susceptibles, and also the rate of non-AIDS mortality among sexually active individuals, m. Different assumptions can be made, but here we assume that the proportion of newly sexually active individuals recruited into each of the two activity groups (high and low) remains constant over time and is equal to the proportion of the population in the high and low-activity groups at $t = 0$. For simplicity, we will ignore all other population heterogeneities such as age and gender, assume proportionate mixing, assume that the period between infection and infectiousness is very short in comparison with the period of infectiousness, assume no sexual activity takes place in the AIDS stage, and assume that individuals do not change activity group over their lifetime.

The equations and parameter values for this model are shown in Panel 8.9 and Model 8.6 (online).

8.8.1.1 The R_0 of HIV infection

We can calculate R_0 for HIV in this model using the equation we derived for R_0 for gonorrhoea in a proportionately mixing population with two activity groups (Equation 8.32). However, we need to adjust the duration of HIV infectiousness because we are explicitly modelling non-AIDS mortality.[33] Let's assume the average life expectancy in the absence of HIV is 50 years and the average age of debut is 15 years. Therefore the average life expectancy at sexual debut is 35 years. Let's also assume the median time from HIV infection to death is 10 years,[30–32] and therefore the duration

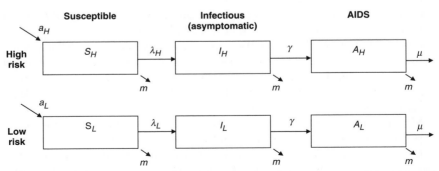

Fig. 8.19 A simple model of HIV transmission and progression. See Panel 8.9 and Model 8.6 (online) for model equations and parameter values.

Panel 8.9 Model equations for simple HIV/AIDS model

The model equations for the high-activity group are shown below. Note that, except for $n_H(0)$, the proportion of individuals in the high-activity group at $t = 0$, the explicit time dependence '(t)' has been omitted to shorten the equations.

$$\frac{dS_H}{dt} = a_H N - \lambda_H S_H - m S_H \tag{8.77}$$

$$\frac{dI_H}{dt} = \lambda_H S_H - \gamma I_H - m I_H \tag{8.78}$$

$$\frac{dA_H}{dt} = \gamma I_H - \mu A_H - m A_H \tag{8.79}$$

$$a_H = a n_H(0) \tag{8.80}$$

$$\lambda_H = c_H \beta_p p \tag{8.81}$$

$$p = g_H i_H + g_L i_L \tag{8.82}$$

$$i_H = \frac{I_H}{U_H} \text{ and } i_L = \frac{I_L}{U_L}$$

$$U_H = S_H + I_H, \text{ and } U_L = S_L + I_L$$

Where
S_H is the number of individuals susceptible to HIV at time t in high-activity group
I_H is the number of individuals infectious with HIV at time t in high-activity group
A_H is the number of individuals with AIDS at time t in high-activity group
N is the total population size
λ_H is the force of HIV infection on the high-activity group at time t
a is the rate of recruitment rate into sexually active age groups, per year
$n_H(0)$ is the proportion of individuals in the high-activity group at $t = 0$
a_H is the recruitment rate into the high-activity group, per year
m is the non-HIV mortality rate among sexually active individuals, per year
γ is progression rate to AIDS, per year
μ is the death rate due to AIDS, per year
c_H is the partner change rate per year in the high-activity group
β_p is the probability of HIV transmission probability per partnership
p is the probability a new partner is HIV infectious

Panel 8.9 Model equations for simple HIV/AIDS model *(continued)*

g_H and g_L are the probability that a sexual partner will be a member of the high and low-activity group, respectively

$i_H(t)$ and $i_L(t)$ are the prevalences of infectious individuals among sexually active individuals in the high and low-activity groups, respectively

U_H and U_L are the numbers of sexually active individuals in the high and low-activity groups, respectively

Where required, the equations for the low-activity group are obtained by replacing the subscript $_H$ with $_L$.

---

of infectiousness is 9 years if we allow one year for the (assumed) sexually inactive AIDS stage. Therefore, assuming these events are distributed exponentially, HIV-infected individuals will leave the infectious stage at a rate which is the sum of the progression rate to AIDS (γ, 1/9 per year) and the non-AIDS mortality rate among sexually active individuals (m, 1/35 per year). The duration of the infectious stage will be $\dfrac{1}{(1/9 + 1/35)} = 7.16$ years.

The mean per-sex act HIV transmission probability over the entire period of HIV infection in low-risk HIV-discordant partnerships in rural Uganda[29] was around 0.0016. If we assume that on average a partnership lasts around 30 sex-acts (averaging over one-off encounters, casual and regular partnerships), the per-partnership transmission probability will be around 0.05, ie $1-(1-0.0016)^{30}$ (see Panel 8.1 and Panel 9.3 for method). So if we assume the average per partner transmission probability is 0.05 and the partner change rates in the high and low-activity groups are 8 and 0.2 per year, respectively, we get the following predictions for the number of secondary infections from a high and low-activity individual in a totally susceptible population:

$$R_H = c_H \beta_p D$$
$$= 8 \times 0.05 \times 7.16$$
$$= 2.86 \qquad\qquad 8.83$$

$$R_L = c_L \beta_p D$$
$$= 0.2 \times 0.05 \times 7.16$$
$$= 0.07 \qquad\qquad 8.84$$

Again, for simplicity, we assume that the per-partnership transmission probability is the same in high and low-activity groups when, in reality, the probabilities may differ. To calculate R_0 we also need to re-calculate the probability that a new sexual partner will be a member of the high and low-activity group. Using Equation 8.20, the partner change rates above and assuming 15 per cent of the population are in the high-activity group we calculate $g_H = 0.88$ and $g_L = 0.12$.

Therefore using Equation 8.32:

$$R_0 = g_H R_H + g_L R_L$$
$$= 0.88 \times 2.86 + 0.12 \times 0.07$$
$$= 2.52 \qquad\qquad 8.85$$

8.8.1.2 Predictions for HIV epidemic

Using this model we get the following predictions for the prevalence and incidence of infection over time and the cumulative number of AIDS deaths. In contrast to the steady rise to an equilibrium prevalence and incidence predicted for short-duration curable STIs (Figure 8.8), the prevalence and incidence of HIV is predicted to rise and then fall (Figure 8.20a). This is because HIV kills, and preferentially kills higher-risk individuals in the population. Therefore, unless new higher-risk individuals are recruited at the same rate they die, the average partner-change rate in the population will fall over time (Figure 8.20b). This reduction in partner change rates can occur even in the absence of explicit safer-sex interventions. If nothing else changes, such as the impact of intervention efforts, HIV prevalence will level off when the annual number of HIV deaths and new HIV infections come into equilibrium (Figure 8.20c).

Falls in HIV prevalence and incidence may also be the result of intervention, but as we see HIV prevalence and incidence are also expected to change due to the natural dynamics of infection, making interpretation of HIV trends difficult.[34] Further, because incidence falls earlier than prevalence (Figure 8.20a), if the early years of the HIV epidemic are missed then it is also possible to see falls in the prevalence of HIV without falls in incidence as was observed in Rakai, Uganda.[35]

Figure 8.20 also shows that in our model HIV prevalence took around 45 years to reach its peak, which is relatively slow compared to the rate at which HIV epidemics have risen in Southern Africa and probably rose in East Africa (Figure 8.21). The HIV epidemic spread earlier in East Africa so HIV surveillance systems tended to miss the rise in prevalence (Figure 8.21, right panel).

The model prediction (the 'numerical solution') for the doubling time of this epidemic in our model can be obtained by examining the time it takes for the number of HIV infectious individuals to increase from 1 to 2. It is about 2.9 years (see Model 8.6, online). We can also make a cruder analytic estimate for the doubling time of the HIV epidemic by assuming there is no heterogeneity in sexual activity. The derivation is shown in Panel 8.10 and the estimated doubling time, t_d, is reasonably close to the numerical estimate:

$$T_d \approx \frac{\ln(2)}{c\beta_p - \gamma - m} = 2.7 \text{ years}$$

The reason for the very rapid spread of HIV in Southern and Eastern Africa is not totally understood, but is likely to have been due to a combination of various biological and behaviour factors, such as low rates of male circumcision combined with high rates of other STIs that are cofactors for HIV transmission. STI cofactors are likely to have been more important for HIV epidemics in resource-poor, than in resource-rich

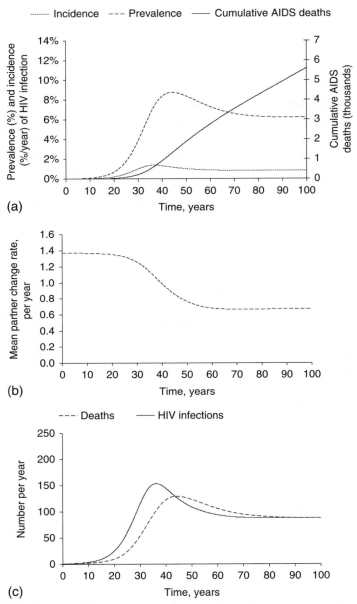

Fig. 8.20 Predictions of (a) the incidence and prevalence of HIV and cumulative AIDS deaths; (b) mean partner change rate in the population; and (c) numbers of new HIV infections and deaths of HIV infecteds. The equations and parameter values for this model are shown in Panel 8.9 and Model 8.6 (online).

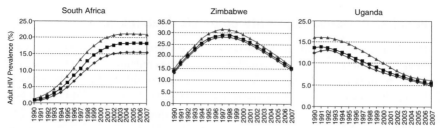

Fig. 8.21 Estimated trend in adult HIV (with high ▲ and low ◆ estimate) prevalence in Southern Africa (15–49 years). From [36–38] Note different scales on y axis.

settings, because STI treatment services are more limited and consequently the prevalence and duration of STI infections were higher.[39] In section 9.4 we use a simple model of HIV/STI co-infection to explore the possible impact of cofactor STIs in increasing rate of spread of HIV, and also the likely impact of the HIV epidemic on the prevalence of cofactor STIs.

In Southern Africa, the effect of population mobility, specifically labour migration, is also thought to have been important in explaining the rapid spread of HIV.[40] One of the effects labour migration is likely to have had is to increase the prevalence of concurrency, or the overlap of sexual partnerships.

8.9 **Concurrency**

The duration and overlap of sexual partnerships are important for understanding the spread of STIs. The most relevant period of time to consider for concurrency is the duration of the infectiousness of the STI, and therefore this period will vary between different STIs. For long duration STIs such as Herpes simplex virus type-2 (HSV-2) or HIV, the infection can spread between subsequent partners over many years, but for shorter-duration infections such as gonorrhoea and during periods of high infectivity of longer-duration STIs such as primary HSV-2 and HIV infection, partnership concurrency is important for STI spread.[41–45]

Partnership concurrency increases the rate of spread of an STI by two mechanisms, firstly by removing the necessity that a partnership is formed with the infected partner before the susceptible partner, and secondly, by reducing the time delay before individuals become exposed to an infectious individual.

To illustrate these two effects Figure 8.22 shows two different scenarios of partnership formation. In both scenarios a man forms partnerships with five women in the same time period, and woman #3 is already infected with an STI from a previous relationship at the start of the partnership. In scenario (a) these five partnerships are formed one after another such that one partnership ends before the next starts (serial monogamy). In scenario (b) these five partnerships overlap completely in time (concurrency).

Panel 8.10 Derivation of HIV epidemic doubling time

If we assume that the partner change rates in the two groups are identical and equal to eight partners per year (the doubling time of the epidemic is primarily determined by the partner change rate in the high-activity group) and that at the start of the epidemic all individuals are essentially susceptible, then from Equation 8.82 $p = \dfrac{I}{U}$ and from Equation 8.81 $\lambda = c\,\beta_p \dfrac{I}{U}$, so the expression for the rate of change in the number of infectious individuals is:

$$\frac{dI}{dt} = \lambda S - \gamma I - mI \tag{8.86}$$

$$= c\beta_p \frac{I}{U} S - \gamma I - mI$$

$$\approx c\beta_p \frac{I}{S} S - \gamma I - mI$$

$$\frac{dI}{dt} \approx (c\beta_p - \gamma - m)I \tag{8.87}$$

Integrating Equation 8.87 to get the number of infectious individuals at time t:

$$I(t) \approx I(0)e^{\Lambda t} \tag{8.88}$$

Where $\Lambda = c\beta_p - \gamma - m$ = the initial growth rate of the epidemic. By definition, at the initial doubling time of the epidemic, T_d, the number of infectious individuals will have doubled. Hence $I(T_d) = 2 \times I(0)$ and therefore:

$$\frac{2I(0)}{I(0)} \approx e^{\Lambda T_d} \tag{8.89}$$

$$2 \approx e^{\Lambda T_d} \tag{8.90}$$

Taking the natural logarithm of both sides of the equation yields:

$$\ln(2) \approx \Lambda T_d \tag{8.91}$$

and rearranging:

$$T_d \approx \frac{\ln(2)}{\Lambda} \tag{8.92}$$

$$T_d \approx \frac{0.69}{8 \times 0.05 - 1/9 - 1/35} \tag{8.93}$$

$$T_d \approx 2.7\,\text{years}$$

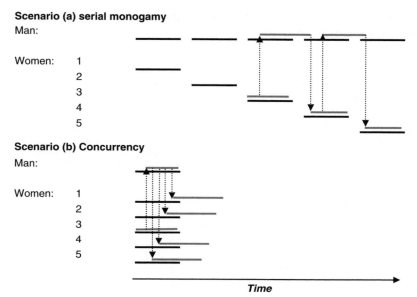

Fig. 8.22 Illustration of effect of partnership concurrency on STI transmission in which a male has partnerships with five women that are formed either (a) serially monogamous or (b) concurrently. Black bars represent time in partnership. Grey bars represent time infected and infectious. Dotted arrows represent transmission event.

In scenario (a) woman #1 and women #2 are completely protected from the infection in woman #3 because woman #1 and woman #2 formed partnerships with the man before woman #3. In contrast, in scenario (b), all women are at risk of infection from the man almost immediately after he is infected.

Concurrency has also allowed the infection to spread much more quickly through the female population in scenario (b) than in scenario (a), because in scenario (a) onward transmission to other women requires partnership dissolution and formation.

The definitions for R_0 that we have derived so far may underestimate the rate of spread of HIV in populations in which concurrency is common. Early analytic work on concurrency using compartmental modelling techniques reformulated the R_0 equation to add an additional term to account for the impact of concurrency, $c\beta_p\tau$ [45]. Where R_0' is the basic reproduction number without concurrency and τ is the average duration of partnerships in the population:

$$R_0 = R_0' + c\beta_p\tau \qquad 8.94$$

This early work showed that the rate of spread of HIV was much quicker in populations with concurrency than without concurrency. Watts and May concluded that in populations with high levels of concurrency, the HIV epidemic would effectively have two rates of spread, one very fast, on the timescale of the time it takes HIV to become infectious after infection, and one much slower, on the time scale of $1/c\beta_p$ and equal to the rate projected by compartmental models that do not take account of concurrency (Figure 8.23).

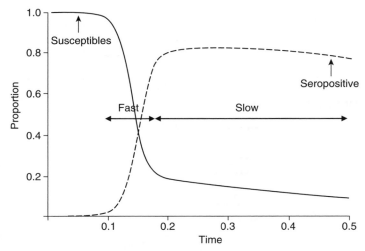

Fig. 8.23 Predictions for the proportion susceptible and seropositive with HIV in a population with high levels of concurrency highlighting the 'Fast' and 'Slow' phases of HIV spread. Adapted from Watts and May 1992.[45]

The finding that partnership concurrency increases the rate of spread of an STI was replicated and extended using a *network modelling* methodology that allows explicit representation of sexual partnerships and their overlap.[43] This work also showed that as the proportion of partnerships that are concurrent increases, a threshold is crossed where a *giant component* is formed, in which the majority of individuals in a population are connected by partnerships. This allows the very rapid spread of highly infectious STIs or STIs with periods of high infectivity.[43] For a review of the relevance of concurrency to STI transmission and control see Morris *et al*.[46]

Next we explore the advantages and disadvantages of *network modelling* and some of the insights this modelling methodology has provided.

8.10 **Network modelling**

The compartmental modelling approach used for the majority of models discussed in this book so far, assume individuals within any pair of population subgroups mix randomly so that each individual in one subgroup has a small and equal chance of contacting every other individual in the other subgroup. This is somewhat unrealistic for human populations because individuals usually contact only a small proportion of individuals with a certain set of characteristics and this simplification of compartmental modelling has some important epidemiological implications. Network models can explicitly incorporate this aspect of human behaviour by modelling permanent or semi-permanent links between individuals so that infection can only be transmitted to a smaller subset of individuals.

Much of the network modelling of infectious diseases is based on research into the mathematical properties of graphs and the social science of human interactions. The network of contacts in human populations (a *contact network*) can be represented as graphs containing *vertices* or *nodes* represented by points, and *edges* or *links* represented by lines (Figure 8.24). These vertices and edges are given different meanings depending on the discipline and research question. In human infectious disease modelling, a vertex typically represents an individual, and an edge typically represents a type of relationship that could lead to transmission of an infection. So for respiratory infections an edge could represent a social relation with a friend or colleague[47] or for a sexually transmitted infection an edge could represent a sexual partnership.[48]

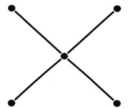

Fig. 8.24 A contact graph of five individuals and four sexual relationships that could lead to transmission of a sexually transmitted infection. Individuals are represented as points or 'vertices' and sexual relationships are represented as lines or 'edges'.

To make this section more understandable, wherever possible 'vertices' are referred to as individuals and 'edges' are referred to as (sexual) partnerships, although these are not necessarily the meanings given to these terms by the authors of all the cited references. See Panel 8.11 for a summary of common network modelling terminology.

Network models can be set up in many different ways. This summary is based on an review by Keeling and Eames.[49] The simplest network models focus on a small number of the aspects of real-world networks, such as the proportion of your partners' partners that are also your partner (*clustering*) or how many partnerships separate two individuals in a network (the *path-length*) whilst ignoring other aspects. More complex network modelling studies allow the simultaneous assessment of the importance of multiple network properties on STI transmission and the simulation of more realistic sexual networks (Figure 8.25).

Random networks are created by connecting individuals irrespective of their spatial or social position. In the simplest models, each individual has the same number of partners. Therefore networks created using this method simulate individuals with homogeneous risk behaviour and there is little clustering.[52] The predictions from these network models showed that the initial growth rate and the number of infected individuals is lower than predicted by compartmental models that assume random mixing. This is because the number of susceptible partners of infectious individuals falls much more quickly in network models because of saturation of local partners, and also because you must have been infected by one of your existing partners, and this infected partner cannot be re-infected immediately.

Lattice models are created by placing individuals on a regular grid in space and linking neighbouring individuals. Therefore all partnerships are restricted to the nearest

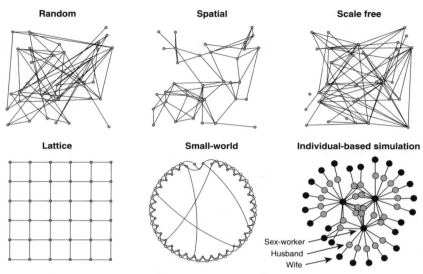

Fig. 8.25 Networks created using different partnership formation rules. Adapted from Keeling and Eames 2005.[49] Each network has 36 individuals (vertices) and approximate average number of partnerships (edges) per person (the 'mean degree') of four, with the exception of the individual-based simulation network that was created using the STDSIM sexual contact formation mechanism[50, 51] and has more individuals and lower mean degree.

neighbours and the network has very long path-lengths. Each individual has the same number of partners but the network is highly clustered, such that the partners' of your partners are very likely to also be your partners. Thus the initial rate of spread of an infection is lower than across random networks because random networks are less clustered and therefore the number of susceptible partners of infectious individuals falls much more slowly.

Small world networks can be created by adding a small number of long range partnerships to a lattice model. This has the effect of allowing infection to reach all parts of the network quickly, greatly reducing the average path-lengths compared to lattice models.[53] Human social networks appear to be 'small-world', the idea often being expressed as there being only '*six degrees of separation*' between any two individuals on the planet.[54] The results from modelling studies on small-world networks have been important for understanding the very rapid spread of infections through human populations and suggest that eliminating infections may be unrealistic restrictions on population movement.

Spatial networks are created by placing individuals in geographic space and connecting them with a probability that depends on the distance between them. The function defining this probability is commonly called a *spatial kernel*. By altering the kernel or the positioning of individuals a wide range of networks can be formed with properties ranging from highly clustered lattices to short path-length random networks.[55–57]

Scale-free networks can be created by connecting individuals with a probability that is directly proportional to their current number of partners. This is called *preferential attachment*. This results in a network in which the number of partners is distributed according to a power law, i.e., the probability of having k partners $P(k)$ is directly proportional to $k^{-\gamma}$. In these networks most individuals have few partners while a few individuals have very many partners.[58] This method of forming networks allows the creation of a 'core' group of highly connected individuals that are important in the spread and persistence of infections as we saw in section 8.4.

The predictions based on scale-free networks go further, however, to suggest that if partnership distributions conform to this power-law and the power, γ, lies between 2 and 3, then the variance (σ^2) of the partnership distribution tends to infinity, and therefore so does R_0 (from $R_0 = \hat{c}\sigma D$ and $\hat{c} = c + \sigma^2/c$, from Equation 8.33 and Equation 8.34). If human sexual behaviour could be adequately described by scale-free networks, then the modelling studies predict that infections could not be eliminated by biomedical interventions that change the transmission probability of the infection or the duration of infectiousness, but that infection could only be eliminated by behaviour change interventions that altered the structure of the network.

Data from Sweden, the UK, and Zimbabwe have been analysed and show that certain aspects of human sexual behaviour data may be described as 'scale-free', specifically, that distributions in the numbers of partners per unit time obey a power law relationship.[4, 59] However, the evidence to support this hypothesis is limited by the range in the available data on the number of partners per unit time (≤ 3 orders of magnitude in these studies) and the small number of high-partner change individuals on which this conclusion is based.[60] Common sense also suggests that there will be some physical maximum to the number of sexual partners an individual could have over any period of time.

Individual-based simulation network models are created by explicitly modelling the entire network of individuals and their partnerships. These models can be used to generate different networks depending on the chosen partnership formation and dissolution rules. Relationship formation and dissolution and infection transitions are typically modelled as chance (stochastic) processes. Individual-based simulation network models are widely used in the modelling of complex ecological systems[61] and their use is becoming more common in epidemiology.[10, 41, 42, 50, 62–70] They tend to be intuitively easier to understand and allow much more realistic partnership networks to be created, but at the cost of increased computation time and, commonly, the loss of mathematical tractability.[49, 71] Alternatively, compartmental *pair-approximation* models can be used that avoid the random mixing assumption and show saturation of local contacts as expected, but can retain the ability to be analysed analytically (Panel 8.11).

Panel 8.11 Pair-wise approximation models

Pair-wise approximation models are created by using the compartmental modelling approach and adding compartments for pairs or triplets.[86, 87] So for example, the number of pairs of individuals in a population in which one individual is infected and one individual is susceptible is recorded as *[SI]* in the same way *S* recorded the number of susceptible individuals in the population. Then, the standard equation for the number of new infections per unit time:

$$\lambda(t)S(t) = c\beta\frac{I(t)}{N}S(t)$$

8.95

is rewritten as:

$$\lambda(t)S(t) = \beta[SI]$$

8.96

The full set of differential equations can be written down in the same way. In this way, pair-approximation models can avoid the random mixing assumption and show saturation of local contacts as expected, but can retain the ability to be analysed analytically. Pair-wise approximation network models have been used to model the spread and control of STIs in heterogeneous populations and in populations in which infected individuals change their behaviour.[55, 86, 88]

Kretzschmar and colleagues use an individual based simulation model to explore the heterosexual spread and control of gonorrhoea and chlamydia in the Netherlands.[66] Contact tracing, subgroup screening, and condom use were compared in an age-structured population with risk heterogeneity. The authors concluded that contact tracing was a very effective prevention strategy, that screening should be targeted to the highly active group, and that age was not a good enough indicator of high-risk behaviour to be able to recommend screening of certain age groups.

Ghani and Garnett created a wide range of networks using individual-based simulation, introduced a gonorrhoea-like infection onto these networks, and used statistical regression techniques to test the association between various measures of the position of individuals in the network and their risks of acquiring and transmitting infection.[42] They found that an individual's risk of both acquiring and transmitting infection depended primarily on their number of partners and partnership concurrency, but that, in addition, local network measures (connectivity to nearby members of the sexual partner network) were more strongly associated with the risk of acquisition of infection and global measures (connectivity to all members of the sexual partner network) were more strongly associated with the risk of transmission of infection.

STDSIM simulates the natural history of and interactions between up to 16 STIs, most often HIV, HSV-2, syphilis, gonorrhoea, chlamydia and chancroid.[50, 70, 72, 73] The formation of partnerships is determined by balancing the demand and supply of males and females[51] allowing for partner age preference.[50] Three types of sexual relationships can be modelled, one-off contact between female sex-workers and male clients, and short and longer-term partnerships that are typically used to represent casual and marital partnerships. An example male sexual life history is shown in Figure 8.26 and the partnership formation mechanism allows for the creation of a wide range of realistic sexual networks (Figure 8.27). *STDSIM* has been used to explore the impact of STI treatment, vaccination and male circumcision for HIV-1 prevention

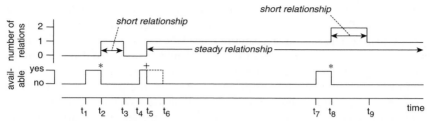

Fig. 8.26 Example of the supply–demand partnership formation mechanism for a male sexual life history in *STDSIM*. A male becomes available for first partnership at time $= t_1$. As he is not found by a female during his 'available period' between t_1 and t_2, he starts searching for a partner himself at t_2 and very soon afterwards starts a short/casual relationship '*' lasts from t_2 to t_3. After a delay he becomes available for partnerships again at t_4 and is found '+' by a female for a long/steady relationship. Concurrency is modelled by allowing individuals to become available for other partnerships before the end of their current partnership, as is shown occurring at t_7 and leading to concurrency between t_8 and t_9. Figure from Korenromp et al, 2000.[50]

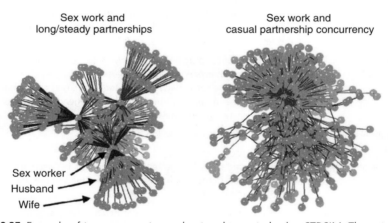

Fig. 8.27 Example of two emergent sexual networks created using STDSIM. The network on the left was created by modelling sex work and long-term (marital) partnerships. The network on the right was created by modelling sex work and casual partnership concurrency. The average path-length is considerably shorter in the network on the left. Figure courtesy of Roel Bakker, Erasmus MC, Rotterdam.

in Africa, the heterogeneous spread of HIV-1 in Africa, and the diverging HIV-1 and HIV-2 prevalence trends in West Africa.[10, 67–70, 74–78]

Boily and colleagues used an individual-based model to generate a wide range of networks and to show the extent to which infection transmission may be affected by varying generally unmeasurable network characteristics such as the mean component and giant component size (called the micro-structure), while keeping fixed generally more measurable network characteristics such as numbers of individuals in different age or activity groups and mixing patterns (called the macro-structure).[79] They found that a wide variety of network micro-structures could be simulated that were consistent with the predefined macro-structure and these differences in micro-structure had a dramatic effect on the establishment, persistence, and spread of infection. They concluded by saying that this illustrates one of the limitations of network modelling and that in the absence of data to more uniquely identify the sexual network, exhaustive sensitivity analysis should be carried out when using network models.

Developing efficient methods for assessing the sensitivity of complex and resource-intensive network models to parameter and structural uncertainty is an area of ongoing research.

Panel 8.12 Network modelling terminology

Bipartite (graph)	Population (graph) that contains individuals of two distinct types, for example males and females, such that no partnerships (edges) connect individuals (vertices) of the same type. For example, a purely heterosexually behaving population of males and females.
Clustering	Can be best summed up as: '*In a highly clustered network a lot of my partners' partners are also my partners.*' Also called 'transitivity' in the social network literature. Increased clustering results in higher numbers of triangles in single-gender networks or squares in two-gender networks.[85]
Component (of a graph)	A set of individuals connected by partnerships.
Connected graph	A graph is said to be 'connected' if a path exists between any two individuals in the graph, so that all individuals in the graph could become infected.
Degree distribution	The distribution of the number of partnerships (edges) per person (vertex) in the population (graph).
Degree of a vertex	The number of partnerships (edges) an individual (vertex) has. Random networks result in binomial or Poisson distributions if n large, but real degree distributions tend to be skewed, see Figure 8.6.
Diameter of graph	The largest *distance* on a graph
Distance	The smallest number of partnerships through the network from one individual to another individual (also called the geodesic path). There may be, and often is, more than one geodesic path between two individuals.

Edge	A partnership. More generally the line connecting two vertices (individuals). The meaning depends on the discipline and research question. Also called a 'bond' in physics, a 'link' in computer science, a 'tie' in sociology, or a 'contact' in epidemiology. There can be more than one type of edge in a graph, for example representing different partnership types, see *valued network*.
Giant component	A giant component exists in a population if the majority of the individuals in a population are connected by partnerships.
Graph	A set of individuals (vertices) and partnerships (edges).
Neighbourhood size	The number of partners of an individual, or the number of vertices with path-length = 1. This may be smaller than the degree distribution if there is more than one edge between two vertices (this may not be relevant for sexual contacts, but could, for example, represent different types of social contacts such as a friend and a work colleague).
Order (of graph)	The number of individuals (vertices) in the graph.
Path	If two individuals can be reached from each other by following partnerships, a *path* exists between them.
Path-length	The *distance* between two individuals.
Preferential attachment	Technique of creating a network, vertex by vertex, by connecting individuals with a probability that is directly proportional to their current number of partners. Can lead to 'scale-free' networks.[58]
Scale free network	Network in which the number of partners is distributed according to a power law.
Size (of graph)	The number of partnerships (edges) in the population (graph).
Valued network	Network in which there are different types of partnerships (edges) between individuals and these are weighted according to their strength such as steady and casual sexual partnerships, see Korenromp *et al.*[50] and Kretzschmar *et al.*[66]
Vertex	An individual. More generally the fundamental unit of a network, also called a site (physics), a node (computer science), or an actor (sociology). Can be more than one type in a network (eg men and women).

8.11 **Summary**

Mathematical modelling has proved to be an enormously useful tool to understand the epidemiology and control of STIs. Modelling has allowed the synthesis of demographic, behavioural and epidemiological data in a single framework, and evaluation of the consistency of these various sources of data. Modelling has helped to identify key behaviours that may be important for understanding the spread of STIs such as risk heterogeneity, mixing patterns and partnership concurrency and, when key data on these behaviours were lacking, guided data collection. Modelling has also allowed us to predict the likely trends in prevalence and incidence of different STIs and the impact of existing and hypothetical control strategies.

Recent advances in computing resources have allowed increasingly complex models to be created. These models have been very useful in allowing more complex research questions to be explored such as the interaction between multiple STIs and HIV, but these complex modelling studies must be designed and analysed with care in order to retain the powerful insights that may be more easily obtained from simpler models.

Unfortunately, with millions of people newly infected with sexually transmitted HIV each year[80] and the global disease burden of other STIs still very high,[39] the mathematical modelling of the transmission and control of sexually transmitted infections will continue to be an active area of research.

See Chapter 9 for details of STI/HIV co-infection modelling and to see how models have been used to help understand the control of sexually transmitted HIV in sub-Saharan Africa.

References

1 Holmes KK, Sparling PF, Stamm W, Piot P, Wasserheit JN, Corey L, et al. Sexually transmitted diseases. 2008. New York: McGraw-Hill. Ref Type: Serial (Book, Monograph).

2 Hethcote H, Yorke J. Lecture notes in biomathematics: gonorrhea transmission and control, vol. 56, S. Levin, ed. 1984. Berlin: Springer-Verlag.

3 Fenton KA, Johnson AM, McManus S, Erens B. Measuring sexual behaviour: methodological challenges in survey research. Sex Transm Infect 2001; 77(2): 84–92.

4 Schneeberger A, Mercer CH, Gregson SA, Ferguson NM, Nyamukapa CA, Anderson RM, et al. Scale-free networks and sexually transmitted diseases: a description of observed patterns of sexual contacts in Britain and Zimbabwe. Sex Transm Dis 2004; 31(6): 380–387.

5 Coffin J, Haase A, Levy JA, Montagnier L, Oroszlan S, Teich N, et al. Human immunodeficiency viruses. Science 1986; 232(4751): 697.

6 Fleming DT, Wasserheit JN. From epidemiological synergy to public health policy and practice: the contribution of other sexually transmitted diseases to sexual transmission of HIV infection. Sex Transm Inf 1999; 75: 3–17.

7 Laga M, Nzila N, Goeman J. The interrelationship of sexually transmitted diseases and HIV infection: implications for the control of both epidemics in Africa. [Review]. AIDS 1991; 5(1): S55–63.

8 Rottingen JA, Cameron DW, Garnett GP. A systematic review of the epidemiologic interactions between classic sexually transmitted diseases and HIV: how much really is known? Sex Transm Dis 2001; 28(10): 579–597.

9 Wasserheit JN. Epidemiological synergy. Interrelationships between human immunodeficiency virus infection and other sexually transmitted diseases. [Review]. Sex Transm Dis 1992; 19(2): 61–77.

10 White RG, Orroth KK, Korenromp EL, Bakker R, Wambura M, Sewankambo NK, et al. Can population differences explain the contrasting results of the Mwanza, Rakai, and Masaka HIV/Sexually Transmitted Disease Intervention Trials?: a modeling study. J Acquir Immune Defic Syndr 2004; 37(4): 1500–1513.

11 Cooke KL, Yorke JA. Some equations modelling growth processes and gonorrhea epidemics. Math Biosc 1973; 16: 75–101.

12 Boily M-C, Masse B. Mathematical models of disease transmission: a precious tool of the study of sexually transmitted diseases. *Canadian Journal of Public Health* 1997; 88: 255–265.

13 Garnett GP, Anderson RM. Balancing sexual partnerships in an age and activity stratified model of HIV transmission in heterosexual populations. *IMA J Math Appl Med Biol* 1994; 11(3): 161–192.

14 Anderson RM, May RM. Spatial, temporal, and genetic heterogeneity in host populations and the design of immunization programmes. *IMA J Math Appl Med Biol* 1984; 1(3): 233–266.

15 Garnett GP, Anderson RM. Contact tracing and the estimation of sexual mixing patterns: the epidemiology of gonococcal infections. *Sex Transm Dis* 1993; 20(4): 181–191.

16 Turner KM, Garnett GP, Ghani AC, Sterne JA, Low N. Investigating ethnic inequalities in the incidence of sexually transmitted infections: mathematical modelling study. *Sex Transm Infect* 2004; 80(5): 379–385.

17 Gupta S, Anderson RM, May RM. Networks of sexual contacts: implications for the pattern of spread of HIV. *AIDS* 1989; 3(12): 181–191.

18 Keeling MJ, Rohani P. Host heterogeneities. In MJ Keeling and P Rohani *Modeling infectious diseases in humans and animals.* 2008. Princeton, NJ and Oxford: Princeton University Press, pp. 54–103.

19 McPherson M, Smith-Lovin L, Cook JM. Birds of a feather: homophily in social networks. *Annual Review of Sociology* 2001; 27(1): 415–444.

20 Garnett GP, Hughes JP, Anderson RM, Stoner BP, Aral SO, Whittington WL, *et al.* Sexual mixing patterns of patients attending sexually transmitted diseases clinics. *Sex Transm Dis* 1996; 23(3): 248–257.

21 Boily M-C, Anderson RM. Sexual contact patterns betwen men and women and the spread of HIV-1 in urban centres in Africa. *IMA J Math Appl Med Biol* 1991; 8: 221–247.

22 Hallett TB, Gregson S, Lewis JJ, Lopman BA, Garnett GP. Behaviour change in generalised HIV epidemics: The impact of reducing cross-generational sex and delaying age at sexual debut. *Sex Transm Infect* 2007; 83:i50–i54.

23 Garnett GP, Swinton J, Brunham RC, Anderson RM. Gonococcal infection, infertility, and population growth: II. The influence of heterogeneity in sexual behaviour. *IMA J Math Appl Med Biol* 1992; 9(2): 127–144.

24 Ross R. The prevention of malaria. Second edition with the addendum on the theory of happening. London: John Murray; 1911.

25 Hethcote HW. Qualitative analysis for communicable disease models. *Math Biosci* 1976; 28: 335–356.

26 Dietz K. The estimation of the basic reproduction number for infectious diseases. *Stat Methods Med Res* 1993; 2(1): 23–41.

27 Boily MC, Baggaley RF, Wang L, Masse B, White RG, Hayes RJ, *et al.* Heterosexual risk of HIV-1 infection per sexual act: a systematic review and meta-analysis of observational studies. *Lancet Infectious Diseases* 2009; 9(2): 118–29.

28 Powers KA, Poole C, Pettifor AE, Cohen MS. Rethinking the heterosexual infectivity of HIV-1: a systematic review and meta-analysis. *Lancet Infectious Diseases* 2008; 8(9): 553–563.

29 Wawer MJ, Gray RH, Sewankambo NK, Serwadda D, Li X, Laeyendecker O, *et al.* Rates of HIV-1 Transmission per Coital Act, by Stage of HIV-1 Infection, in Rakai, Uganda. *J Infect Dis* 2005; 191(9): 1403–1409.

30 CASCADE. Time from HIV-1 seroconversion to AIDS and death before widespread use of highly-active antiretroviral therapy: a collaborative re-analysis. Collaborative Group on AIDS Incubation and HIV Survival including the CASCADE EU Concerted Action. Concerted Action on SeroConversion to AIDS and Death in Europe. *Lancet* 2000; 355(9210):1131–1317.

31 Morgan D, Mahe B, Okongo MJ, Lubega R, Whitworth JA. HIV-1 infection in rural Africa: is there a difference in median time to AIDS and survival compared with that in industrialized countries? *AIDS* 2002; 16:597–603.

32 Todd J, Glynn JR, Marston M, Lutalo T, Biraro S, Mwita W, *et al.* Time from HIV seroconversion to death: a collaborative analysis of eight studies in six low and middle-income countries before highly active antiretroviral therapy. *AIDS* 2007; 21 Suppl 6: S55–63.

33 Anderson R, May R. Social heterogeneity and sexually transmitted diseases. In R Anderson and R May, *Infectious diseases. Dynamics and control.* 1991. Oxford: Oxford University Press; pp. 228–303.

34 Garnett GP, Gregson S, Stanecki KA. Criteria for detecting and understanding changes in the risk of HIV infection at a national level in generalised epidemics10.1136/sti.2005.016022. *Sex Transm Infect* 2006; 82(suppl 1):i48–51.

35 Wawer MJ, Serwadda D, Gray RH, Sewankambo NK, Li C, Nalugoda F, *et al.* Trends in HIV-1 prevalence may not reflect trends in incidence in mature epidemics: data from the Rakai population-based cohort, Uganda. *AIDS* 1997; 11(8):1023–1030.

36 UNAIDS/WHO. *UNAIDS/WHO Epidemiological Fact Sheet, 2008 Update, South Africa.* 2008. Geneva: UNAIDS/WHO.

37 UNAIDS/WHO. *UNAIDS/WHO Epidemiological Fact Sheet, 2008 Update, Zimbabwe.* 2008. Geneva: UNAIDS/WHO.

38 UNAIDS/WHO. *UNAIDS/WHO Epidemiological Fact Sheet, 2008 Update, Uganda.* 2008. Geneva: UNAIDS/WHO.

39 WHO. *Global prevalence and incidence of selected curable sexually transmitted infections: overview and estimates.* 2001. Geneva: WHO.

40 Coffee MP, Lurie M, Garnett GP. Modelling the impact of migration on the HIV epidemic in South Africa. *AIDS* 2007; 21: 343–350.

41 Doherty IA, Shiboski S, Ellen JM, Adimora AA, Padian NS. Sexual bridging socially and over time: a simulation model exploring the relative effects of mixing and concurrency on viral sexually transmitted infection transmission. *Sex Transm Dis* 2006; 33(6): 368–373.

42 Ghani AC, Garnett GP. Risks of acquiring and transmitting sexually transmitted diseases in sexual partner networks. *Sex Transm Dis* 2000; 27(10):579–587.

43 Morris M, Kretzschmar M. Concurrent partnerships and the spread of HIV [see comments]. *AIDS* 1997; 11(5):641–648.

44 Morris M, Kretzschmar M. *A microsimulation study of the effect of concurrent partnerships on the spread of HIV in Uganda.* 2000. PA: Population Research Institute.

45 Watts CH, May RM. The influence of concurrent partnerships on the dynamics of HIV/AIDS. *Math Biosci* 1992; 108:89–104.

46 Morris M, Goodreau S, Moody J. Sexual networks, concurrency and STD/HIV. In Holmes KK, ed., *Sexually transmitted diseases.* 2008. New York: McGraw-Hill; pp. 118–125.

47 Halloran ME, Longini IM, Jr., Nizam A, Yang Y. Containing bioterrorist smallpox. *Science* 2002; 298(5597):1428–1432.

48 Garnett GP, Anderson RM. Sexually transmitted diseases and sexual behavior: insights from mathematical models. *J Infect Dis* 1996; 174 Suppl 2:S150–161.

49 Keeling MJ, Eames KT. Networks and epidemic models. *J R Soc Interface* 2005; 2(4): 295–307.

50 Korenromp EL, Van Vliet C, Bakker R, De Vlas SJ, Habbema JDF. HIV spread and partnership reduction for different patterns of sexual behaviour - a study with the microsimulation model STDSIM. *Mathematical Population Studies* 2000; 8(2):135–173.

51 Le Pont F, Blower SM. The supply and demand of sexual behavior: implications for heterosexual HIV epidemics. *J Acq Imm Def Syndr* 1991; 4:987–999.

52 Diekmann O, De Jong MCM, Metz JAJ. A deterministic epidemic model taking account of repeated contacts between the same individuals. *Journal of Applied Probability* 1998; 35(2):448–462.

53 Watts DJ, Strogatz SH. Collective dynamics of 'small-world' networks. *Nature* 1998; 393(6684):440–442.

54 Wikipedia. Six degrees of separation. Accessed 4 January 2010.

55 Eames KTD, Keeling MJ. Modeling dynamic and network heterogeneities in the spread of sexually transmitted diseases10.1073/pnas.202244299. *PNAS* 2002; 99(20): 13330–13335.

56 Keeling M. The implications of network structure for epidemic dynamics. *Theor Popul Biol* 2005; 67:1–8.

57 Read JM, Keeling MJ. Disease evolution on networks: the role of contact structure. *Proc R Soc Lond B Biol Sci* 2003; 270(1516):699–708.

58 Barabasi AL, Albert R. Emergence of scaling in random networks. *Science* 1999; 286(5439):509–512.

59 Liljeros F, Edling CR, Amaral LA, Stanley HE, Aberg Y. The web of human sexual contacts. *Nature* 2001; 411(6840):907–908.

60 Jones JH, Handcock MS. Social networks: sexual contacts and epidemic thresholds. *Nature* 2003; 423(6940):605 6; discussion 606.

61 Grimm V, Railsback SF. *Individual-based modeling and ecology.* Princeton, NJ: Princeton University Press; 2005.

62 Chick SE, Adams AL, Koopman JS. Analysis and simulation of a stochastic, discrete-individual model of STD transmission with partnership concurrency. *Math Biosci* 2000; 166(1):45–68.

63 Ghani AC, Swinton J, Garnett GP. The role of sexual partnership networks in the epidemiology of gonorrhea. *Sex Trans Dis* 1997; 24(1):45–56.

64 Goodreau SM. Assessing the effects of human mixing patterns on human immunodeficiency virus-1 interhost phylogenetics through social network simulation. *Genetics* 2006; 172(4):2033–2045.

65 Handcock MS, Jones JH. Likelihood-based inference for stochastic models of sexual network formation. *Theor Popul Biol* 2004; 65(4):413–422.

66 Kretzschmar M, Van Duynhoven YT, Severijnen AJ. Modeling prevention strategies for gonorrhea and chlamydia using stochastic network simulations. *Am J Epidemiol* 1996; 144(3):306–317.

67 Freeman EE, White RG, Bakker R, Orroth KK, Weiss HA, Buve A, *et al.* Population-level effect of potential HSV2 prophylactic vaccines on HIV incidence in sub-Saharan Africa. *Vaccine* 2009; 27:940–946.

68 White RG, Orroth KK, Glynn JR, Freeman EE, Bakker R, Habbema JDF, *et al.* Treating curable sexually transmitted infections to prevent HIV in Africa: still an effective control strategy? *J Acquir Immune Defic Syndr* 2008; 47:940–946.

69 White RG, Freeman EE, Orroth KK, Bakker R, Weiss HA, O'Farrell N, *et al.* Population-level effect of HSV-2 therapy on the incidence of HIV in sub-Saharan Africa. *Sex Trans Inf* 2008; 84(S2):12–18.

70 White RG, Glynn JR, Orroth KK, Freeman EE, Bakker R, Weiss HA, *et al.* Male circumcision for HIV prevention in sub-Saharan Africa: who, what and when? *AIDS* 2008; 22(14):1841–1850.

71 May RM. Uses and abuses of mathematics in biology. *Science* 2004; 303(5659):790–793.

72 Korenromp EL, Van Vliet C, Grosskurth H, Gavyole A, Van der Ploeg CPB, Fransen L, *et al.* Model-based evaluation of single-round mass STD treatment for HIV control in a rural African population. *AIDS* 2000; 14:573–593.

73 Van der Ploeg CPB, Van Vliet C, De Vlas SJ, Ndinya-Achola Jeckoniah O, Fransen Lieve, Van Oortmarssen Gerrit J, *et al.* STDSIM: a microsimulation model for decision support in STD control. *Interfaces* 1998; 28:84–100.

74 Korenromp EL, White RG, Orroth KK, Bakker R, Kamali A, Serwadda D, *et al.* Determinants of the impact of sexually transmitted infection treatment on prevention of HIV infection: a synthesis of evidence from the Mwanza, Rakai, and Masaka Intervention Trials. *J Infect Dis* 2005; 191(Suppl 1):S168–178.

75 Orroth KK, Freeman E, Bakker R, Buve A, Glynn J, Boily M-C, *et al.* Understanding differences across the contrasting epidemics in East and West Africa: results from a simulation model of the Four Cities Study. *STI* 2007; 83:i5–i16.

76 Schmidt WP, Schim VLM, Aaby P, Whittle H, Bakker R, Buckner M, *et al.* Behaviour change and competitive exclusion can explain the diverging HIV-1 and HIV-2 prevalence trends in Guinea-Bissau. *Epidemiol Infect* 2008; 136(4):551–561.

77 Freeman E, Orroth K, White RG, Glynn JR, Bakker R, Boily M-C, *et al.* The proportion of new HIV infections attributable to HSV-2 increases over time: simulations of the changing role of sexually transmitted infections in sub-Saharan African HIV epidemics. *STI* 2007; 83:i17–i24.

78 Orroth KK, White RG, Korenromp EL, Bakker R, Changalucha J, Habbema JD, *et al.* Empirical observations underestimate the proportion of human immunodeficiency virus infections attributable to sexually transmitted diseases in the Mwanza and Rakai sexually transmitted disease treatment trials: simulation results. *Sex Transm Dis* 2006; 33(9): 536–544.

79 Boily MC, Asghar Z, Garske T, Ghani AC, Poulin R. Influence of selected formation rules for finite population networks with fixed macrostructures: implications for individual-based model of infectious diseases. *Mathematical Population Studies* 2007; 14(4):237–267.

80 UNAIDS/WHO. *AIDS epidemic update 2007.* Geneva: UNAIDS/ WHO.

81 Kaplan EH. Modeling HIV infectivity: must sex acts be counted? *J Acquir Immune Defic Syndr* 1990; 3(1):55–61.

82 Garnett GP, Anderson RM. Strategies for limiting the spread of HIV in developing countries: conclusions based on studies of the transmission dynamics of the virus. *J Acquir Immune Defic Syndr Hum Retrovirol* 1995; 9(5):500–513.

83 Pinkerton SD, Abramson PR. Occasional condom use and HIV risk reduction. *J Acquir Immune Defic Syndr Hum Retrovirol* 1996; 13(5):456–460.

84 Yorke J, Hethcote H, Nod A. Dynamics and control of the transmission of gonorrhea. *Sex Transm Dis* 1978; 5:51–56.

85 Lind PG, Gonzalez MC, Herrmann HJ. Cycles and clustering in bipartite networks. *Phys Rev E Stat Nonlin Soft Matter Phys* 2005; 72(5 Pt 2):056127.

86 Ferguson NM, Garnett GP. More realistic models of sexually transmitted disease transmission dynamics: sexual partnership networks, pair models, and moment closure. *Sex Transm Dis* 2000; 27(10):600–609.

87 Keeling MJ, Rand DA, Morris AJ. Correlation models for childhood epidemics. *Proc Biol Sci* 1997; 264(1385):1149–1156.

88 Lloyd-Smith JO, Getz WM, Westerhoff HV. Frequency-dependent incidence in models of sexually transmitted diseases: portrayal of pair-based transmission and effects of illness on contact behaviour. *Proc Biol Sci* 2004; 271(1539):625–634.

Chapter 9

Special topics in infectious disease modelling

9.1 Overview and objectives

We conclude this book by discussing four specific topics which highlight some of the insights into the dynamics of infections that models have provided: modelling vaccination and the effects of boosting and serotype replacement, modelling the transmission dynamics of diseases with long incubation periods, modelling HIV/STI coinfection and a case study describing how HIV modelling studies have evolved with the HIV epidemic.

By the end of this chapter you should:

- Be aware of how, for some infections, the introduction of vaccination can lead to changes in the dynamics through reducing the amount of boosting of infection or through serotype replacement;

- Understand how changes in the risk of infection for *M. tuberculosis* have affected the underlying dynamics of tuberculosis in Western populations and the implications for control;

- Understand how coinfection with other sexually transmitted infections may have influenced the spread of HIV, and how the spread of HIV may have reduced the prevalence of other sexually transmitted infections;

- Understand how HIV modelling studies have evolved with the HIV epidemic.

9.2 The effect of vaccination on the dynamics of infections

In Chapter 5, we discussed how changes in the amount of transmission following the introduction of vaccination among young children may lead to increases in the number of new infections occurring in adults. We discuss two specific examples for which vaccination can lead to other changes in the dynamics of infections.

9.2.1 Varicella vaccination and boosting

Chickenpox is caused by the varicella zoster virus; following infection, the virus remains latent in an individual and can reactivate many years later to cause varicella zoster ('shingles'). As discussed in Panel 7.7, there are several concerns regarding the introduction of varicella vaccination (see review in Edmunds and Brisson[1]); for convenience, we summarize them briefly here. First, by reducing the prevalence of infectious persons, vaccination reduces the opportunity for individuals to be exposed, and could lead to increases in the number of infections among adults, who have an increased risk of complications following infection. Second, the reduced circulation of varicella because of a vaccination programme could lead to an increase in the number of cases of zoster, given that exposure to the virus can boost the immune system of individuals who have been previously infected, reducing their chances of developing zoster ('shingles').[2, 3] Third, vaccination may lead to an increased occurrence of so-called 'breakthrough varicella', which is defined as a mild form of varicella which occurs among vaccine failures following infection.

The potential for increases in the number of zoster cases following the introduction of vaccination, and the other complications, has been explored by several studies.[2, 4–6] Figure 9.1 summarizes the findings of Brisson et al.,[4] who used an age-structured model to examine the potential impact of several strategies in Canada, e.g. routine vaccination of 1-year-olds with or without routine vaccination of 11-year-olds. This study illustrated that if exposure to varicella cases does not boost a person's immunity to zoster, then the annual number of zoster cases will probably decrease after varicella vaccination is introduced among 1-year-olds. On the other hand, if vaccination provides 2 or 20 years of immunity to zoster, then the introduction of varicella vaccination is likely to lead to increases in the annual number of zoster cases. This study also explored the sensitivity of predictions of the impact of vaccination to assumptions about contact between individuals (see Panel 7.6).

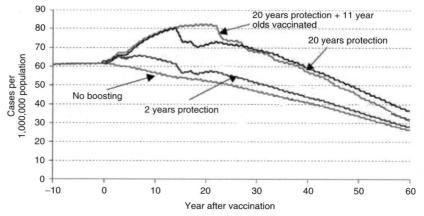

Fig. 9.1 Predictions of the annual number of zoster cases following the introduction of varicella vaccination in year 0 from the study of Brisson et al., assuming that exposure to a varicella case either does not boost an individual's immunity, or, on average, provides 2 or 20 years of protection against zoster.[4] The vaccine coverage is assumed to be 90 per cent (among those aged 12 months, unless otherwise stated), and the efficacy is 93 per cent, declining over time. Reproduced with permission from Brisson et al, 2000.[4]

The USA was the first country to introduce routine varicella vaccination for those aged between 12 months and 13 years although, as yet,[7, 8] it appears to be too early to determine whether predictions from these models will be realized.[9]

9.2.2 Serotype replacement

Reductions in the transmission following the introduction of vaccination are also relevant for pneumococcal disease. Pneumococcal conjugate vaccination has been introduced recently into the routine schedule for infants and the elderly in several European countries and the US. [10] There are about 90 serotypes for *Streptococcus pneumoniae* (pneumococci). Pneumococci are normally carried in the nasopharynx and, whilst they usually cause no symptoms, they can lead to invasive disease, including bacteraemic pneumonia, bacteraemia and meningitis.[11] Thus, carriers rather than diseased individuals are mainly responsible for transmitting pneumococci. The vaccines which have been licensed to date in the UK[11] for the elderly and children protect against 23 and 7 serotypes respectively.

By reducing the amount of transmission of the serotypes included in the vaccine, the introduction of vaccination could lead to an increase in prevalence and transmission of pneumococcal serotypes which are not included in the vaccine.[12, 13] Such increases have been observed in several places.[14, 15] They depend on many factors, including the amount of competition for colonization between different serotypes and differences between the protection provided against different serotypes.[12, 16] Many of these aspects are poorly understood, although some of their implications have been explored using theoretical models.[12, 16]

For example, Figure 9.2 shows predictions obtained by Lipsitch[12, 16] using a model which assumed that there is relatively little competition between two serotypes (carriage with a given serotype reduces the probability of acquiring the other serotype by 30 per cent). For simplicity, these serotypes are referred to as serotype 1 and 2. This shows that if the vaccine provides complete protection against one serotype, then, as the vaccination coverage increases, the proportion of individuals carrying serotype one or both serotypes decreases and the prevalence of individuals carrying serotype 2 should increase (Figure 9.2a). On the other hand, if the vaccine also provides 80 per cent protection against serotype 2, then the prevalence of both serotypes 1 and 2 should decrease as the vaccination coverage increases, and if the vaccination coverage is sufficiently high, the prevalence of carriage should be zero (Figure 9.2b).

9.3 Diseases with long incubation periods: tuberculosis

9.3.1 The long-term dynamics

Much of the discussion in this book has been on the long term dynamics and control of acute infections, for which the incubation period is short (measured in days or months). In this section, we will be considering tuberculosis, for which the incubation period is measured in years.

Tuberculosis disease is caused by the tubercle bacillus *Mycobacterium tuberculosis*. It usually affects the lungs, although other organs can be involved and the disease is

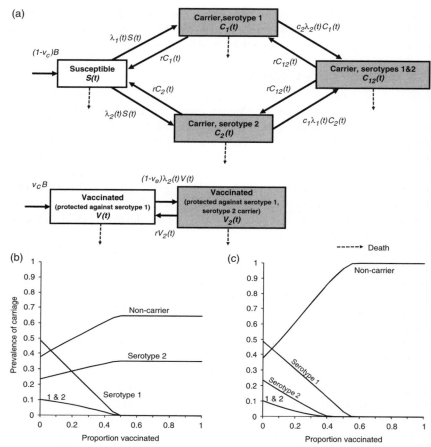

Fig. 9.2 (a) General structure of the model of Lipsitch.[12] (b) and (c) Predictions from the model of Lipsitch[12] of the equilibrium proportions of individuals carrying serotypes 1, serotype 2, both serotypes or neither serotype for different levels of vaccination coverage. Predictions in (b) assume that vaccination provides complete protection against carriage only for serotype 1; predictions in (c) are based on the assumption that vaccination provides complete protection against carriage for serotype 1 and 80 per cent protection for serotype 2. The basic reproduction numbers for serotypes 1 and 2 are assumed to be 2.2 and 1.6 respectively. See Lipsitch[12] for further details of the model and Model 9.1 (online) for an example of its formulation. (b) and (c) are adapted from Lipsitch, 1997.[12]

described as being either 'pulmonary' (respiratory) or 'extrapulmonary', depending on the site affected. *M. tuberculosis* is transmitted most commonly through coughing by a case with infectious or 'open' pulmonary tuberculosis.

In Western populations, the long-term trends in tuberculosis differ from the cyclic patterns seen for the immunizing infections (Figure 9.3a): aside from the increases seen during the two World Wars, the mortality rates declined since 1850, as did the notifications since records began. Treatment became available during the early 1950s; hence the mortality rates reliably reflected the trend in incidence before then. The annual risk of infection also declined during the twentieth century (Figure 9.3b,c),

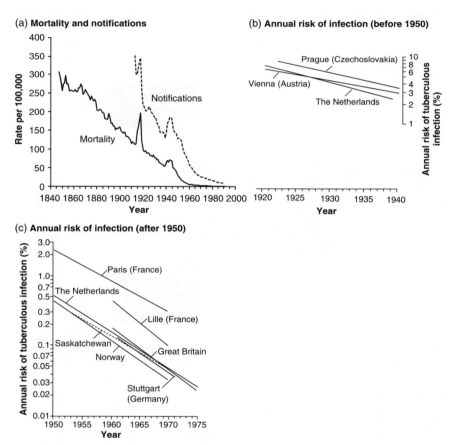

Fig. 9.3 (a) Summary of the overall mortality and notification rates for respiratory tuberculosis among males in England and Wales since 1850. The mortality rates are standardized to the population in 1901; the notification rates are the crude rates. Data sources Registrar General annual reports.[28] (b) and (c) Estimates of the annual risk of tuberculous infection in several Western populations obtained by Styblo *et al.* Reproduced with permission from Styblo K. 1991.[23]

from about 12 per cent in the early 1900s, to about 2 per cent and <0.1 per cent by 1950 and 1980 respectively.[17–20] This decline probably resulted from many factors, in particular, reductions in the number of individuals effectively contacted by each infectious person.[21, 22] This reduction, in turn, resulted from reductions in crowding in living conditions or removal of infectious cases to sanatoria (before 1950), shortening the duration of infectiousness through treatment (from 1950), and improvements in general hygiene (e.g. the discouragement of spitting behaviour).

This long-term decline in the infection risk in Western populations means that the proportion of individuals that were infected by given ages decreased over time. Such decreases are analogous to the increases in the proportion of individuals that were predicted to reach older ages still susceptible to immunizing infections, following the reductions in the force of infection that were discussed in relation to vaccination programmes in section 5.3.2.

However, the effect of such changes in the infection risk are more complicated for tuberculosis than for the immunizing infections, given that, in contrast with these

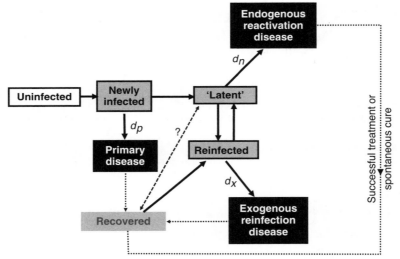

Fig. 9.4 Schematic diagram of the natural history of tuberculosis. Black boxes reflect categories for diseased individuals; medium grey boxes reflect categories containing individuals who are infected. Not all cases are treated successfully or cure spontaneously, as reflected by use of a dotted arrow from the boxes reflecting diseased individuals to the recovered category. Note that recovery from disease does not necessarily mean recovery from infection. The shading for the 'Recovered' compartment differs from that of the other compartments involving individuals who are infected but not diseased, since the immunity associated with treatment/recovery after disease is poorly understood, and it is not known as to how it differs for individuals who are in the 'latent' category. Note that for tuberculosis, the term 'latent' is used in a different way from the way it is used for acute immunizing infections, since individuals who have 'latent' infection can go on to develop either infectious or non-infectious disease. The letters d_p, d_x and d_n represent the different risks of developing disease soon after infection, reinfection or through reactivation respectively.

Panel 9.1 Estimates of the risk of developing tuberculosis disease soon after recent initial infection, reinfection and through reactivation

The first analyses of these risks, which were carried out by Sutherland et al.[24] (Figure 9.5a) estimated that the five-year cumulative risk of disease following infection or reinfection were 22.9 and 9.2 per cent respectively. The annual risk of disease through endogenous reactivation for individuals (re)infected >5 years previously was 0.023 per cent. These risks imply that infection provides about 60 per cent protection against disease following reinfection.

Subsequent analyses, based on data from England and Wales, have revised this estimate of the protection downwards to 16–41 per cent,[25] with the cumulative five-year risk of disease following infection and re-infection being 13.8 and 8.3 per cent respectively.

---

infections, tuberculosis disease can occur either soon after first infection ('primary' disease) or many years later through 'endogenous reactivation' of the earlier infection, or following a new (exogenous) reinfection[23] (Figure 9.4). Also the risks of developing disease through these various mechanisms differ, and the protection provided by either previous infection, treatment of the infection or disease is poorly understood (see below and Panel 9.1).[24, 25] Other complications in the epidemiology of tuberculosis include the fact that the lifetime risk of disease given infection is about 10 per cent on average, although it depends on age.[26] In addition, the proportion of disease that is infectious is age-dependent.[27]

As demonstrated extensively, first by Styblo and Sutherland[17, 24, 29, 30] and then by others,[25] the decline in the risk of tuberculous infection in Western populations has led to declines in the proportion of individuals who experienced disease attributable to recent reinfection, and to changes in the proportion experiencing disease attributable to reactivation and recent first infection (Figure 9.5a).

For example, in 1952, the annual numbers of cases among 45–49-year-olds in The Netherlands was about 60 per 100,000, with about two-thirds of the cases being attributed by the modelling work of Sutherland et al[24, 29, 30] to recent (exogenous) reinfection, a quarter being attributed to reactivation and the remainder to recent primary infection (Figure 9.5a). By 1967, however, the annual numbers of cases had declined to about 20 per 100,000, with over half of them being attributed to reactivation (Figure 9.5a). Throughout this time, the actual amount of disease attributable to recent (primary) infection was predicted to have remained at a similar level ($\approx$10 per 100,000).

How did the decline in the risk of M. tuberculosis infection lead to these changes?

The decline in the amount of disease attributable to reinfection is largely attributable to the fact that the decline in the infection risk reduced the opportunity for reinfection. For example, individuals alive in 1952 were less likely to be reinfected than those alive in 1967. A further contributing factor was the decline in the proportion of individuals who had been infected, and who, by definition, could be reinfected. For example, the declining risk over time meant that about 93% of 47 year olds alive

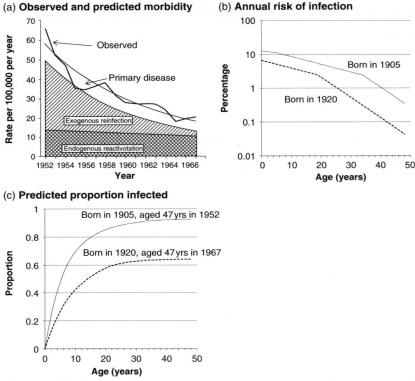

Fig. 9.5 (a) Estimated contribution of recent (primary) infection, reinfection and endogenous reactivation disease to the total morbidity from pulmonary tuberculosis among 45–49-year-olds (males and females combined) in The Netherlands, produced by the study of Sutherland et al.[29] Reproduced with permission from Canetti et al, 1972.[29] (b) Predictions of the annual risk of tuberculous infection experienced in each year of life until age 50 years for individuals born in 1905 and 1920 in The Netherlands, based on estimates from Styblo et al.[17] These individuals would have been aged 47 years in 1952 and 1967, and hence would have been in the youngest and oldest cohorts shown in Figure a). For a given year, the infection risk is assumed to be the same for all individuals irrespective of age. (c) Predictions of the proportion of individuals born in 1905 and 1920 in The Netherlands who were infected with M tuberculosis by the time they reached different ages, calculated using the infection risks in (b) and the methods described in section 9.3.1.1. See Model 9.2, online.

in 1952 had been infected, as compared with about 64% of 47 year olds alive in 1967 (see Figure 9.5c and Section 9.3.1.1).

The stable amount of disease due to primary infection that is predicted in Figure 9.5a is due to the fact that the proportion of 45–49-year-old individuals that had never been infected, and who were therefore at risk of primary infection increased between 1952 and 1967 (Figure 9.5c). However since the risk of infection also decreased during this time (from about 0.4 per cent to 0.05 per cent respectively), the number of new infections *per capita* remained relatively unchanged in this age group.

9.3.1.1 Example: calculating the proportion of individuals who have been infected by different ages

In general, the proportion of individuals who are infected by their a^{th} birthday in year t ($z_{a,t}$) can be calculated using the expression:

$$z_{a,t} = 1 - (1-\lambda_{t-a})(1-\lambda_{t-a+1})(1-\lambda_{t-a+2})...(1-\lambda_{t-2})(1-\lambda_{t-1}) \qquad 9.1$$

where λ_t is the risk of infection in year t.

This equation follows from the facts that:

i) The proportion $z_{a,t}$ is equivalent to $1 - s_{a,t}$, where $s_{a,t}$ is the proportion of individuals who escaped infection in each year of life until their a^{th} birthday in year t.

ii) The proportion who escape infection in the first year of life (i.e. in year $t-a$) equals 1−risk of infection in the first year of life = $1 - \lambda_{t-a}$

iii) The proportion who have still escaped infection by their second birthday is given by

(1−risk of infection in the first year of life, i.e., in year $t-a$)

×

(1−risk of infection in the 2nd year of life, i.e., in year $t-a+1$)

$$= (1-\lambda_{t-a})(1-\lambda_{t-a+1})$$

By analogy, the proportion who escape infection by their third birthday is given by $(1-\lambda_{t-a})(1-\lambda_{t-a+1})(1-\lambda_{t-a+2})$. Extending this logic to the ath birthday gives the result: $s_{a,t} = (1-\lambda_{t-a})(1-\lambda_{t-a+1})(1-\lambda_{t-a+2})...(1-\lambda_{t-2})(1-\lambda_{t-1})$. Combining this expression for $s_{a,t}$ with statement i) leads to Equation 9.1.

The following table summarizes the risk of tuberculous infection in The Netherlands for selected years between 1905 and 1952:[23]

Year	1905	1906	1907	1908	..	1948	1949	1950	1951	1952
	0.1284	0.1251	0.1220	0.1190	..	0.0070	0.0061	0.0053	0.0046	0.0040

We illustrate how these equations can be applied by calculating the proportion of 47 year olds (i.e. the midpoint of the age range 45–49 years) who would have been infected by 1952, in The Netherlands ($z_{47,1952}$). These individuals would have been born in 1905 and, according to the above table, would have experienced an infection risk of 12.84%, 12.51%, 12.20% in their first, second and third years of life respectively.

Applying Equation 9.1 leads to the following estimates: $z_{47,1952} =$

$$1 - (1-0.1284)(1-0.1251)(1-0.1220)...(1-0.0053)(1-0.0046)(1-0.0040) = 0.926$$

In contrast, those aged 47 years in 1967 would have experienced a 7 per cent risk of infection in their first year of life (i.e. in 1920)-see Figure 9.5b. Analogous calculations suggest that the proportion that were infected by age 47 years was about 0.64.

9.3.1.2 Example: calculating the proportion of individuals that are at risk of exogenous disease by age 47 years

Suppose that the risk of developing disease as a result of reinfection is greatest during the first five years after reinfection. The proportion of 47-year-olds in 1952 who experience this high risk can then be calculated using the following equation:

Proportion of individuals who had been infected by age 42 in the year 1947

×

Risk of being reinfected between the year 1947 and 1952

Assuming, for simplicity, that the risk of reinfection equals the risk of first infection (see below and Panel 9.1), this expression is given by the following:

$$z_{42,1947}\{1-(1-\lambda_{1948})(1-\lambda_{1949})(1-\lambda_{1950})(1-\lambda_{1951})(1-\lambda_{1952})\} \qquad 9.2$$

where $z_{42,1947}$ is the proportion of 42 year olds in 1947 that had been infected, and λ_t is the risk of infection in year t. The term in curly brackets in Equation 9.2 is obtained by using an analogous argument to that used to obtain Equation 9.1. As shown in Figure 9.5c, $z_{42,1947} = 0.923$ (obtained by reading off the proportion of those born in 1905 who were infected by age 42 years). Applying Equation 9.2 and the values for the risk of infection for The Netherlands leads to the following value for the proportion of 47 year olds in 1952 that had been reinfected:

$$0.923\{1-(1-0.007)(1-0.0061)(1-0.0053)(1-0.0046)(1-0.0040)\}$$
$$= 0.0247 \qquad 9.3$$

Analogous calculations imply that the proportion of 47-year-olds that had been reinfected during the preceding five years in 1967 was about 0.002.

Given estimates of the numbers of individuals in a given age group a at a given time t that have been recently infected ($I_{a,t}$), reinfected ($R_{a,t}$) or who are in the 'latent' category and are at risk of reactivation ($L_{a,t}$), based on calculations which are similar to those above, the overall numbers of incident tuberculosis cases in age group a at time t can be calculated using the expression:

$$I_{a,t}d_p + L_{a,t}d_n + R_{a,t}d_x \qquad 9.4$$

where d_p, d_n and d_x are the risks of developing disease soon after first infection, through reactivation and following reinfection respectively. In the absence of empirical estimates of the risk of disease given recent reinfection (d_x), researchers have typically estimated the size of this risk, together with that of d_p and d_n, by fitting predictions of the numbers of new cases based on Equation 9.4 for several different age groups and time periods for a given setting to observed tuberculosis notification data (Panel 9.1). Since it is not known what protection infection provides against reinfection, researchers typically assume that the risk of reinfection equals the risk of first infection. In this instance, the quantity $1-d_x/d_p$, which is used in Panel 9.1, is best interpreted as the protection provided by previous infection against the combined risk of reinfection and subsequent disease.

As we shall see below, the relative proportions of disease attributable to recent infection, reinfection and reactivation determine the impact of control.

9.3.2 **Predicting the impact of control for tuberculosis**

As discussed in Chapter 4, for acute immunizing infections, the size of the net reproduction number correlates with the trend in incidence: the incidence increases and decreases if it is above and below one respectively. We also saw that the basic reproduction number for the immunizing infections is typically used to calculate the herd immunity threshold, and therefore the proportion of the population at which an intervention should be targeted in order to control transmission.

The application of these concepts for tuberculosis is complicated by the long time interval between infection and disease onset and the fact that the number of individuals effectively contacted by each person may change between an individual being infected and transmitting to others. Therefore, the trend in tuberculosis incidence at a given time is influenced by transmission which occurred many years previously, and the size of the net reproduction number at a given time need not reflect the trend in incidence at that time. Consequently, the relationship between R_0 and the net reproduction number for tuberculosis is not clear, and this complicates the applicability of the herd immunity threshold concept for tuberculosis. The same applies for other infections with long incubation periods, such as HIV (see Chapter 8).

Instead, the impact of control for tuberculosis has often been estimated using transmission models.[31–35] The relative importance of disease attributable to recent infection or reinfection strongly determines the impact of those interventions which aim to interrupt transmission, such as increased case detection. For example, if a large proportion of disease is attributable to reactivation, then such control strategies will have little impact in the short-term, since much of the burden is attributable to infection events which occurred many years previously.

This is illustrated in Figure 9.6, which provides estimates of the impact of different levels of case detection in settings in which the annual numbers of new cases per 100,000 population had either already been declining by 4 per cent per year or had been stable over time, as estimated by the modelling study of Dye *et al.*[31] This study used an age-structured model to explore the impact of the World Health Organization DOTS (Directly Observed Treatment, Short-course) control strategy, involving passive case detection and a short-course treatment regimen.

In settings in which the annual numbers of new cases, and therefore the risk of infection, had already been decreasing over time by about 4 per cent per year, increasing case detection to the WHO target of 70 per cent was predicted to accelerate this decline to about 8 per cent per year. Such a setting is similar to that shown in Figure 9.6b, where much of the disease among adults is due to reactivation: the high infection risk in the past meant that many of these individuals were infected when young and the current low risk of (re)infection means that few will have been recently reinfected.

On the other hand, in settings in which the annual numbers of new cases per 100,000 population has been stable over time, the same strategy was predicted to lead to an average decline in the annual numbers of new cases of about 11 per cent per year. Such settings are similar to parts of Africa, before the HIV epidemic, where the risk of tuberculous infection may have remained unchanged over time[36] and a large

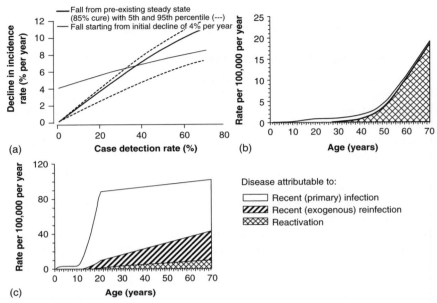

Fig. 9.6 (a) Predicted effects of increased case detection obtained by the study of Dye et al.[31] on the decline in the incidence (defined by the study as the annual number of new cases per 100,000 population) of tuberculosis for settings in which the incidence of tuberculosis has been declining by about 4 per cent per year or it was stable over time. Reproduced with permission from Dye et al, 1998.[31] (b) and (c) Estimates of the annual number of cases of infectious pulmonary tuberculosis per 100,000 population in settings with a (b) declining infection risk (taken to be The Netherlands in 1990) and (c) a 1 per cent annual infection risk. The disease risks and the proportion of disease that is infectious (sputum positive) are assumed to be identical to those in Vynnycky and Fine.[25] The shaded areas reflect the proportion of disease that is attributable to recent (primary) infection, re-infection and reactivation. (See model 9.3, online).

proportion of disease among all cases is likely to be due to recent transmission. The high proportion of disease due to recent transmission is due to the fact that the risk of infection is sufficiently high both for a large proportion of adults to have been infected in the past and for them to have been recently reinfected (Figure 9.6c).

In many countries, the epidemiology of tuberculosis has changed as a result of the HIV epidemic. This, in turn, has probably affected the distribution of disease attributable to recent infection, reinfection and reactivation, and therefore the impact of control, given that the risk of developing tuberculosis disease depends on CD4 count, which decreases with the duration for which individuals have been HIV-positive. However, it is presently not known whether HIV has a different effect on the risks of developing disease following recent first infection, reinfection or through reactivation. Given the large proportion of tuberculosis cases that are presently HIV-positive and that their lives will be prolonged because of antiretrovirals, elucidation of these factors is important for predicting the impact of HIV on the incidence of tuberculosis and the effect of control. Panel 9.2 discusses a study which has explored one aspect of the control of tuberculosis, namely the effect of antiretrovirals for HIV on the incidence of tuberculosis.

Panel 9.2 Predicting the effect of antiretrovirals for HIV on the incidence of tuberculosis

Several studies have used models to look at the impact of antiretroviral therapy for HIV on tuberculosis trends.[35, 106]

The first study by Williams and Dye in 2003[106] linked data on the decline of CD4 counts to data on the overall risk of tuberculosis at different stages of immuno-suppression, to infer the relative risk of tuberculosis among HIV-positive individuals, compared with those who are HIV-negative (Figure 9.7a). In the absence of reliable data, this risk was not stratified according to the mechanism by which individuals developed tuberculosis. Antiretroviral therapy among HIV-positive individuals was assumed to reduce the risk of tuberculosis to the level of that shortly after seroconversion (Figure 9.7b).

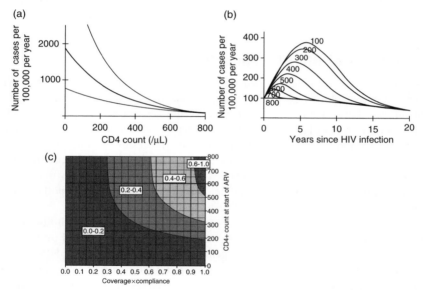

Fig. 9.7 Predictions and assumptions of the model of Williams and Dye[106] based on the assumption that the incidence of TB after HIV seroconversion is 100 per 100,000 per year. (a) Possible relationship between the association between annual incidence of TB and CD4 count, inferred by Williams and Dye.[106] The heavy line reflects the expected values; the light lines reflect the confidence limits. (b) Effect of providing antiretrovirals at different stages of immuno-suppression (indicated by the numbers above the curves) on the incidence of TB, assuming that the incidence of TB after seroconversion is 100 per 100,000 per year, assumed by Williams and Dye. (c) Predicted reduction in the incidence of tuberculosis (indicated by the numbers within the shaded areas) resulting from providing antiretrovirals at different CD4 counts. All three figures were reproduced with permission from Williams and Dye, 2003.[106]

Panel 9.2 Predicting the effect of antiretrovirals for HIV on the incidence of tuberculosis *(continued)*

The study pessimistically concluded that a large proportion of tuberculosis cases could be prevented using antiretroviral therapy only if it was provided shortly after HIV seroconversion and the levels of coverage and compliance were to be high (Figure 9.7c). For example, even if ARVs were provided when CD4 counts had reached 500cells/μL, the tuberculosis incidence would only be halved over a period of 20 years with an 85 per cent effective coverage.

Other, more recent, modelling studies which stratified individuals into those who have been recently infected, re-infected or are at risk of developing disease through reactivation, reached conclusions which are slightly more optimistic than those of Williams and Dye, namely that antiretrovirals may lead to a reduction in the notifications of tuberculosis.[35] It is thus likely that the effect of antiretrovirals will depend on whether the effect of HIV on the risk of disease differs according to the mechanism by which individuals develop TB, which is as yet, poorly understood.

9.4 Models of HIV/STI coinfection

In this section we continue the discussion of HIV and use a simple model of HIV/STI coinfection to explore the possible impact of cofactor STIs (cSTIs) in increasing the rate of spread of sexually transmitted HIV. We also describe some of the other cSTI/HIV coinfection modelling studies that have been carried out to help understand the epidemiology and control of sexually transmitted HIV in sub-Saharan Africa.

The interactions between classical STIs and HIV have been the subject of repeated review over the past couple of decades.[37–40] There is now a large body of evidence from laboratory, clinical and epidemiological studies supporting the hypothesis, first voiced in 1984, that classical STIs may facilitate the spread of HIV.[41]

For the HIV-uninfected individual, cofactor STIs increase susceptibility to HIV infection owing to breaks in the skin caused by ulcers or increased presence of T-lymphocytes and macrophages in the genital tract which are targets for HIV. For the HIV-infected individual, cofactor STIs increase transmission of HIV as STIs frequently cause increased shedding of HIV in the genital tract. These effects are collectively known as STI cofactor effects. The magnitude of an STI cofactor effect is defined as the multiple by which HIV transmission will be increased in the presence of the cofactor STI.

However, translating the relative risks of cofactor STIs for HIV transmission that are measured in epidemiological studies into per-partnership or per-act transmission probabilities, and that are needed to predict the impact of cSTIs on HIV transmission using mathematical models, is not straightforward.[42–44] Typically the actual exposure period with ulcers or inflammation is not measured in epidemiological studies and the exposure period is frequently much longer than the actual duration of ulcers or inflammation caused by the STI (measured using survey questions such as '*Have you had genital ulcers in the last X months?*'). This differential misclassification bias will lead to an underestimate of the true per-contact relative risk.[43] Conversely, even though most epidemiological studies adjust for confounding as best they can, the estimated effects are likely to be subject to residual confounding by poorly measured aspects of sexual risk behaviour in the study subjects, or unmeasured risk behaviours of their sexual partners.[42] Residual confounding would lead to an overestimate of the true relative risk.

The per-act cofactor effect for genital ulcer disease (GUD) has been estimated from empirical data to be in the range of 50–300 for female to male transmission and 10–50 for male to female transmission for ulcerative STI.[43] Recognizing that these estimates may suffer from the biases listed above, if we assume the per-act cofactor effect for female to male and male to female transmission combined is 10 and that GUD was only present for 25 per cent of the three month period in which an ulcer was reported, then a *per-contact* cofactor of 10 is equivalent to a *per-partnership* cofactor of around 3.1 (see Panel 9.3).

Panel 9.3 Calculation of the per-partnership STI cofactor effects on HIV transmission

HIV transmission probability per act without GUD	0.0016
Per-act GUD cofactor magnitude	10
Observation period	3 months
Number of acts in observation period	30 (10/mth)
% of observation period with GUD	25%
Transmission probability in observation period without GUD	0.047
Transmission probability in observation period with GUD	0.145
Relative risk	3.1

Where:

Transmission probability in observation period without GUD

$$= 1 - (1 - 0.0016)^{30} = 0.047$$

Transmission probability in observation period with GUD

$$= 1 - (1 - 0.0016)^{30*75\%}(1 - 0.0016 * 10)^{30*25\%} = 0.145$$

We can predict the impact of cSTIs on the spread of HIV by adapting our simple HIV/AIDS model (section 8.8) to explicitly model the transmission of a cofactor STI as shown in Figure 9.8. The model equations and parameter values are shown in Panel 9.4.

9.4.1 Predictions for the impact of cofactor STIs on the HIV epidemic

The relatively slow rise in the prevalence and incidence of HIV we predicted in section 8.8 using the HIV/AIDS model without a cofactor STI is reproduced in Figure 9.9a for comparison. The addition of a cofactor STI greatly increases the rate of spread of HIV (Figure 9.9b) such that the HIV epidemic now peaks at around 20 years after its introduction, rather than around 45 years after introduction.

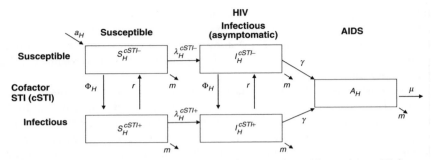

Fig. 9.8 A simple model of HIV transmission and progression with a cofactor STI for HIV transmission. The figure illustrates the high-activity group in the model only. See Panel 9.4 and Model 9.4 (online) for model equations and parameter values.

The model predicts (the numerical solution) that the addition of the cofactor STI reduced the doubling time of the HIV epidemic from 2.9 years to 1.1 years. You can check this using Model 9.4 to see the time it takes for the number of HIV infectious individuals to increase from 1 to 2.

The interaction between HIV and other sexually transmitted infections is complex. Note that our model also predicted that the prevalence of the cofactor STI may fall during an HIV epidemic (Figure 9.9c) in line with the predictions of other modelling studies.[45] This is because HIV will tend to preferentially kill the more sexually active members of the population, and these individuals are also more likely to be infected with other STIs because of the common risk-behaviour. In Uganda, a historically high HIV prevalence population, an empirical analysis suggests cSTI rates may have fallen during the HIV epidemic.[46] However, it is difficult to disentangle the effects of HIV-attributable mortality, reduction in social disruption caused by the civil war in Uganda, volitional behaviour change due to safer-sex campaigns and improvements in STI treatment services, on STI trends.

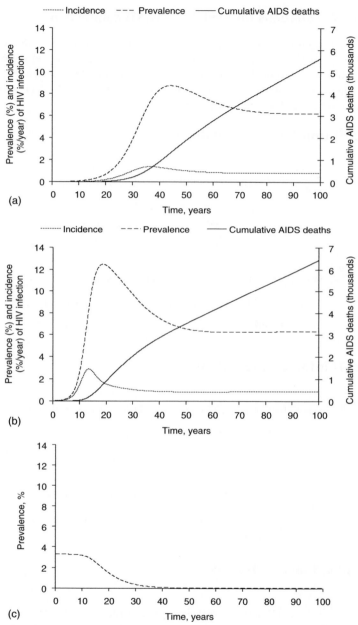

Fig. 9.9 HIV epidemic with and without STI cofactor. Predictions of (a) the incidence and prevalence of HIV and cumulative AIDS deaths without STI cofactor, (b) the incidence and prevalence of HIV and cumulative AIDS deaths with STI cofactor, (c) the prevalence of the cofactor STI in model with STI cofactor. The model is run for 50 years before introducing HIV to allow the cSTI to reach equilibrium (i.e. $t = -50$ to $t = 0$), and then for another 100 years. See Panel 9.4 and Model 9.4 (online) for model equations and parameter values.

Panel 9.4 Equations for model of HIV/STI coinfection

The model equations for the high-activity group are shown below. Note that, except for $n_H(-50)$, the proportion of individuals in the high-activity group at $t = -50$, the explicit time dependence '(t)' has been omitted to shorten the equations. The model is started at $t = -50$ to allow the cofactor STI (cSTI) to reach equilibrium before HIV is introduced at $t = 0$.

For cSTI uninfected individuals:

$$\frac{dS_H^{cSTI-}}{dt} = +\text{Recruited} + \text{cSTIRecovered} - \text{HIVInfected}$$
$$- \text{cSTIInfected} - \text{OtherDeaths}$$
$$= +a_H N + rS_H^{cSTI+} - \lambda_H^{cSTI-} S_H^{cSTI-} - \Phi_H S_H^{cSTI-} - mS_H^{cSTI-} \qquad 9.5$$

$$\frac{dI_H^{cSTI-}}{dt} = +\text{HIVIntro} + \text{HIVInfected} + \text{cSTIRecovered} -$$
$$\text{cSTIInfected} - \text{cSTIUninfectAIDSCases} - \text{OtherDeaths}$$
$$= +HIVIntro + \lambda_H^{cSTI-} S_H^{cSTI-} + rI_H^{cSTI+} - \Phi_H I_H^{cSTI-} - \gamma I_H^{cSTI-} - mI_H^{cSTI-} \qquad 9.6$$

For cSTI infected individuals:

$$\frac{dS_H^{cSTI+}}{dt} = +\text{cSTIInfected} - \text{cSTIRecovered} - \text{HIVInfected} - \text{OtherDeaths}$$
$$= +\Phi_H S_H^{cSTI-} - rS_H^{cSTI+} - \lambda_H^{cSTI+} S_H^{cSTI+} - mS_H^{cSTI+} \qquad 9.7$$

$$\frac{dI_H^{cSTI+}}{dt} = +\text{cSTIInfected} + \text{HIVInfected} - \text{cSTIRecovered} -$$
$$\text{cSTIInfectedAIDSCases} - \text{OtherDeaths}$$
$$= +\Phi_H I_H^{cSTI-} + \lambda_H^{cSTI+} S_H^{cSTI+} - rI_H^{cSTI+} - \gamma I_H^{cSTI+} - mI_H^{cSTI+} \qquad 9.8$$

For individuals with AIDS:

$$\frac{dA_H}{dt} = +\text{cSTIUninfectedAIDScases} + \text{cSTIInfectedAIDSCases} -$$
$$\text{AIDSDeaths} - \text{OtherDeaths}$$
$$= +\gamma I_H^{cSTI-} + \gamma I_H^{cSTI+} - \mu A_H - mA_H \qquad 9.9$$

Panel 9.4 Equations for model of HIV/STI coinfection *(continued)*

Where

S_H^{cSTI-} is the number of individuals HIV-uninfected and cSTI-uninfected at time t in high-activity group

S_H^{cSTI+} is the number of individuals HIV-uninfected and cSTI-infected at time t in high-activity group

I_H^{cSTI-} is the number of individuals who are HIV-infectious and cSTI-uninfected at time t in high-activity group

I_H^{cSTI+} is the number of individuals who are HIV-infectious and cSTI-infected at time t in high-activity group

A_H is the number of individuals with AIDS at time t in high- activity group

N is the total population size

λ_H^{cSTI-} is the force of HIV infection on cSTI-uninfected individuals at time t in high-activity group

λ_H^{cSTI+} is the force of HIV infection on cSTI-infected individuals at time t in high-activity group

Φ_H is the force of cSTI infection on individuals at time t in high-activity group

a is the rate of recruitment into sexually active age groups, per year

$n_H(-50)$ is the proportion of individuals in the high-activity group at $t = -50$

$a_H = a n_H(-50)$, is the recruitment rate into the high-activity group, per year

m is the non-HIV mortality rate among sexually active individuals, per year

γ is progression rate to AIDS, per year

μ is the death rate due to AIDS, per year

r is recovery rate from cSTI infection, per year

HIVIntro introduces an HIV infected person at $t = 0$.

The force of cofactor STI infection

The force of cofactor STI infection on individuals in the high-activity group Φ_H will depend on the partner change rate, c_H, the transmission probability per partnership, β_{cSTI}, and the probability a partner is infected, P_{cSTI}. For simplicity, because we assume no sexual activity during AIDS and because this stage is relatively short, we don't track cSTI status in the AIDS stage. Note that we now make a distinction between the transmission probability of the cofactor STI, β_{cSTI} and the transmission probability of HIV, β_{HIV}.

$$\Phi_H = c_H \beta_{cSTI} P_{cSTI} \qquad\qquad 9.10$$

Where

c_H is the partner change rate per year in high-activity group

β_{cSTI} is the cSTI transmission probability

P_{cSTI} is the probability partners are infected with cSTI and this is the weighted average of the cSTI prevalence among sexually active individuals in the high, f_H, and low, f_L activity groups (see Equation 8.18).

$$P_{cSTI} = g_H f_H + g_L f_L \qquad\qquad 9.11$$

Panel 9.4 Equations for model of HIV/STI coinfection *(continued)*

Where g_H and g_L are the probability that a sexual partner will be a member of the high and low-activity group, respectively,

$$f_H = \frac{S_H^{cSTI+} + I_H^{cSTI+}}{U_H}$$

9.12

$$U_H = S_H^{cSTI-} + I_H^{cSTI-} + S_H^{cSTI+} + I_H^{cSTI+}$$

9.13

Where U_H is the number of sexually active individuals in the population in the high-activity group at time *t*.

The equations for the low-activity group can be written by replacing the $_H$ subscript with $_L$.

The force of HIV infection

In our model the force of HIV infection will depend on whether one or both of the partners are infected with the cofactor-STI. Alternative assumptions can be made, but here we assume the per-partnership STI cofactor for HIV acquisition and separately HIV transmission, x, is = 3.1 (Panel 9.3). β_{HIV} is the probability of transmission of HIV infection during a sexual partnership if neither partner is cSTI-infected. Therefore if one partner is cSTI-infected, the transmission probability in an HIV-discordant partnership is $x\beta_{HIV}$ and if both partners are cSTI-infected the transmission probability in an HIV-discordant partnership is $x^2\beta_{HIV}$.

There are four equations for the force of HIV infection to consider. One for each activity group and cSTI-status of HIV-susceptible partner, ie λ_H^{cSTI-}, λ_H^{cSTI+}, λ_L^{cSTI-} and λ_L^{cSTI+}.

Focusing first on the equation for HIV infection on cSTI-uninfected individuals in the high-activity group, λ_H^{cSTI-} (Equation 9.14). This is equal to their partner change rate, c_H, the HIV transmission probability (without STI-cofactors), β_{HIV} and the probability that a partner is HIV-infected multiplied by the magnitude of the STI-cofactor effect if a HIV-infected partner is also coinfected with the cSTI.

This probability is calculated by the terms between the square brackets in Equation 9.14. It depends on whether the partner is selected from the high or low-activity group (but as we assume proportionate mixing this is just g_H or g_L), and whether the selected partner is HIV-infectious and cSTI-uninfected or HIV-infectious and cSTI-infected. These probabilities will vary between the two activity groups. If the selected partner is HIV-infectious and cSTI-infected then the HIV transmission probability is multiplied by the magnitude of the STI-cofactor effect, x.

$$\lambda_H^{cSTI-} = c_H \beta_{HIV} \left[g_H(q_H^{HIV+cSTI-} + q_H^{HIV+cSTI+}x) + g_L(q_L^{HIV+cSTI-} + q_L^{HIV+cSTI+}x) \right]$$

9.14

Where

$$q_H^{HIV+cSTI-} = \frac{I_H^{cSTI-}}{U_H}, \text{ and } q_H^{HIV+cSTI+} = \frac{I_H^{cSTI+}}{U_H}$$

$$q_L^{HIV+cSTI-} = \frac{I_L^{cSTI-}}{U_L}, \text{ and } q_L^{HIV+cSTI+} = \frac{I_L^{cSTI+}}{U_L}$$

Panel 9.4 Equations for model of HIV/STI coinfection *(continued)*

The equation for the force of HIV infection on a cSTI-uninfected individual in the low-activity group, λ_L^{cSTI-}, can be derived in the same way and is identical to Equation 9.14 except the partner change rate is c_L.

By slightly adapting Equation 9.14 we can write down the force of HIV infection on cSTI-infected individuals in the high-activity group, λ_H^{cSTI+} (Equation 9.15). We can use the same logic as above but need to account for the fact that the HIV-uninfected partner is already infected with the cSTI. λ_H^{cSTI+} is equal to the product of

1. the partner change rate, c_H,

2. the HIV transmission probability (with the STI-cofactor), $\beta_{HIV} x$, and

3. the probability that the selected partner is HIV infected multiplied by the magnitude of the STI-cofactor effect if the HIV-infected partner is also coinfected with the cSTI. Note that because the HIV-uninfected partner is already cSTI-infected, the HIV transmission probability will be $\beta_{HIV} x$ if their partner is HIV-infectious and STI-uninfected and $\beta_{HIV} x^2$ if the partner is HIV-infectious and STI-infected.

$$\lambda_L^{cSTI+} = c_H \beta_{HIV} x \left[g_H (q_H^{HIV+cSTI-} + q_H^{HIV+cSTI+} x) + g_L (q_L^{HIV+cSTI-} + q_L^{HIV+cSTI+} x) \right] \quad 9.15$$

Similarly, the equation for the force of infection on a cSTI-infected individual in the low-activity group, λ_L^{cSTI+}, can be derived in the same way and is identical to Equation 9.15 except the partner change rate is C_L.

9.4.2 The changing role of curable STI treatment for HIV prevention

Many cSTI/HIV coinfection modelling studies have been carried out to help understand the potential impact of the control of cofactor sexually transmitted infections on HIV transmission in sub-Saharan Africa.

Modelling has helped better understand the seemingly contrasting results of three first randomized controlled trials of STI treatment for HIV prevention in sub-Saharan Africa. Early modelling studies of the interaction between HIV and other STIs showed that the role of STIs, particularly STIs causing genital ulcers, was likely to be critical in the rapid spread of HIV in sub-Saharan Africa[47, 48] and a community randomized-controlled trial in Mwanza, Tanzania showed that improved clinic-based syndromic STI treatment reduced the incidence of HIV infection by around 38 per cent (95 per cent confidence interval = 15 to 55 per cent) among the general population.[49–51] Soon after however, trials of STI mass treatment in Rakai, Uganda, and of an information, education, and communication intervention with and without improved syndromic STI treatment in Masaka, Uganda, showed no significant effect on the incidence of HIV infection,[52, 53] despite similar reductions in the prevalence of curable STIs in all three sites. Detailed data analysis and modelling of the interventions and the populations in which the trials took place showed that population differences in sexual behaviour, curable STI rates, and HIV epidemic stage could explain most of the contrast in HIV impact observed between the three trials, and concluded that STI management is likely to be an effective HIV prevention strategy in populations with a high prevalence of curable STIs, particularly in an early HIV epidemic.[46, 54]

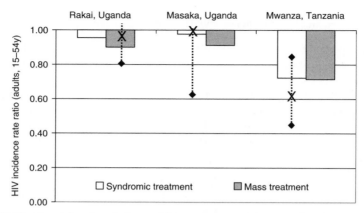

Fig. 9.10 Simulated (bars) and observed (X's with 95 per cent confidence intervals) impact of syndromic and mass STI treatment interventions on HIV incidence in three populations in East Africa. Adapted from White *et al*,2004.[54]

Figure 9.10 illustrates this by showing the model prediction that the impact of either syndromic or mass STI treatment on HIV incidence would have been larger in the early HIV epidemic in Mwanza, than in the later HIV epidemics in Rakai or Masaka in Uganda.[54]

Modelling studies have suggested that the impact of STI treatment on HIV incidence will depend on the characteristics of the population,[55, 56] the characteristics of those reached,[57] and the stage of the HIV epidemic.[58, 59]

Modelling was also helpful in highlighting that the proportion of HIV incidence due to curable STIs (the population attributable fraction, or 'PAF') was likely to fall as the HIV epidemic matures. This is because AIDS mortality and behaviour change (if it had occurred) reduced curable STI rates, and because, as HIV prevalence increases, a larger proportion of HIV transmission occurs outside higher-risk groups, in groups with lower rates of curable STIs.[58, 59] Conversely, later in the HIV epidemic, the proportion of HIV incidence due to the incurable STI *Herpes simplex* Virus type-2 (HSV-2) would rise, due to the fall in classical STI rates and increased HSV-2 ulceration among immuno-compromised HIV-infected individuals.[60–63] This is illustrated using the predicted trends in the PAFs of herpes simplex virus type 2 and chancroid on HIV incidence in four cities in sub-Saharan Africa in Figure 9.11.[60]

Although these studies suggest that the relative impact of curable STI treatment will be lower later in generalized HIV epidemics, other work has shown that curable STI treatment may remain cost-saving in generalized epidemics because the absolute impact remains high.[64]

Recently, the potential of HSV-2 treatment as an HIV prevention strategy has been explored. However, in general, the modelling work has suggested that a substantial

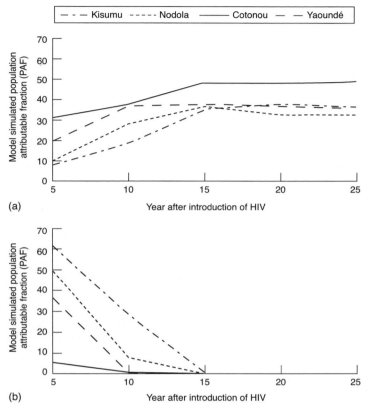

Fig. 9.11 Simulated proportion of new adult (15–49 years) HIV infections due to (a) herpes simplex virus type 2 (b) chancroid in four cities in sub-Saharan Africa, by year after the introduction of HIV. Model: STDSIM. Reproduced from Freeman *et al*, 2007.[60]

impact of HSV-2 therapy on population HIV incidence is unlikely because it would require high coverage and long-duration therapy, or very high symptom recognition and treatment-seeking behaviour,[65, 66] and all three of randomized controlled trials of herpes suppressive therapy failed to show an impact on the HIV transmission.[67–69] This lack of impact may be because any STI cofactor effect is small, because there was insufficient herpes suppression due to inadequate drug dosage or adherence, or because the mechanism of action of acyclovir does not adequately control the effect of HSV-2 on HIV transmission.[67, 69]

More encouragingly, Figure 9.12 shows some initial modelling results that suggest that an effective prophylactic HSV-2 vaccine, if developed, could have a substantial impact on HIV incidence.[70]

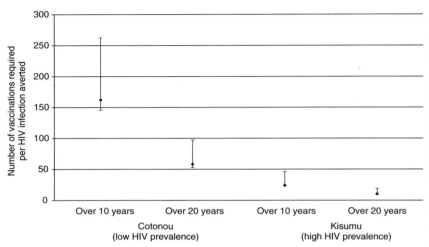

Fig. 9.12 Simulated number of vaccinations per HIV infection averted over 10 and 20 years using a hypothetical prophylactic HSV-2 vaccine, in a low and high HIV prevalence African city (all ages). The modelled scenario assumes an increase from 0 to 70 per cent in vaccine coverage over 5 years in 14–29-year-olds using a vaccine with 10-year duration of effect on susceptibility and reactivation in males and females. Three scenarios are shown corresponding to the 'weak' (30%, T), 'moderate' (75 per cent, ♦) and 'strong' (90 per cent, ⊥) vaccine efficacy. See Freeman *et al*, 2009[70] for full details.

9.5 Case study: how models of the control of sexually transmitted HIV in sub-Saharan Africa have evolved with the epidemic

In this section we describe how mathematical modelling studies of the sexual transmission of HIV have evolved in line with our increasing understanding of its spread and control.

Studies in the late 1980s and early 1990s tended to be more theoretical, identifying the importance of the various risk factors for the transmission of HIV, such as partner change rates, heterogeneity in risk behaviour and mixing between risk groups.[71–75]

These early studies were crucial in showing how little was known about the identified risk factors and in guiding the subsequent data collection. Models in the early literature were also presented with the intention that they could be used in the future to estimate the impact of control strategies, initially primarily as a tool for HIV researchers,[71, 74] but later for use by policy makers.[47, 75] The early modelling studies showed that the impact of interventions on HIV incidence would be non-linear (as for most infectious disease control) and that the stage of the HIV epidemic would be important. Impact on HIV incidence would be larger when the basic reproduction number (R_0) of HIV was close to unity, than at higher reproductive potentials.[76, 77]

It also showed that intervention early in the epidemic and targeted at higher-risk individuals would be most effective.[78–80] The focus of many of these modelling studies was on sub-Saharan Africa as it became apparent that this was the most severely affected region. However, as early as 1990, modelling studies had suggested that HIV was already so widespread in parts of sub-Saharan Africa, that large-scale behaviour change in the general population and greatly increased resources would be required to control the HIV epidemic.[79, 81]

As scientific understanding of the risk factors for HIV transmission improved and the data required to parameterize and validate these models became more readily available, modelling was increasingly used to predict the impact of more realistic prevention strategies, to interpret the results of empirical HIV control trials, and to warn of potentially perverse outcomes of HIV prevention activities.

Modelling work showed the potential role of other sexually transmitted infections (STIs), particularly STIs causing genital ulcers, in the rapid spread of HIV in sub-Saharan Africa as described in section 9.4.2. With the advent of treatment for HIV, mathematical modelling has been used to explore the impact of antiretroviral treatment (ART) on HIV incidence. Early work showed that without reduction in infectiousness and in risk behaviour, ART would tend to increase HIV incidence[82, 83] as HIV-infected individuals would remain healthy and sexually active for longer. However, as ART has been shown to reduce viral load considerably and therefore should reduce the infectiousness of HIV-infected individuals, more recent work has focused on the critical importance of risk-compensation (the possible increase in risk behaviour due to reduction in the perceived severity of the consequences of HIV infection),[84, 85] the benefits of integrating HIV prevention and treatment activities,[86, 87] and the potential of universal voluntary HIV testing and ART.[88] The work by Baggaley and colleagues illustrated an understandable, but potentially worrying, effect of HIV treatment programmes, which is that population HIV prevalence will increase due to falling mortality rates (Figure 9.13, left).

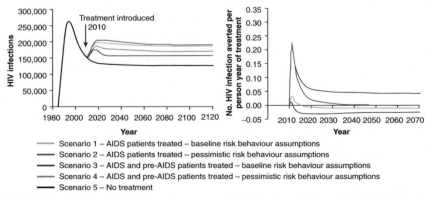

Fig. 9.13 Predicted total number of prevalent HIV infections (left) and incident HIV infections averted per person-year of treatment (right) over time in a high prevalence mature sub-Saharan Africa epidemic for various assumptions of behaviour change of treated patients and treatment targeting. From Baggaley *et al*, 2006.[87]

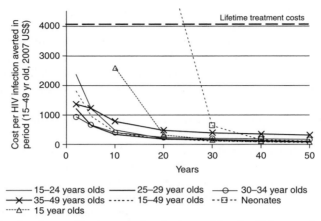

Fig. 9.14 Simulated cost-effectiveness of male-circumcision for HIV prevention in sub-Saharan Africa, by target age group. Cost required to avert one HIV infection in adults aged 15–49 years, over time in 2007US$. For comparison, an adjusted estimate of the lifetime treatment costs of an HIV infection in sub-Saharan Africa[103] is shown as a horizontal dashed line. Reproduced from White *et al*, 2008.[100]

As such, a rapid rise in prevalence when treatment programmes are initiated should be regarded as an indicator of the likely success of a treatment programme, rather than a failure. More pessimistically, the study by Baggaley and colleagues suggested that HIV treatment was unlikely to have much effect on the prevention of new HIV infections, because of increases in the sexual activity of treated patients and the development of resistance (Figure 9.13, right).

Male circumcision is likely to have been very important in explaining the heterogeneous spread of HIV in sub-Saharan Africa.[89–92] Three individual randomized controlled trials in Africa have shown male circumcision to reduce HIV-incidence in males by 50–60 per cent.[93–95] Modelling work has been very useful in projecting the potential population-level impact implied by these individual-level trial findings. The predictions of these modelling studies have been very consistent,[96–100] primarily because the impacts of the empirical trials were so similar. Overall, modelling studies suggest that circumcision could prevent 6 million HIV infections over 20 years in sub-Saharan Africa and will be cost-saving because of the reduction of future antiretroviral treatment costs: see [96, 101, 102] and Figure 9.14.

Unfortunately, with 2.8 million men, women and children newly infected with HIV each year in sub-Saharan Africa,[104] the mathematical modelling of HIV control will continue to be an active area of research for the foreseeable future.

9.6 **Summary**

This chapter has highlighted several topics in infectious disease modelling, namely vaccination and the role of boosting and serotype replacement, diseases with long incubation periods, modelling HIV/STI coinfection, and a case study describing how HIV modelling studies have evolved with the HIV epidemic.

The introduction of vaccination for varicella can have important implications for chickenpox, for which a reduction in the incidence of the infection reduces the opportunity for boosting. Such increases can lead to increases in the burden of zoster. Likewise, the introduction of vaccination for pneumococcal disease, whilst reducing the reduction in transmission of a vaccine-specific serotype, can lead to an increase in the incidence of a serotype which had not been included in the vaccine. At the time of writing, these predictions have yet to be realized.

Some of these issues are also relevant for tuberculosis, for which the risk of infection in Western populations has declined over time, which has led to changes in the proportion of disease attributable to recent infection, reinfection and reactivation. The relative contribution of these disease mechanisms has important implications for the impact of control, and this is likely to have changed with the HIV pandemic.

We have seen how coinfection with other sexually transmitted infections may have increased the rate the spread of HIV in populations with poor STI services, and how the spread of HIV may have reduced the prevalence of other sexually transmitted infections.

Finally, we concluded with a description of how models of the transmission and control of HIV have evolved along with our understanding of the natural history of HIV and with the research and public health questions that needed to be addressed.

References

1 Edmunds WJ, Brisson M. The effect of vaccination on the epidemiology of varicella zoster virus. *J Infect* 2002; 44(4):211–219.

2 Thomas SL, Wheeler JG, Hall AJ. Contacts with varicella or with children and protection against herpes zoster in adults: a case–control study. *Lancet* 2002; 360(9334):678–682.

3 Brisson M, Gay NJ, Edmunds WJ, Andrews NJ. Exposure to varicella boosts immunity to herpes-zoster: implications for mass vaccination against chickenpox. *Vaccine* 2002; 20 (19–20):2500–2507.

4 Brisson M, Edmunds WJ, Gay NJ, Law B, De Serre G. Modelling the impact of immunization on the epidemiology of varicella zoster virus. *Epidemiol Infect* 2000; 125(3):651–669.

5 Garnett GP, Grenfell BT. The epidemiology of varicella-zoster virus infections: the influence of varicella on the prevalence of herpes zoster. *Epidemiol Infect* 1992; 108(3): 513–528.

6 Ferguson NM, Anderson RM, Garnett GP. Mass vaccination to control chickenpox: the influence of zoster. *Proc Natl Acad Sci USA* 1996; 93(14):7231–7235.

7 Recommendations for the use of live attenuated varicella vaccine. American Academy of Pediatrics Committee on Infectious Diseases. *Pediatrics* 1995; 95(5):791–796.

8 Prevention of varicella: recommendations of the Advisory Committee on Immunization Practices (ACIP). Centers for Disease Control and Prevention. *MMWR Recomm Rep* 1996; 45(RR–11):1–36.

9 Marin M, Meissner HC, Seward JF. Varicella prevention in the United States: a review of successes and challenges. *Pediatrics* 2008; 122(3):e744–e751.

10 Pebody RG, Hellenbrand W, D'Ancona F, Ruutu P. Pneumococcal disease surveillance in Europe. *Euro Surveill* 2006; 11(9):171–178.

11 Department of Health. Pneumococcal. Pneumococcal meningitis notifiable. Immunisation against infectious disease 2006. *The Green Book*. London: Department of Health; 2007, pp. 295–311.

12 Lipsitch M. Vaccination against colonizing bacteria with multiple serotypes. *Proc Natl Acad Sci USA* 1997; 94(12):6571–6576.

13 O'Brien KL, Dagan R. The potential indirect effect of conjugate pneumococcal vaccines. *Vaccine* 2003; 21(17–18):1815–1825.

14 Singleton RJ, Hennessy TW, Bulkow LR *et al*. Invasive pneumococcal disease caused by nonvaccine serotypes among alaska native children with high levels of 7-valent pneumococcal conjugate vaccine coverage. *JAMA* 2007; 297(16):1784–1792.

15 Gonzalez BE, Hulten KG, Lamberth L, Kaplan SL, Mason EO, Jr. Streptococcus pneumoniae serogroups 15 and 33: an increasing cause of pneumococcal infections in children in the United States after the introduction of the pneumococcal 7-valent conjugate vaccine. *Pediatr Infect Dis J* 2006; 25(4):301–305.

16 Lipsitch M. Bacterial vaccines and serotype replacement: lessons from *Haemophilus influenzae* and prospects for *Streptococcus pneumoniae*. *Emerg Infect Dis* 1999; 5(3): 336–345.

17 Styblo K, Meijer J, Sutherland I. Tuberculosis Surveillance Research Unit Report No. 1: the transmission of tubercle bacilli; its trend in a human population. *Bull Int Union Tuberc* 1969; 42:1–104.:1–104.

18 Sutherland I, Bleiker MA, Meijer J, Styblo K. The risk of tuberculous infection in The Netherlands from 1967 to 1979. *Tubercle* 1983; 64(4):241–253.

19 Vynnycky E, Fine PE. The annual risk of infection with *Mycobacterium tuberculosis* in England and Wales since 1901. *Int J Tuberc Lung Dis* 1997; 1(5).

20 Sutherland I, Styblo K, Sampalik M, Bleiker MA. [Annual risks of tuberculosis infection in 14 countries according to the results of tuberculosis surveys from 1948 to 1952]. *Bull Int Union Tuberc* 1971; 45:80–122.:80–122.

21 Borgdorff MW, Nagelkerke NJ, van SD, Broekmans JF. Transmission of tuberculosis between people of different ages in The Netherlands: an analysis using DNA fingerprinting. *Int J Tuberc Lung Dis* 1999; 3(3):202–206.

22 Vynnycky E, Fine PE. Interpreting the decline in tuberculosis: the role of secular trends in effective contact. *Int J Epidemiol* 1999; 28(2).

23 Styblo K. Epidemiology of tuberculosis. [24]. 1991. The Hague, The Netherlands, KNCV. Selected papers.

24 Sutherland I, Svandova E, Radhakrishna S. The development of clinical tuberculosis following infection with tubercle bacilli. 1. A theoretical model for the development of clinical tuberculosis following infection, linking from data on the risk of tuberculous infection and the incidence of clinical tuberculosis in the Netherlands. *Tubercle* 1982; 63(4):255–268.

25 Vynnycky E, Fine PE. The natural history of tuberculosis: the implications of age-dependent risks of disease and the role of reinfection. *Epidemiol Infect* 1997; 119(2).

26 Vynnycky E, Fine PE. Lifetime risks, incubation period, and serial interval of tuberculosis. *Am J Epidemiol* 2000; 152(3):247–263.

27 Murray CJL, Styblo K, Rouillon A. Tuberculosis. In: Jamison DT, Mosley WH, Measham AR, Bobadilla JL, eds, *Disease Control Priorities in Developing Countries*. Oxford Universty Press; 1993, pp. 233–259.

28 Registrar General. *Annual report of the Registrar General of births, deaths and marriages in England and Wales.* 1939. London, England, Her Majesty's Stationery Office.

29 Canetti G, Sutherland I, Svandova E. Endogenous reactivation and exogenous reinfection: their relative importance with regard to the development of non-primary tuberculosis. *Bull Int Union Tuberc* 1972; 47:116–34:116–134.

30 Sutherland I, Svandova E, Radhakrishna S. Alternative models for the development of tuberculosis disease following infection with tubercle bacilli. *Bull Int Union Tuberc* 1976; 51(1):171–179.

31 Dye C, Garnett GP, Sleeman K, Williams BG. Prospects for worldwide tuberculosis control under the WHO DOTS strategy. Directly observed short-course therapy. *Lancet* 1998; 352(9144):1886–1891.

32 Waaler HT, Gothi GD, Baily GV, Nair SS. Tuberculosis in rural South India. A study of possible trends and the potential impact of antituberculosis programmes. *Bull World Health Organ* 1974; 51(3):263–271.

33 Murray CJ, Salomon JA. Modeling the impact of global tuberculosis control strategies. *Proc Natl Acad Sci USA* 1998; 95(23):13881–13886.

34 Schulzer M, Fitzgerald JM, Enarson DA, Grzybowski S. An estimate of the future size of the tuberculosis problem in sub-Saharan Africa resulting from HIV infection. *Tuber Lung Dis* 1992; 73(1):52–58.

35 Bacaer N, Ouifki R, Pretorius C, Wood R, Williams B. Modeling the joint epidemics of TB and HIV in a South African township. *J Math Biol* 2008; 57(4):557–593.

36 Bleiker MA, Styblo K. The annual tuberculous infection rate and its trend in developing countries. *Bull Int Union Tuberc* 1978; 53:295–299.

37 Laga M, Nzila N, Goeman J. The interrelationship of sexually transmitted diseases and HIV infection: implications for the control of both epidemics in Africa. [Review]. *AIDS* 1991; 5(1):S55–63.

38 Fleming DT, Wasserheit JN. From epidemiological synergy to public health policy and practice: the contribution of other sexually transmitted diseases to sexual transmission of HIV infection. *Sex Transm Inf* 1999; 75:3–17.

39 Rottingen JA, Cameron DW, Garnett GP. A systematic review of the epidemiologic interactions between classic sexually transmitted diseases and HIV: how much really is known? *Sex Transm Dis* 2001; 28(10): 579–597.

40 Wasserheit JN. Epidemiological synergy. Interrelationships between human immunodeficiency virus infection and other sexually transmitted diseases. [Review]. *Sex Transm Dis* 1992; 19(2): 61–77.

41 Piot P, Quinn TC, Taelman H *et al.* Acquired immunodeficiency syndrome in a heterosexual population in Zaire. *Lancet* 1984; 2(8394): 65–69.

42 Korenromp EL, De Vlas S, Nagelkerke N, Habbema J. Estimating the magnitude of STD cofactor effects on HIV transmission – how well can it be done? *STD* 2001; 28(11): 613–621.

43 Hayes RJ, Schulz KF, Plummer FA. The cofactor effect of genital ulcers on the per-exposure risk of HIV transmission in sub-Saharan Africa. [Review]. *J Trop Med Hyg* 1995; 98(1):1–8.

44 Boily M, Anderson M. Human immunodeficiency virus transmission and the role of other sexually transmitted diseases: measures of association and study design. *Sexually Transmitted Diseases* 1996; 23:312–332.

45 Boily M-C, Masse B. Mathematical models of disease transmission: A precious tool of the study of sexually transmitted diseases. *Canadian Journal of Public Health* 1997; 88:255–265.

46 Orroth K, Korenromp E, White R *et al.* Higher risk behaviour and rates of sexually transmitted diseases in Mwanza compared to Uganda may help explain HIV prevention trial outcomes. *AIDS* 2003; 17(18):2653–2660.

47 Van der Ploeg CPB, Van Vliet C, De Vlas SJ *et al.* STDSIM: a microsimulation model for decision support in STD control. *Interfaces* 1998; 28:84–100.

48 Robinson NJ, Mulder DW, Auvert B, Hayes RJ. Proportion of HIV infections attributable to other sexually transmitted diseases in a rural Ugandan population: simulation model estimates. *International Journal Of Epidemiology* 1997; 26(1):180–189.

49 Grosskurth H, Mosha F, Todd J *et al.* Impact of improved treatment of sexually transmitted diseases on HIV infection in rural Tanzania: randomised controlled trial. *Lancet* 1995; 346(8974):530–536.

50 Hayes R, Grosskurth H, ka-Gina G. Impact of improved treatment of sexually transmitted diseases on HIV infection in rural Tanzania: randomised controlled trial [Letter to Lancet]. *Lancet* 1995; 346:1159–1160.

51 Habbema JDF, De Vlas SJ. Impact of improved treatment of sexually transmitted disease on HIV infection [letter; comment]. *Lancet* 1995; 346(8983):1157–1158.

52 Kamali A, Quigley M, Nakiyingi J *et al.* Syndromic management of sexually-transmitted infections and behaviour change interventions on transmission of HIV-1 in rural Uganda: a community randomised trial. *Lancet* 2003; 361(9358):645–652.

53 Wawer MJ, Sewankambo NK, Serwadda D *et al.* Control of sexually transmitted diseases for AIDS prevention in Uganda: a randomised community trial. *Lancet* 1999; 353(9152):645–652.

54 White RG, Orroth KK, Korenromp EL *et al.* Can population differences explain the contrasting results of the Mwanza, Rakai, and Masaka HIV/Sexually Transmitted Disease Intervention Trials?: A modeling study. *J Acquir Immune Defic Syndr* 2004; 37(4):1500–1513.

55 Korenromp EL, Van Vliet C, Grosskurth H *et al.* Model-based evaluation of single-round mass STD treatment for HIV control in a rural African population. *AIDS* 2000; 14:573–593.

56 Korenromp EL, White RG, Orroth KK *et al.* Determinants of the Impact of sexually transmitted infection treatment on prevention of HIV infection: a synthesis of evidence from the Mwanza, Rakai, and Masaka intervention trials. *J Infect Dis* 2005; 191(Suppl 1): S168–178.

57 Boily M-C, Lowndes CM, Alary M. Complementary hypothesis concerning the community sexually transmitted disease mass treatment puzzle in Rakai, Uganda. *AIDS* 2000; 14(16):2583–2592.

58 Korenromp E, Bakker R, De Vlas S *et al.* The effect of HIV, behaviour change, and STD syndromic management on STD epidemiology in sub-Saharan Africa: simulations of Uganda. *STI* 2002; 78(Suppl 1):i55–63.

59 Korenromp E, Bakker R, De Vlas S *et al.* HIV dynamics and behaviour change as determinants of the impact of sexually transmitted disease treatment on HIV transmission in the context of the Rakai trial. *AIDS* 2002; 16:2209–2218.

60 Freeman E, Orroth K, White RG *et al.* The proportion of new HIV infections attributable to HSV-2 increases over time: simulations of the changing role of sexually transmitted infections in sub-Saharan African HIV epidemics. *STI* 2007; 83:i17–24.

61 Abu-Raddad LJ, Magaret AS, Celum C *et al.* Genital herpes has played a more important role than any other sexually transmitted infection in driving HIV prevalence in Africa. *PLoS ONE* 2008; 3(5):e2230.

62 Blower S, Ma L. Calculating the contribution of herpes simplex virus type 2 epidemics to increasing HIV incidence: treatment implications. *Clin Infect Dis* 2004; 39(Suppl 5): S240–247.

63 Korenromp E, Bakker R, De Vlas S, Robinson N, Hayes R, Habbema J. Can behaviour change explain increases in the proportion of genital ulcers attributable to herpes in sub-Saharan Africa? A simulation modelling study. *Sex Transm Dis* 2002; 29(4):228–238.

64 White RG, Orroth KK, Glynn JR *et al*. Treating curable sexually transmitted infections to prevent HIV in Africa: still an effective control strategy? *J Acquir Immune Defic Syndr* 2008; 47:346–353.

65 White RG, Freeman EE, Orroth KK *et al*. Population-level effect of HSV-2 therapy on the incidence of HIV in sub-Saharan Africa. *Sex Trans Inf* 2008; 84(S2):12–18.

66 Baggaley RF, Griffin JT, Chapman R *et al*. Estimating the public health impact of the effect of herpes simplex virus suppressive therapy on plasma HIV-1 viral load. *AIDS* 2009; 23(8):1005–1013.

67 Celum C, Wald A, Hughes J *et al*. Effect of aciclovir on HIV-1 acquisition in herpes simplex virus 2 seropositive women and men who have sex with men: a randomised, double-blind, placebo-controlled trial. *Lancet* 2008; 371(9630):2109–2119.

68 Celum C, Wald A, Lingappa Jr *et al*. Twice-daily acyclovir to reduve HIV-1 transmission from HIV-1/NHSV-1 co-infected persons within HIV-1 discordant couples: a randomized, double-blind, placebo controlled trial. Submitted.

69 Watson-Jones D, Weiss HA, Rusizoka M *et al*. Effect of Herpes Simplex Suppression on Incidence of HIV among Women in Tanzania. *N Engl J Med* 2008; 358(15):1560–1571.

70 Freeman EE, White RG, Bakker R *et al*. Population-level effect of potential HSV2 prophylactic vaccines on HIV incidence in sub-Saharan Africa. http://dx.doi.org/10.1016/j.vaccine.2008.11.074. *Vaccine* 2009; 27:940–946.

71 Hyman J, Stanley E. Using mathematical models to understand the AIDS epidemic. *Math Biosc* 1988; 90:415–473.

72 Van Druten JA, Reintjes AG, Jager JC *et al*. HIV infection dynamics and intervention experiments in linked risk groups. *Stat Med* 1990; 9(7):721–736.

73 Anderson RM, Gupta S, May RM. Potential of community-wide chemotherapy or immunotherapy to control the spread of HIV-1. *Nature* 1991; 350(6316):356–359.

74 Bailey N. Core-group dynamics and public health action. In Kaplan E, Brandeau M, eds, New York: Raven Press Ltd; 1994.

75 Rehle TM, Saidel TJ, Hassig SE, Bouey PD, Gaillard EM, Sokal DC. AVERT: a user-friendly model to estimate the impact of HIV/sexually transmitted disease prevention interventions on HIV transmission. *AIDS* 1998; 12(Suppl 2):S27–35.

76 Morris M, Dean L. Effect of sexual behavior change on long-term human immunodeficiency virus prevalence among homosexual men. *Am J Epidemiol* 1994; 140(3):217–232.

77 Rowley JT, Anderson RM. Modeling the impact and cost-effectiveness of HIV prevention efforts. *AIDS* 1994; 8(4):539–548.

78 Garnett GP, Anderson RM. Strategies for limiting the spread of HIV in developing countries: conclusions based on studies of the transmission dynamics of the virus. *J Acquir Immune Defic Syndr Hum Retrovirol* 1995; 9(5):500–513.

79 Stover J, O'Way P. Impact of interventions on reducing the spread of HIV in developing countries: computer simulation applications. *African Journal of Medical Practice* 1995; 2(4):110–120.

80 Over M, Piot P. Human immunodeficiency virus infection and other sexually transmitted diseases in developing countries: public health importance and priorities for resource allocation. *The Journal of Infectious Diseases* 1996; 174(Suppl):S162–175.

81 Auvert B, Moore M, Bertrand WE *et al.* Dynamics of HIV infection and AIDS in central African cities. *Int J Epidemiol* 1990; 19(2):417–428.

82 Gupta S, Anderson R, May RM. Mathematical models and the design of public health policy: HIV and antiviral therapy. *SIAM Review* 1993; 35:1–16.

83 Garnett GP, Anderson RM. Antiviral therapy and the transmission dynamics of HIV-1. *J Antimicrob Chemother* 1996; 37(Suppl.B):135–150.

84 Blower S, Gershengorn H, Grant RM. A tale of two futures: HIV and antiretroviral therapy in San Francisco. *Science* 2000; 287:650–654.

85 Gray RH, Xianbin Li, Wawer MJ *et al.* Stochastic simulation of the impact of antiretroviral therapy and HIV vaccines on HIV transmission; Rakai Uganda. *AIDS* 2003; 17:1941–1951.

86 Salomon JA, Hogan DR, Stover J *et al.* Integrating HIV prevention and treatment: from slogans to impact. *PLoS Medicine* 2005; 2(1):50–56.

87 Baggaley RF, Garnett GP, Ferguson NM. Modelling the impact of antiretroviral use in resource-poor settings. *PLoS Med* 2006; 3(4):e124.

88 Granich RM, Gilks CF, Dye C, De Cock KM, Williams BG. Universal voluntary HIV testing with immediate antiretroviral therapy as a strategy for elimination of HIV transmission: a mathematical model. *Lancet* 2009 Jan 3; 373(9657):48–57.

89 Moses S, Bradley JE, Nagelkerke NJ, Ronald AR, Ndinya-Achola JO, Plummer FA. Geographical patterns of male circumcision practices in Africa: association with HIV seroprevalence. *Int J Epidemiol* 1990; 19(3):693–697.

90 Weiss H, Quigley M, HAYES R. Male circumcision and risk of HIV infection in sub-Saharan Africa: a systematic review and meta-analysis. *AIDS* 2000; 14(15):2361–2370.

91 Buve A, Carael M, Hayes RJ *et al.* The multicentre study on factors determining the differential spread of HIV in four African cities: summary and conclusions. *AIDS* 2001; 15(Suppl 4):S127–131.

92 Orroth KK, Freeman E, Bakker R *et al.* Understanding differences across the contrasting epidemics in East and West Africa: results from a simulation model of the Four Cities Study. *STI* 2007; 83:i15–16.

93 Auvert B, Taljaard D, Lagarde E, Sobngwi-Tambekou J, Sitta R, Puren A. Randomized, controlled intervention trial of male circumcision for reduction of HIV infection risk: the ANRS 1265 Trial. *PLoS Med* 2005; 2(11):e298.

94 Bailey RC, Moses S, Parker CB *et al.* Male circumcision for HIV prevention in young men in Kisumu, Kenya: a randomised controlled trial. *Lancet* 2007; 369(9562):643–656.

95 Gray RH, Kigozi G, Serwadda D *et al.* Male circumcision for HIV prevention in men in Rakai, Uganda: a randomised trial. *Lancet* 2007; 369(9562):657–666.

96 Williams BG, Lloyd-Smith JO, Gouws E *et al.* The potential impact of male circumcision on HIV in Sub-Saharan Africa. *PLoS Med* 2006; 3(7):e262.

97 Hallett TB, Singh KJ, Smith JA, White RG, Abu-Raddad L, Garnett GP. Understanding the impact of male circumcision interventions on the spread of HIV in Southern Africa. *PLoS ONE* 2008; 3(5):e2212.

98 Gray R, Azire J, Serwadda D *et al.* Male circumcision and the risk of sexually transmitted infections and HIV in Rakai, Uganda. *AIDS* 2004; 18(18):657–666.

99 Nagelkerke NJ, Moses S, De Vlas SJ, Bailey RC. Modelling the public health impact of male circumcision for HIV prevention in high prevalence areas in Africa. *BMC Infect Dis* 2007; 7(1):16.

100 White RG, Glynn JR, Orroth KK *et al.* Male circumcision for HIV prevention in sub-Saharan Africa: who, what and when? *AIDS* 2008; 22(14):1841–1850.

101 Auvert B *et al.* Cost of the roll-out of male circumcision in sub-Saharan Africa. In Fourth International AIDS Society Conference, 2007. Sydney, Australia.

102 Expert Group on Modelling the Impact and Cost of Male Circumcision for HIV Risk Reduction. Informing decision making on male circumcision for HIV prevention in high HIV prevalence settings: what mathematical modelling can contribute. *PLoS Med* 2009; 6(9):e1000109.

103 Stover J, Bertozzi S, Gutierrez JP *et al.* The global impact of scaling up HIV/AIDS prevention programs in low- and middle-income countries. *Science* 2006; 311(5766): 1474–1476.

104 UNAIDS. *AIDS epidemic update 2007.* Geneva, UNAIDS/ WHO, 2007.

105 Kritzinger FE, den BS, Verver S *et al.* No decrease in annual risk of tuberculosis infection in endemic area in Cape Town, South Africa. *Trop Med Int Health* 2009; 14(2):136–142.

106 Williams BG, Dye C. Antiretroviral drugs for tuberculosis control in the era of HIV/AIDS. *Science* 2003; 301(5639):1535–1537.

Further reading

Modelling/statistical texts

Anderson RM and May RM. *Infectious diseases of Humans. Dynamics and control.* 1991; Oxford University Press. An excellent summary of the modelling work conducted on both respiratory and vector-borne diseases until 1991.

Benjamin M. Bolker. *Ecological models and data in R.* 2008; Princeton, NJ: Princeton University Press. Provides an introduction to setting up models and analysing data using the programming language R.

Daley DJ. *Epidemic modelling: introduction.* 1999; Cambridge University Press, Cambridge Studies in Mathematical Biology: 15.

Diekmann O and Heesterbeek H. *Mathematical epidemiology of infectious diseases. Model building, analysis and interpretation.* 2000; Chichester: Wiley. A good introduction to the principles of mathematical modelling and dynamics of infectious diseases; particularly useful for those interested in the mathematical theory. Also includes exercises with solutions.

Farrington CP. *Modelling epidemics.* 2008; The Open University. Milton Keynes. Excellent short book on the basics of infectious disease epidemiology and modelling. Used as part of the Open University course on Infectious Diseases.

Grimm V and Railsback SF. *Individual-based modeling and ecology.* 2005; Princeton, NJ: Princeton University Press. Provides a good introduction to individual-based models.

Isham V and Medley G. (eds) *Models for infectious human diseases. Their structure and relation to data.* 1996; Cambridge: Publications of the Newton Institute. Summary of papers presented during a workshop on infectious disease modelling.

Keeling MEJ and Rohani P. *Modeling infectious diseases in humans and animals.* 2008; Princeton, NJ: Princeton University Press. Excellent overview of both the methods for modelling infectious diseases and the application of infectious disease modelling; especially useful for readers who wish to go beyond a basic introduction.

May RM and MacLean A. *Theoretical ecology, 3rd edn.* 2007; Oxford University Press. Provides a good introduction to the dynamics of ecological systems.

Newman MEJ, Barabási AL and Watts DJ. *The structure and dynamics of networks.* 2006; Princeton University Press. An excellent annotated collection of papers on network modelling and research.

Nowak M and May RM. *Virus dynamics.* 2000; Oxford University Press. Short, useful book on modelling within-host viral dynamics, primarily illustrated using HIV/AIDS and hepatitis B.

Scott ME and Smith G. *Parasitic and infectious diseases: epidemiology and ecology.* 1994; San Diego, CA: Academic Press.

Infectious disease epidemiology/general epidemiology

Giesecke J. *Modern infectious disease epidemiology.* 2002; Arnold. Provides a good overview of infectious disease epidemiology.

Nelson KE and Williams CM. *Infectious disease epidemiology.* 2006; Oxford University Press.

Rothman KJ and Greeenland S. *Modern epidemiology, 2nd edn.* 1997; Lippincott Williams & Williams. Contains the chapter by Halloran "Concepts on infectious disease epidemiology" which was not included in the third edition. However, the second edition can be picked up cheaply second hand.

General mathematics topics covered in the text

There are numerous texts on differential equations, matrices, integration etc. For a general introduction to specific topics, readers may find it helpful to refer to the Schaum Outlines series, for example:

Bronson R and Costa GB. *Schaum's Outline of differential equations.* 2006; McGraw Hill.

Appendix

A.1 Differential equations

A.1.1 Writing down differential equations using the formal definition of the rate of change

The differential equations for the number of susceptible individuals can also be obtained by using the approach used to write down difference equations and considering the formal definition of the rate of change of a given quantity (see Section 3.3). The rate of change in the number of susceptible individuals, for example, is given by the following expression:

$$\frac{S(t+\delta t)-S(t)}{\delta t} \text{ as } \delta t \text{ approaches zero} \qquad \text{A.1}$$

We begin by noting that the number of susceptible individuals at time $t + \delta t$, $S(t + \delta t)$ is given by the difference between the number of individuals who were susceptible at time t and the number who were newly infected between time t and $t + \delta t$, i.e.:

$$S(t+\delta t)= \text{number of susceptible individuals at time } t \,(S(t))-$$
$$\text{the number of susceptible individuals who are}$$
$$\text{newly infected between time } t \text{ and } t+\delta t$$

However, the second term in this expression, that is, the number of susceptible individuals who are newly infected between time t and $t + \delta t$, is given by the number of individuals who are newly infected per unit time ($\lambda(t)S(t)$) multiplied by the size of the time step (δt). For example, if 10 individuals are newly infected each second, then 20 individuals should be newly infected every two seconds. This expression holds as long as the time step is so small that $\lambda(t)S(t)$ does not change over the time step.

Using this fact in the above expression, we see that the number of susceptible individuals at time $t + \delta t$ is given by:

$$S(t+\delta t)= S(t)- \lambda(t)S(t)\delta t \qquad \text{A.2}$$

Rearranging this expression, we see that:

$$S(t+\delta t)- S(t)=-\lambda(t)S(t)\delta t \qquad \text{A.3}$$

Dividing both sides of the equation by δt, we see that:

$$\frac{S(t+\delta t)-S(t)}{\delta t}=-\lambda(t)S(t) \qquad\qquad \text{A.4}$$

If δt is taken to be 'infinitessimally' small, the left-hand side of this equation can be replaced by $\frac{dS(t)}{dt}$, and we obtain the following expression for the *rate of change in the number* of susceptible individuals over time:

$$\frac{dS(t)}{dt}=\frac{S(t+\delta t)-S(t)}{\delta t}=-\lambda(t)S(t) \qquad as\,\delta t \to 0 \qquad \text{A.5}$$

i.e. the *rate of change in the number* of susceptible individuals at time t is equal to (minus) the product of the force of infection at time t, and the number of susceptible individuals at time t. The differential equations for the rate of change in the number of pre-infectious, infectious or immune individuals can be obtained in an analogous way.

A.1.2 Illustration of the result that the equation $\frac{dQ(t)}{dt}=-kQ(t)$ solves to give $Q(t)=Q(0)e^{-kt}$

We will illustrate this result by differentiating the expression $Q(t)=Q(0)e^{-kt}$ and showing that it leads to the equation $\frac{dQ(t)}{dt}=-kQ(t)$.

As discussed in Basic maths section B.3 e^{-kt} is given by the following expression:

$$e^{-kt}=1-kt+\frac{(-kt)^2}{2!}+\frac{(-kt)^3}{3!}+\frac{(-kt)^4}{4!}+\frac{(-kt)^5}{5!}+ \qquad \text{A.6}$$

and the derivative of e^{-kt} equals $-ke^{-kt}$ (Basic maths section B.5, point 3).

Differentiating the $Q(t)=Q(0)e^{-kt}$ expression using the rules of differentiation (Basic maths section B5 point 3), we obtain the following expression:

$$\frac{dQ(t)}{dt}=-kQ(0)e^{-kt} \qquad\qquad \text{A.7}$$

Since $Q(t)=Q(0)e^{-kt}$, we obtain our desired result:

$$\frac{dQ(t)}{dt}=-kQ(t) \qquad\qquad \text{A.8}$$

If we substitute $+k$ for $-k$ where appropriate throughout the above equations, we obtain the analogous result that the solution to the equation $\frac{dQ(t)}{dt}=kQ(t)$ is $Q(t)=Q(0)e^{kt}$.

A.1.3 **Illustration of the result that the average life expectancy = 1/mortality rate**

This result can be proved formally using the facts that if individuals die at a constant rate m, then

a) The number of individuals who were present in the population at time $t = 0$, who are still alive at time t is given by the expression $N(0)e^{-mt}$ where $N(0)$ is the number of individuals who were alive at time 0 (Equation 3.15).

b) The number of individuals who die at time t is $mN(0)e^{-mt}$ (i.e. the mortality rate multiplied by the population size at time t).

c) The average time until individuals die (the life expectancy) is given by the formal mathematical definition of the average (see also Equation 5.9 for the average age at infection) as:

$$\frac{\int_0^\infty mtN(0)e^{-mt}dt}{\int_0^\infty mN(0)e^{-mt}dt}$$

A.9

Using the rules of integration (see Basic maths section B.6), the numerator of this expression is given by $N(0)/m$ and the denominator equals $N(0)$. Dividing the numerator by the denominator leads to the result that the life expectancy equals $1/m$.

This result can be generalized to obtain the result that the average time until an event occurs = 1/average rate at which the event occurs.

A.2 **The dynamics of infections**

A.2.1 **Illustration of the result that when the number of infectious individuals in a population peaks for an immunizing infection, the proportion of the population that is susceptible equals $1/R_0$**

To prove this result, we consider the differential equations describing the rate of change in the number of infectious individuals for a Susceptible–Infectious–Recovered (SIR) model:

$$\frac{dI(t)}{dt} = \beta S(t)I(t) - rI(t)$$

A.10

When the number of infectious individuals increases, the rate of change in the number of infectious individuals (i.e. Equation A.10) is greater than zero:

$$\beta S(t)I(t) - rI(t) > 0$$

A.11

This equation is equivalent to the following:

$$I(t)(\beta S(t) - r) > 0$$

A.12

Since $I(t) > 0$ (because the number of infectious individuals is always greater than zero), the term in brackets must also be greater than zero. For example, if the product of two terms is greater than zero, and one of the two terms is greater than zero, then the other term must be greater than zero. We can therefore say that:

$$\beta S(t) - r > 0 \qquad \text{A.13}$$

After rearranging this expression and dividing by β, we obtain the following:

$$S(t) > \frac{r}{\beta} \qquad \text{A.14}$$

Dividing both sides of this equation by the population size, N, we obtain the following equation:

$$\frac{S(t)}{N} > \frac{r}{N\beta} \qquad \text{A.15}$$

Note that the left-hand side of this equation equals the proportion of the population that is susceptible (i.e. the number of individuals that are susceptible divided by the population size). Note that the right-hand side of this equation equals $1/R_0$, since $R_0 = \dfrac{\beta N}{r}$ (see Equation 4.2). Using this result in Equation A.15 we obtain the following equation for the proportion of the population that is susceptible when the number of infectious persons is increasing:

$$\frac{S(t)}{N} > \frac{1}{R_0} \qquad \text{A.16}$$

By applying similar logic, we obtain the result that when the number of infectious persons is declining ($\dfrac{dI(t)}{dt} < 0$), the proportion of the population that is susceptible is $< 1/R_0$. Also when the number of infectious persons is at a peak (i.e. when the number of infectious persons is neither increasing or decreasing, and so $\dfrac{dI(t)}{dt} = 0$), the proportion of the population that is susceptible is equal to $1/R_0$.

The above proof has considered the relationship between the total number of infectious persons and the proportion of the population that is susceptible. It also generally holds for the *incidence* of infectious persons and the proportion of the population that is susceptible, although the time at which the incidence peaks may differ vary slightly from the time at which the proportion of the population that is susceptible equals $1/R_0$, depending on the rate at which individuals recover from being infectious.

A.2.2 Derivation that the threshold condition $R_0 = \beta ND > 1$ must hold for the number of infectious persons to increase once an infectious person enters a totally susceptible population, using a susceptible–pre-infectious–infectious–recovered (SEIR) model

The derivation of this result is analogous to that in Section 4.2.2.1, except that we will consider the differential equations for the rate of change in the number of individuals who are infected, but not yet infectious, i.e. the pre-infectious ($E(t)$), and infectious individuals ($I(t)$).

Note that if the number of new infections and infectious persons increases following the introduction of an infectious case into a totally susceptible population then the rate of change in the number of pre-infectious and infectious individuals must be 'positive', i.e. $\dfrac{dE(t)}{dt} > 0$ and $\dfrac{dI(t)}{dt} > 0$

As discussed in Chapter 2, the expressions for the rate of change in the number of pre-infectious and infectious individuals for an SEIR model are given by:

$$\frac{dE(t)}{dt} = \beta S(t)I(t) - fE(t) \qquad\qquad \text{A.17}$$

$$\frac{dI(t)}{dt} = fE(t) - rI(t) \qquad\qquad \text{A.18}$$

where f is the rate at which pre-infectious individuals become infectious.

For the rate of change in the number of pre-infectious individuals (described in A.17) to be positive, the number of new infections which occur in the population per unit time ($\beta S(t)I(t)$) has to exceed the number of pre-infectious individuals who become infectious per unit time ($fE(t)$), i.e.:

$$\beta S(t)I(t) > fE(t) \qquad\qquad \text{A.19}$$

Similarly, for the rate of change in the number of infectious individuals to be positive (described in A.18), the number of pre-infectious individuals who become infectious per unit time ($fE(t)$) has to exceed the number of infectious individuals who recover per unit time ($rI(t)$), i.e.:

$$fE(t) > rI(t) \qquad\qquad \text{A.20}$$

Combining the logic in Equations A.19 and A.20, we see that the number of individuals who are newly infected per unit time must also be larger than the number of individuals who recover per unit time, i.e.:

$$\beta S(t)I(t) > rI(t) \qquad\qquad \text{A.21}$$

This expression is identical to Equation 4.3, and so we can complete the remainder of the proof using the steps after this expression in the main text.

A.2.3 Proof of the result that when the number of infectious individuals in the population peaks and troughs for an immunizing infection, the proportion of the population that is susceptible equals $1/R_0$

To prove this result we consider the differential equations describing the rate of change in the number of susceptible individuals for a susceptible–infectious–recovered (SIR) model.

$$\frac{dI(t)}{dt} = \beta S(t)I(t) - rI(t) \qquad\qquad \text{A.22}$$

When the number of infectious individuals is at a peak, the rate of change in the number of infectious individuals (i.e. A.22) equals zero:

$$\beta S(t)I(t) - rI(t) = 0 \qquad\qquad\text{A.23}$$

This equation is equivalent to the following:

$$I(t)(\beta S(t) - r) = 0 \qquad\qquad\text{A.24}$$

Since $I(t)$ is not equal to zero at a peak, the term in brackets must equal zero:

$$\beta S(t) - r = 0 \qquad\qquad\text{A.25}$$

After rearranging this expression and dividing by β, we obtain the following:

$$S(t) = \frac{r}{\beta} \qquad\qquad\text{A.26}$$

Dividing both sides of this equation by the population size, N, we obtain the following equation:

$$\frac{S(t)}{N} = \frac{r}{N\beta} \qquad\qquad\text{A.27}$$

Note that the left-hand side of this equation equals the proportion of the population that is susceptible (i.e. the number of individuals that are susceptible divided by the population size). Substituting for $R_0 = \dfrac{\beta N}{r}$ (see Equation 4.2) into Equation A.27, we obtain the following equation for the proportion of the population that is susceptible at a peak:

$$\frac{S(t)}{N} = \frac{1}{R_0} \qquad\qquad\text{A.28}$$

A.2.4 The mathematical theory for why the number of infectious individuals increases at an approximately constant rate during the early stages of an epidemic

As shown in Section 3.5.1, if some quantity Q changes at a constant rate, k, the differential equation for the rate of change in that quantity has the following form:

$$\frac{dQ(t)}{dt} = kQ(t) \qquad\qquad\text{A.29}$$

To show that the number of infectious individuals increases at a constant rate during the early stages of an epidemic, we simply need to show that the equation for the rate of change in the number of infectious individuals has a similar form to this equation, i.e. the right-hand side of the equation is some constant (size to be determined) multiplied by the number of infectious individuals ($I(t)$).

The following are the differential equations for the rate of change in the number of infectious individuals for the simplest (SIR) model whereby individuals are assumed to be infectious immediately after infection:

$$\frac{dI(t)}{dt} = \beta S(t)I(t) - rI(t)$$

A.30

where β is the rate at which two specific individuals come into effective contact, $r\,(=1/(\text{duration of infectiousness}, D)$ is the rate at which infectious individuals recover to become immune and $S(t)$ is the number of susceptible individuals at time t.

During the early stages of an epidemic, whilst very few susceptible individuals have been infected, the size of the susceptible population is very similar to the population size (N). Using this approximation, we can rewrite Equation A.30 as follows:

$$\frac{dI(t)}{dt} \approx \beta NI(t) - rI(t)$$
$$\approx (\beta N - r)I(t)$$

A.31

The expression $(\beta N - r)$ is constant, and thus Equation A.31 is similar in form to Equation A.29, suggesting that the number of infectious individuals changes at an approximately constant rate during the early stages of an epidemic.

A.2.5 Derivation of the equation $R_0 = 1 + \Lambda D$

As shown in section A.2.4, the rate of change in the number of infectious individuals during the early stages of an epidemic is given by the expression:

$$\frac{dI(t)}{dt} \approx (\beta N - r)I(t)$$

Setting the growth rate Λ equal to $(\beta N - r)$, we obtain the following:

$$\Lambda = \beta N - r$$

A.32

Factoring out r from the right-hand side of this equation and using the relationship $R_0 = \beta N / r$ (see Equation 4.2) this equation can be written as follows:

$$\Lambda = r\left(\frac{\beta N}{r} - 1\right) = r(R_0 - 1)$$

A.33

Assuming that the duration of infectiousness, D, equals $1/r$, this equation simplifies to the following:

$$\Lambda = \frac{R_0 - 1}{D}$$

A.34

After some rearranging, we obtain the following equation:

$$R_0 = 1 + \Lambda D \qquad \text{A.35}$$

The derivation of the other equations in Table 4.1 is analogous (although it requires some more complicated manipulation.)

A.2.6 Proof of the result that the estimated growth rate of an epidemic should be similar if cases are under-reported

If we can only observe a fraction (e.g. 20 per cent) of the cases over time, then a plot of the log of the observed number of cases also follows a straight line, and the gradient of this line equals the growth rate of the epidemic (see e.g. Figure 4.10).

This result follows from the fact that the number observed cases at time t, $O(t)$ is given by the expression:

$$O(t) = pI(t) \qquad \text{A.36}$$

where p is the proportion of infectious individuals in the population which are reported.

Using the result that during the early stages of an epidemic $I(t) \approx I(0)e^{\Lambda t}$ (Equation 4.8), we obtain the following result:

$$O(t) \approx pI(0)e^{\Lambda t} \qquad \text{A.37}$$

Taking the natural logs of both sides of Equation A.37, we see that:

$$\ln\{O(t)\} \approx \ln\{pI(0)e^{\Lambda t}\} \qquad \text{A.38}$$

By the law of logarithms (Basic maths section B.4), this equation simplifies to:

$$\ln\{O(t)\} \approx \ln\{pI(0)\} + \Lambda t \qquad \text{A.39}$$

This equation is that of a straight line when plotted on the x-axis (Basic maths section B.2) and the gradient of this line equals Λ, i.e. the growth rate of the epidemic. Consequently, if we plot the natural log of $O(t)$ against time, we should see a straight line, which has a gradient of Λ.

A.2.7 Mathematical proof of the result that at a peak or trough in the number of infectious persons for an immunizing infection, the proportion of individuals that are susceptible equals $1/R_0$, accounting for births into and deaths out of the population

To obtain this result, we use the differential equations for an SIR model, accounting for births into and deaths out of the population:

$$\frac{dS(t)}{dt} = bN - \beta I(t)S(t) - mS(t) \qquad \text{A.40}$$

$$\frac{dI(t)}{dt} = \beta I(t)S(t) - rI(t) - mI(t)$$

A.41

$$\frac{dR(t)}{dt} = rI(t) - mR(t)$$

A.42

For simplicity, we will consider the situation in which the birth rate equals the death rate (i.e. $b=m$). Since, in this instance, the population size remains unchanged, we will denote the population size using the symbol 'N', rather than $N(t)$.

We begin by noting that, after extending the proof in Section 4.2.2.1, the basic reproduction number for an immunizing infection in this population is given by the expression:

$$R_0 = \frac{\beta N}{r + m}$$

At a peak or trough in the number of infectious persons, the rate of change in the number of infectious individuals is zero, i.e. Equation A.41 equals zero, as follows:

$$\beta I(t)S(t) - rI(t) - mI(t) = 0$$

A.43

Rearranging this equation, we obtain the following:

$$I(t)(\beta S(t) - r - m) = 0$$

A.44

At a peak or trough in the number of infectious persons, the number of infectious individuals cannot be equal to zero, which implies that the term in brackets must be equal to zero, i.e.:

$$\beta S(t) - r - m = 0$$

A.45

Rearranging this equation, we obtain the following expression for the number of susceptible individuals at time t:

$$S(t) = \frac{r + m}{\beta}$$

A.46

The proportion of the population that is susceptible, $s(t)$, is given by Equation A.46, divided by the population size, N:

$$s(t) = \frac{r + m}{\beta N}$$

A.47

Substituting for $R_0 = \frac{\beta N}{r + m}$ into Equation A.47 leads to the result that at a peak or trough in the number of infectious persons $s(t) = 1/R_0$. Note that $s(t) = 1/R_0$ when the incidence of infection (and therefore, for acute infections, the incidence of infectious persons) is at a peak or trough, since the force of infection is directly proportional to the number of infectious persons (see equation 2.5).

A.3 **Age patterns**

A.3.1 **Proof of the result that for a population with an exponential age distribution, the average force of infection (λ), the average life expectancy and R_0 are related through the expression $R_0 = 1 + \lambda L$**

This relationship can be obtained by considering the differential equations for the rate of change in the number of susceptible, infectious and immune discussed in Appendix section A.2.7 for an SIR model, accounting for births into and deaths out of the population. In the long-term, the rate of change in the number of susceptible, infectious and immune individuals equals zero since the cycles in incidence damp out (see Figure 4.17), i.e. $\dfrac{dS(t)}{dt} = \dfrac{dI(t)}{dt} = \dfrac{dR(t)}{dt} = 0$

We begin by noting that the rate of change in the number of susceptible individuals can be written as follows:

$$\frac{dS(t)}{dt} = bN(t) - \lambda(t)S(t) - mS(t) \qquad \text{A.48}$$

For simplicity, we will assume that the population size ($N(t)$) remains unchanged over time and so the birth rate equals the death rate ($b=m$). Since we are considering the long-term equilibrium values of all these variables, we will drop the 't' from the notation. Setting Equation A.48 equal to zero, and after rearranging this expression we obtain the following result:

$$bN - S(\lambda + m) = 0 \qquad \text{A.49}$$

Dividing this equation by the population size, and rearranging the resulting expression, we obtain the following:

$$\frac{S}{N} = \frac{b}{(\lambda + m)} \qquad \text{A.50}$$

or, since the birth rate equals the death rate (i.e. $b=m$):

$$\frac{S}{N} = \frac{m}{(\lambda + m)} \qquad \text{A.51}$$

In the long term, the rate of change in the number of infectious individuals equals zero, i.e. $\dfrac{dI(t)}{dt} = 0$ (see above). As shown in Appendix section A2.7, when $\dfrac{dI(t)}{dt} = 0$, the proportion of the population that is susceptible equals $1/R_0$ i.e. $\dfrac{S(t)}{N(t)} = \dfrac{1}{R_0}$. Substituting for $\dfrac{S}{N} = \dfrac{1}{R_0}$ into Equation A.51 we obtain the following:

$$\frac{1}{R_0} = \frac{m}{(\lambda + m)} \qquad \text{A.52}$$

Rearranging this equation leads to the result:

$$R_0 = \frac{\lambda}{m} + 1$$

A.53

The average life expectancy, L, is related to the average mortality rate m through the expression:

$$L = \frac{1}{m}$$

A.54

Using this result in Equation A.53, we obtain the following:

$$R_0 = \lambda L + 1$$

A.55

Similarly, substituting for $m = 1/L$ into equation A.51 leads to the equation:

$$\frac{S}{N} = \frac{1}{\lambda L + 1}$$

A.3.2 Proof of the result that for a population with a rectangular age distribution, the average force of infection (λ), the average life expectancy and R_0 are related through the expression $R_0 = \lambda L$

We obtain this result by using the finding that in the long term, for an endemic immunizing infection and assuming that individuals mix randomly, the proportion of the population that is susceptible (s) and R_0 are related through the equation $s = 1/R_0$ (Table 4.3) or conversely:

$$R_0 = 1/s$$

A.56

We begin by obtaining an equation for the proportion of the population that is susceptible in terms of λ.

For a population with a rectangular age distribution, the overall proportion of the population that is susceptible is given by the following expression:

The sum (or integral) of the number of individuals that are susceptible

at each age a

÷

Total population size

A.57

Assuming that the population remains site unchanged over time, the total population size is given by the following expression, where N_0 is the number of individuals that are born each year:

Total population size $= N_0 L$

A.58

As discussed in section 5.2.2, the proportion of individuals of a given age a that are susceptible is given by the expression:

$$s(a) = e^{-\lambda a}$$

A.59

The total number of individuals of age a that are susceptible is therefore given by $N_0\,e^{-\lambda a}$ and the total number of individuals in the population that are susceptible is then given by the equation:

$$\text{Total number susceptible} = N_0 \int_0^L e^{-\lambda a} da = \frac{N_0(1-e^{-\lambda L})}{\lambda} \qquad \text{A.60}$$

Using the results from Equations A.58 and A.60 in Expression A.57, we obtain the following equation for the overall average proportion of the population that is susceptible, s:

$$s = \frac{N_0(1-e^{-\lambda L})}{\lambda L N_0} = \frac{(1-e^{-\lambda L})}{\lambda L} \qquad \text{A.61}$$

Substituting this equation for s into Equation A.56 leads to the result:

$$R_0 = \frac{\lambda L}{1-e^{-\lambda L}} \qquad \text{A.62}$$

For realistic values for the life expectancy (L) and the force of infection, $e^{-\lambda L} \approx 0$, and so the denominator of this expression is approximately equal to 1. This leads to the following approximation for R_0:

$$R_0 \approx \lambda L \qquad \text{A.63}$$

Likewise, the numerator in equation A.61 is approximately equal to one, and therefore $s \approx \dfrac{1}{\lambda L}$.

A.3.3 Proof of the result that, for a population with a rectangular age distribution, the long-term average force of infection and R_0 are related through the expression

$$R_0 = \frac{\lambda' L}{(1-v)(1-e^{-\lambda' L})}$$

We obtain this result by using the finding that in the long term, for an endemic immunizing infection and assuming that individuals mix randomly, the proportion of the population that is susceptible (s) and R_0 are related through the equation $s = 1/R_0$ (Table 4.3) or conversely:

$$R_0 = 1/s$$

Note that, if we assume that individuals mix randomly, this relationship holds even when a proportion of individuals (<herd immunity threshold) has been vaccinated. This follows from the fact that this relationship is derived by using the result that $R_n = R_0 s$ (see sections 1.3 and 4.2.2.2), and if individuals mix randomly, this relationship holds—irrespective of whether or not individuals have been vaccinated.

We begin by calculating the total number of susceptible individuals in the population.

Assuming that a proportion v of individuals are immunized at age a_v, we can adapt the expressions for the proportion of individuals that are susceptible to infection at age a, that were discussed in section 5.2.2 to obtain the following expressions for the number of individuals of age a that are susceptible to infection in the long-term after the introduction of vaccination:

$$S(a) = \begin{cases} N_0 e^{-\lambda' a} & a < a_v \\ N_0 (1-v) e^{-\lambda' a} & a \geq a_v \end{cases}$$

A.64

Here N_0 is the number of individuals that are born each year. The equation for individuals aged over a_v years can be derived by using the following logic:

Number susceptible at age a =

Number who were susceptible at age a_v $(= N_0 e^{-\lambda' a_v})$

×

Proportion that were vaccinated at age a_v $(= (1-v))$

×

Proportion who escaped infection between age a and age a_v $(= e^{-\lambda'(a-a_v)})$

The total number of individuals that are susceptible (S) can be obtained by integrating Equation A.64 between 0 and the life expectancy, L:

$$S = \int_0^{a_v} N_0 e^{-\lambda' a} da + \int_{a_v}^{L} N_0 (1-v) e^{-\lambda' a} da$$

A.65

After some manipulation, we obtain the following expression for S:

$$S = \frac{N_0}{\lambda'} \{ 1 - v e^{-\lambda' a_v} - (1-v) e^{-\lambda' L} \}$$

A.66

For a population with a rectangular age distribution, the total population size equals $N_0 L$ (see also Panel 7.4) and therefore the overall proportion of the population that is susceptible is given by the equation:

$$\frac{S}{N} = \frac{N_0}{L\lambda' N_0} \{ 1 - v e^{-\lambda' a_v} - (1-v) e^{-\lambda' L} \} = \frac{1 - v e^{-\lambda' a_v} - (1-v) e^{-\lambda' L}}{\lambda' L}$$

A.67

Using the result that R_0 is related to the overall proportion of the population that is susceptible (s) through the equation $R_0 = 1/s$ (Table 4.3), we obtain the following equation relating R_0 and λ':

$$R_0 = \frac{\lambda' L}{1 - v e^{-\lambda' a_v} - (1-v) e^{-\lambda' L}}$$

A.68

If individuals are vaccinated at birth, then substituting for $a_v = 0$ into Equation A.68 leads to the result:

$$R_0 = \frac{\lambda' L}{(1-v)(1 - e^{-\lambda' L})}$$

A.69

A.3.4 **Proof of the result that, for a population with an exponential age distribution, the long-term average force of infection and R_0 are related through the expression**
$$R_0 = \frac{\lambda' L}{(1-v)}$$

To obtain this result, we adapt logic used for a population with a rectangular age distribution (Appendix section A.3.3).

We begin by noting that, for this population, assuming that a proportion v of individuals are immunized at age a_v, the number of individuals that are susceptible at age a is given by the following equation:

$$S(a) = \begin{cases} N_0 e^{-(\lambda'+m)a} & a < a_v \\ N_0(1-v)e^{-(\lambda'+m)a} & a \geq a_v \end{cases}$$
A.70

where m is the average mortality rate, N_0 is the number of individuals that are born each year and therefore $N_0 e^{-ma}$ is the number of individuals of age a (see also section 3.5.1).

The total number of individuals that are susceptible (S) can be obtained by integrating Equation A.70 between 0 and infinity (see the note about use of infinity below):

$$S = \int_0^{a_v} N_0 e^{-(\lambda'+m)a} da + \int_{a_v}^{\infty} N_0(1-v)e^{-(\lambda'+m)a} da$$
A.71

After some manipulation, we obtain the following expression for S:

$$S = \frac{N_0 \left[1 - ve^{-(\lambda'+m)a_v}\right]}{\lambda' + m}$$
A.72

For a population with an exponential age distribution, the total population size given by the equation $N = N_0/m$ which is obtained by integrating the expression $N(a) = N_0 e^{-ma}$ between 0 and infinity. Dividing Equation A.72 by the equation $N = N_0/m$ leads to the following equation for the proportion of the population that is susceptible:

$$\frac{S}{N} = \frac{N_0 m\left[1 - ve^{-(\lambda'+m)a_v}\right]}{(\lambda'+m)N_0} = \frac{m\left[1 - ve^{-(\lambda'+m)a_v}\right]}{(\lambda'+m)}$$
A.73

Using the result $R_0 = 1/s$ and the relationship $L = 1/m$ leads to the following equation for R_0:

$$R_0 = \frac{1 + \lambda' L}{1 - ve^{-(\lambda'+m)a_v}}$$
A.74

If individuals are only vaccinated at birth, then substituting for $a_v = 0$ leads to the following equation:

$$R_0 = \frac{1 + \lambda' L}{1 - v}$$
A.75

The use of infinity in deriving the above results

Note that the theoretical upper age limit of a population with an exponential age distribution is infinity. The results above could have been obtained by setting a realistic value for the upper limit, although this would have required more manipulation of the equations than was used in the explanation provided here.

A.3.5 Proof of the result that the average age at infection in the long-term after the introduction of infants for a population with an exponential age distribution is given by the equation $A' = \dfrac{A}{(1-v)}$

To obtain this result from the equation $A' = \dfrac{1}{\lambda' + m}$ we begin by noting that R_0 and λ' are related through the equation $R_0 = \dfrac{\lambda' L + 1}{(1-v)}$ (Equation 5.29), which is equivalent to the following equation:

$$R_0 = \frac{\lambda' + m}{m(1-v)} \qquad\qquad \text{A.76}$$

assuming that the life expectancy and the average mortality rate are related through the equation $L = 1/m$.

Rearranging Equation A.76, we obtain the following expression for $A' = \dfrac{1}{\lambda' + m}$:

$$A' = \frac{1}{\lambda' + m} = \frac{1}{mR_0(1-v)} \qquad\qquad \text{A.77}$$

As discussed in Appendix section A3.1 $R_0 = 1 + \dfrac{\lambda}{m}$, or equivalently, $R_0 = \dfrac{\lambda + m}{m}$.

Substituting the latter expression for R_0 into Equation A.77, we obtain the following equation for $A' = \dfrac{1}{\lambda' + m}$:

$$A' = \frac{1}{\lambda' + m} = \frac{1}{m\dfrac{\lambda + m}{m}(1-v)} = \frac{1}{(\lambda + m)(1-v)} \qquad\qquad \text{A.78}$$

As discussed in Table 5.1, the average age at infection before the introduction of vaccination in a population with an exponential age distribution is given by the equation:

$$A = \frac{1}{\lambda + m} \qquad\qquad \text{A.79}$$

Using the result $A = \dfrac{1}{\lambda + m}$ in Equation A.78 leads to the intended result:

$$A' = \frac{A}{(1-v)} \qquad\qquad \text{A.80}$$

A.4 **Stochastic modelling**

A.4.1 **Derivation of the result that** $1-(1-p)^{I_t} \approx pI_t$

The expression $(1-p)^{I_t}$ can be expanded to give the expression:

$$(1-p)^{I_t} = 1 - pI_t + \frac{I_t(I_t-1)p^2}{2} - \frac{I_t(I_t-1)(I_t-2)}{3!}p^3 + \qquad \text{A.81}$$

When either p or I_t are very small, terms involving p^2, p^3 and higher order terms in p in Equation A.81 are negligible in comparison with the first two terms. In this situation, we can see that Equation A.81 is approximately equal to $1-pI_t$ as follows:

$$(1-p)^{I_t} \approx 1 - pI_t \qquad \text{A.82}$$

This equation can be rearranged to give the following result:

$$1-(1-p)^{I_t} \approx pI_t \qquad \text{A.83}$$

If the size of the time step is very small, then the probability of an effective contact between two specific individuals per time step is approximately equal to the (*per capita*) rate at which two specific individuals come into effective contact, i.e. β, and therefore:

$$1-(1-p)^{I_t} \approx \beta I_t \qquad \text{A.84}$$

A.4.2 **An illustration of Method 3**

Table 6.2 and Figure 6.8 summarize the results of simulating the introduction of one infectious person into a totally susceptible population consisting of 10 individuals, using a value for β of 0.1/day and an average duration of infectiousness of 2 days (which is equivalent to a recovery rate of 0.5/day). These parameters are equivalent to assuming that R_0 is 2. The calculations during the first time step are summarized below.

First time step

Step 1: Calculate M_0, the total hazard rate for individuals to change their current status

At the start of the simulations, there are 10 susceptible individuals, 1 infectious individual and 0 immune individuals.

The rate at which individuals who can become newly infected (and, in this model, infectious) during the next time step is given by $\beta S(0)I(0) = 0.1 \times 10 \times 1 = 1$ per day.

The rate at which individuals can recover and become immune during the next time step is given by $rI(0) = 0.5 \times 1 = 0.5$ per day.

Thus M_0 is given by $1+0.5 = 1.5$ per day.

> ### Step 2: Draw a random number, n_1, to determine the time T at which the next transition occurs.
>
> In this instance, the random number $n_1 = 0.46$ was drawn and the equation $T = -ln(n_1)/M_0$ gives the result that the next transition occurs at time $T = 0.518$ days.
>
> ### Step 3: Calculate the probability that each type of transition occurs next and specify the range in which a number drawn at random will have to lie for the next transition to be of a given type.
>
> The probability that one susceptible individual becomes infected is given by $\beta S(0)I(0)/M_0 = 1/1.5 = 0.667$.
>
> The probability that one infectious individual recovers and becomes immune is given by $rI(0)/M_0 = 0.5/1.5 = 0.337$.
>
> It would therefore be sensible to specify that if the random number lies in the interval $(0, 0.667)$, then the next event will be an infection event, and otherwise, one infectious individual will recover and become immune.
>
> ### Step 4: Draw a uniform random number n_2 to determine the type of transition event which occurs next
>
> In this example, the random number drawn is 0.56. As this lies between 0 and 0.667, the next event will be the infection of 1 susceptible individual.
>
> ### Step 5: Update the number of individuals in each category
>
> At time $T = 0.518$ days, there are nine susceptible individuals, one infectious individual and 0 immune individuals.
>
> Return to step 1 etc.

A.5 Age-dependent contact patterns

A.5.1 Derivation of the mathematical approaches for calculating R_0

A.5.1.1 Derivation of the simultaneous equations approach

Equations 7.37 and 7.38 can be derived by using the result discussed in section 7.5.2 that, if infectious individuals are introduced into a population in which individuals mix according to some WAIFW matrix and there is an unlimited supply of susceptible individuals, then after several generations have occurred:

A. The number of secondary infectious persons which result from each infectious person equals R_0 (Figure 7.14).

B. The age distribution of the infectious persons in each generation converges to some distribution (Figure 7.15), e.g. a fraction x are young and a fraction $1-x$ are old.

For illustrative purposes, we consider a scenario in which there are 100 infectious individuals in the kth generation.

Statement A implies that there will be $100R_0$ infectious individuals in generation $k + 1$.

According to statement B, there will be $100x$ and $100(1 - x)$ infectious children and adults respectively in generation k. Using the assumption that each infectious person leads to R_0 secondary infectious persons, there will be $100R_0x$ and $100R_0(1 - x)$ infectious children and adults respectively in generation $k + 1$.

We can obtain another expression for the number of infectious children in generation $k + 1$ in terms of the R_{yy}, R_{yo}, R_{oy} and R_{oo} values in the Next Generation Matrix and, after equating this expression to $100R_0x$, we can obtain Equation 7.37 as follows.

For example, the number of infectious children in generation $k + 1$ ($100R_0x$) is given by the sum of the number generated by each of the $100x$ children in generation k ($= 100xR_{yy}$) and the number generated by each of the $100(1 - x)$ adults in generation k ($= 100(1 - x)R_{oy}$), i.e.:

$$100xR_{yy} + 100(1 - x)R_{yo}$$

Equating this expression to $100R_0x$, which, as we saw above, also equals the number of infectious children in generation $k+1$, we obtain the following:

$$100xR_{yy} + 100(1 - x)R_{yo} = 100R_0x \qquad \text{A.85}$$

Cancelling the common factor 100 from both sides of this equation leads to Equation 7.37.

We can use an analogous argument to obtain Equation 7.38.

A.5.1.2 Derivation of the matrix determinant approach for calculating R_0

We can obtain Equation 7.40 by rearranging Equations 7.37 and 7.38 in several stages as follows.

Dividing Equations 7.37 and 7.38 by $1-x$, we obtain the following equations:

$$R_{yy}\frac{x}{1-x} + R_{yo} = R_0\frac{x}{1-x} \qquad \text{A.86}$$

$$R_{oy}\frac{x}{1-x} + R_{oo} = R_0 \qquad \text{A.87}$$

Equations A.86 and A.87 can be rearranged to give the following expressions for $\dfrac{x}{1-x}$:

$$\frac{x}{1-x} = \frac{R_{yo}}{R_0 - R_{yy}} \qquad \text{A.88}$$

$$\frac{x}{1-x} = \frac{R_0 - R_{oo}}{R_{oy}} \qquad \text{A.89}$$

Equating Equation A.88 to Equation A.89, we obtain the following equation:

$$\frac{R_{yo}}{R_0 - R_{yy}} = \frac{R_0 - R_{oo}}{R_{oy}}$$

Rearranging this equation, we obtain the following result:

$$R_{yo}R_{oy} = (R_0 - R_{oo})(R_0 - R_{yy})$$

which, after further rearranging, leads to Equation 7.40.

A.6 **Sexually transmitted infections**

A.6.1 **Other methods to calculate R_0 in a population with heterogeneity in sexual activity and proportionate mixing**

(a) Calculate R_0 using the matrix determinant approach

For our model population with two sexual activity groups, R_0 is the maximum value that satisfies the following equation (see section 7.5.3):

$$(R_{HH} - R_0)(R_{LL} - R_0) - R_{LH}R_{HL} = 0 \qquad \text{A.90}$$

where R_{HH} is the number of secondary infections generated by an infected high-activity member in high-activity members, R_{HL} is the number of secondary infections generated by an infected low-activity member in high-activity members, R_{LH} is the number of secondary infections generated by an infected high-activity member in low-activity members, and R_{LL} is the number of secondary infections generated by an infected low-activity member in low-activity members.

R_{HH}, R_{HL}, R_{LH} and R_{LL} together make up our next generation matrix $\begin{pmatrix} R_{HH} & R_{HL} \\ R_{LH} & R_{LL} \end{pmatrix}$

Using Equation 8.21 and 8.22 we know that in a completely susceptible population, a high-activity member generates R_H (3.93) infections and a low-activity member generates R_L (0.18) infections. As we assume proportionate mixing, using Equation 8.20 we also know that 31 per cent (g_H) of these infections will be transmitted to high-activity members and 69 per cent (g_L) will be transmitted to low-activity members, so we can write:

$$R_{HH} = R_H g_H$$
$$R_{HL} = R_L g_H$$
$$R_{LH} = R_H g_L$$
$$R_{LL} = R_L g_L$$

Substituting these expressions into Equation A.90 we obtain the following expression that R_0 has to satisfy:

$$(R_H g_H - R_0)(R_L g_L - R_0) - R_H g_L R_L g_H = 0 \qquad \text{A.91}$$

Multiplying out this expression and cancelling, we see that R_0 has to satisfy the following expression:

$$R_0^2 - R_0 R_H g_H - R_0 R_L g_L = 0 \qquad \text{A.92}$$

which simplifies to:

$$R_0(R_0 - (R_H g_H + R_L g_L)) = 0 \qquad \text{A.93}$$

To satisfy this equation R_0 must equal 0, or:

$$\begin{aligned} R_0 &= g_H R_H + g_L R_L \\ &= 0.31 \times 3.93 + 0.69 \times 0.18 \\ &= 1.36 \end{aligned}$$

(b) Calculate R_0 using the dominant eigenvalue of the next generation matrix.

Using the simulation approach outlined in Section 7.5.3 to calculate R_0 we need to calculate the next generation matrix, or the number of secondary cases in the high and low-activity groups that result from an infected high or low-activity individual. Again we use the results of Equation 8.20, 8.21 and 8.22 to write down the next generation matrix:

$$
\begin{array}{cc}
 & \begin{array}{c} \text{Activity group of} \\ \text{infectious individual} \\ \text{High} \quad \text{Low} \end{array} \\
\begin{array}{cc} \text{Activity group of} & \text{High} \\ \text{susceptible individual} & \text{Low} \end{array} &
\begin{pmatrix} R_{HH} & R_{HL} \\ R_{LH} & R_{LL} \end{pmatrix}
\end{array}
$$

$$
= \begin{pmatrix} R_H g_H & R_L g_H \\ R_H g_L & R_L g_L \end{pmatrix}
$$

$$
= \begin{pmatrix} 3.93 \times 0.31 & 0.18 \times 0.31 \\ 3.93 \times 0.69 & 0.18 \times 0.69 \end{pmatrix}
$$

$$
= \begin{pmatrix} 1.23 & 0.06 \\ 2.70 & 0.12 \end{pmatrix} \qquad \text{A.94}
$$

By simulation R_0 can be calculated to be 1.36.

Basic maths

B.1 **Overview**

This chapter revises the following basic concepts in mathematics that are used in various sections of the book:

1) The equation of a straight line
2) The constant 'e'
3) Logarithms
4) Differentiation
5) Integration
6) Matrices

B.2 **The equation of a straight line**

The equation of a straight line is as follows:

$$y = mx + c$$

B1

where m is the gradient of the line (the amount by which the line goes up, divided by the amount by which it goes across) and c is the constant value at which the line crosses the vertical y axis, i.e. when $x = 0$ (see Figure B.1).

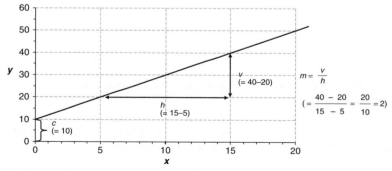

Fig. B1 The equation of a straight line. In this example, $m = 2$ (i.e. the line goes up 20 units for each 10 units that the line goes across horizontally) and $c = 10$ (i.e. the line crosses the vertical y axis when $y = 2$. The equation in this example is $y = 2x + 10$.

B.3 **The constant 'e'**

'*e*' is a mathematical constant, named after the famous Swiss mathematician, Euler. It has many useful properties and is used extensively in mathematics and in the biological and physical sciences.

It is formally defined as the following infinite sum:

$$1+\frac{1}{1!}+\frac{1}{2!}+\frac{1}{3!}+\frac{1}{4!}+\frac{1}{5!}+...\frac{1}{n!}+...$$

This expression can also be written using the shorthand notation $\sum_{z=0}^{\infty}\frac{1}{z!}$. Taken to five decimal places, *e* equals 2.71828. *e* raised to the power of any number *t* is equal to the following expression:

$$e^t =1+t+\frac{t^2}{2!}+\frac{t^3}{3!}+\frac{t^4}{4!}+\frac{t^5}{5!}+...$$

Using shorthand notation, this expression would be written as $\sum_{z=0}^{\infty}\frac{t^z}{z!}$.

Similarly, *e* raised to the power of the product of any two numbers, e.g. e^{kt} could be written as:

$$e^{kt} =1+kt+\frac{(kt)^2}{2!}+\frac{(kt)^3}{3!}+\frac{(kt)^4}{4!}+\frac{(kt)^5}{5!}+...$$

It could also be written as:

$$e^{kt} =1+kt+\frac{k^2t^2}{2!}+\frac{k^3t^3}{3!}+\frac{k^4t^4}{4!}+\frac{k^5t^5}{5!}+...$$

e^{-kt} would be written as follows:

$$e^{-kt} =1-kt+\frac{(-kt)^2}{2!}+\frac{(-kt)^3}{3!}+\frac{(-kt)^4}{4!}+\frac{(-kt)^5}{5!}+...+\frac{(-kt)^n}{n!}+...$$

This equation can be simplified to the following:

$$e^{-kt} =1-kt+\frac{k^2t^2}{2!}-\frac{k^3t^3}{3!}+\frac{k^4t^4}{4!}-\frac{k^5t^5}{5!}+...+\frac{(-1)^n k^n t^n}{n!}+...$$

Figure B2 shows the shape of e^{kt}, as *t* varies, for different values for negative and positive values of *k*.

e is used to define the exponential distribution, which is sometimes used to characterize the age distribution of some populations (see Figure 3.7). The left-hand figure in Figure B2 illustrates the typical shape of this distribution.

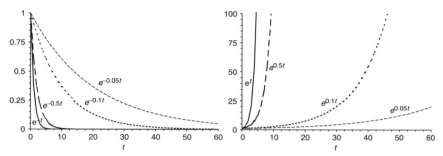

Fig. B2 Plot of the lines e^{kt} against t for negative and positive values of k.

B.4 **Logarithms**

The *logarithm* (or 'log') of a number is the power (or value) to which a number (called the *base*) must be raised to equal that number.

We first consider logarithms to base 10.

As $10^2 = 100$, we can write $\log_{10} 100 = 2$, since 2 is the power to which 10 (the base) must be raised to give 100. The table below shows the logarithms to base 10 of numbers ranging from 0.01 to 10,000. Note that logarithms (logs) are only defined for POSITIVE values of x.

x	0.01	0.1	1	10	100	1000	10000
$\log_{10} x$	−2	−1	0	1	2	3	4

In general, if $x = a^y$ then $\log_a x = y$.

To get back from y to x, we need to raise the base to the power of y. This operation is called 'taking the exponent' or 'taking anti-logarithms'.

Example

$\log_{10} 100 = 2$ since 10 must be raised to the power 2 in order to get 100.

$\log_2 8 = 3$ since 2 must be raised to the power 3 in order to get 8.

$\log_e(e^{-\lambda a}) = -\lambda a$, since the power to which the mathematical constant, e must be raised to get $e^{-\lambda a}$ is $-\lambda a$.

$\log_e(e^{\Lambda t}) = \Lambda t$, since the power to which e must be raised to get $e^{\Lambda t}$ is Λt.

Note that $\log_e x$ is usually written as *ln(x)* and this is referred to as the *natural log* of x.

Logarithms have several other useful properties:

$$\text{(a) } \log_b x^a = a \log_b x$$

$$\text{(b) } \log_b(ax) = \log_b(a) + \log_b(x)$$

> **Example**
>
> $\log_{10}(100) = 2$ since $10^2 = 100$.
> This result is consistent with rule (a), which says that $\log_{10}(10^2) = 2\log_{10}10 = 2 \times 1$.
> According to rule (b), $\log_{10}(10 \times 10) = \log_{10}(10) + \log_{10}(10) = 1 + 2 = 2$.
> Also, $\log_{10}(100) = 2$, since 10 must be raised to the power 2 to obtain 100.

Exercise B1

a) Express the following using logarithmic notation:

$$\text{(a)} \quad 10^6 = 1,000,000 \qquad \text{(b)} \quad 10^4 = 10,000$$

$$\text{(c)} \quad 10^{-3} = 0.001 \qquad \text{(d)} \quad p^q = r$$

b) Express the following using exponential notation:

$$\text{(e)} \quad \log_{10}100,000 = 5 \qquad \text{(f)} \; p = \log_q r$$

B.5 **Differentiation**

There are several rules for differentiating equations which can be seen in any standard text on calculus. They are included here for convenience.

1. The sum of the derivatives of several expressions is equal to the derivative of the sum of all the expressions.

For example, if a population consists of only three types of individuals, namely those who are susceptible to infection, those who are infectious and those who are immune and no individual can belong to more than one type at any time, then the rate of change in the total population size is the same as the sum of the rate of change in the number of susceptible individuals, the rate of change in the number of infectious individuals and the rate of change in the number of immune individuals.

Using mathematical notation, this is equivalent to saying that:

$$\frac{dN(t)}{dt} = \frac{dS(t)}{dt} + \frac{dI(t)}{dt} + \frac{dR(t)}{dt}$$

where $N(t)$ is the total population at time t, $S(t)$ is the number of susceptible individuals at time t, $I(t)$ is the number of infectious individuals at time t and $R(t)$ is the number of immune ('recovered') individuals at time t, and $N(t) = S(t) + I(t) + R(t)$.

2. The derivative of an expression (e.g. $y(t)$) multiplied by a constant (e.g. k) is just the constant multiplied by the derivative of that function i.e. $\dfrac{d}{dt}[ky(t)] = k\dfrac{dy(t)}{dt}$

The logic behind this rule is illustrated in the following figure, which shows the situation in which $y(t)$ is just the straight line $y(t)=t$. The gradient of the line $y(t)$ is just one (i.e. 20/20); the gradient of the line $y(t)=2t$ is 2 (i.e. 40/20); the gradient of the line $y(t)=3t$ is 3 (i.e. 60/20) and so on.

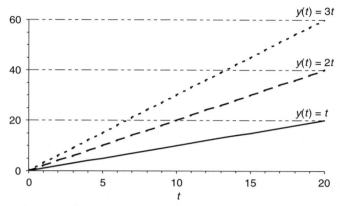

Fig. B3 Plots of the lines $y(t) = t$, $y(t) = 2t$, $y(t) = 3t$.

3. The derivative, with respect to t, of an expression $y(t) = t^n$ is nt^{n-1}.

This particular rule, used in combination with all the previous rules, means that we can differentiate 'any' expression, e.g. $2t^3 + t^2$ or $5t^8 - 3t^2$ etc. This is helpful, since many expressions can be written as the sum of some simpler expression. For example, the formal definition of the expression e^{kt} (where k is a constant) is:

$$e^{kt} = 1 + kt + \frac{(kt)^2}{2!} + \frac{(kt)^3}{3!} + \frac{(kt)^4}{4!} + \frac{(kt)^5}{5!} + \dots$$

B2

It can be shown (see below) that the derivative of the expression e^{kt} is given by ke^{kt}, i.e.:

$$\frac{d}{dt}\left[e^{kt}\right] = ke^{kt}$$

For example, applying the rule that the derivative of the expression with respect to t of an expression t^n is nt^{n-1}, we see that the derivative of e^{kt} is:

$$\frac{d}{dt}[e^{kt}] = k + \frac{2k^2 t}{2!} + \frac{3k^3 t^2}{3!} + \frac{4k^4 t^3}{4!} + \dots + \frac{nk^n t^{n-1}}{n!} + \dots$$

B3

After cancelling out common terms in the denominator and numerator of each term on the right-hand side, Equation B3 simplifies to:

$$\frac{d}{dt}[e^{kt}] = k + k^2 t + \frac{k^3 t^2}{2!} + \frac{k^4 t^3}{3!} + \dots + \frac{k^n t^{n-1}}{(n-1)!} + \dots$$

B4

Taking out a common factor of k from each term within the brackets, Equation B4 becomes:

$$\frac{d}{dt}[e^{kt}] = k\left\{1 + kt + \frac{k^2 t^2}{2!} + \frac{k^3 t^3}{3!} + \dots + \frac{k^{n-1} t^{n-1}}{(n-1)!} + \dots\right\}$$

B5

However, the term in curly brackets in Equation B5 equals e^{kt} (see Equation B2) and so Equation B5 simplifies to the following

$$\frac{d}{dt}[e^{kt}] = ke^{kt}$$

B6

By analogy, the derivative of e^{-kt} (see section B.3) equals $-ke^{-kt}$.

4 (a) The derivative of the product of two expressions $f(t)$ and $g(t)$ i.e. $f(t)g(t)$ is given by the expression $\dfrac{df(t)}{dt}g(t) + f(t)\dfrac{dg(t)}{dt}$

Example

Suppose we wish to differentiate the expression $y(t) = te^{kt}$.

If we use $f(t) = t$ and $g(t) = e^{kt}$, then $\dfrac{df(t)}{dt} = 1$ and $\dfrac{dg(t)}{dt} = ke^{kt}$.

Applying the above rule leads to the following expression for $\dfrac{dy(t)}{dt}$:

$$\frac{dy(t)}{dt} = \frac{df(t)}{dt}g(t) + f(t)\frac{dg(t)}{dt} = 1 \times e^{kt} + tke^{kt} = (1 + tk)e^{kt}$$

B7

---

4 (b) The derivative of the quotient of two expressions $f(t)$ and $g(t)$, i.e. $\dfrac{f(t)}{g(t)}$ is given by the expression $\dfrac{\dfrac{df(t)}{dt}g(t) - f(t)\dfrac{dg(t)}{dt}}{(g(t))^2}$

Example

Suppose we wish to differentiate the expression $y(t) = \dfrac{t}{1 + t^3}$.

If we use $f(t) = t$ and $g(t) = 1 + t^3$, then $\dfrac{df(t)}{dt} = 1$ and $\dfrac{dg(t)}{dt} = 3t^2$.

Applying the above rule leads to the following expression for $\dfrac{dy(t)}{dt}$:

$$\frac{dy(t)}{dt} = \frac{\dfrac{df(t)}{dt}g(t) - f(t)\dfrac{dg(t)}{dt}}{(g(t))^2} = \frac{1 \times (1 + t^3) - t3t^2}{(1 + t^3)^2} = \frac{-2t^3}{(1 + t^3)^2}$$

B8

Exercise B2

Write down the derivatives with respect to t (or the rate of change of y with respect to t) of the expressions:

$$(a)\ y = 28t + 30 \quad (b)\ y = 5t^2 e^{-5t} \quad (c)\ y = 3e^t$$

$$(d)\ y = 2t^4 - 6t^8 \quad (e)\ y = t^{-7} + t^2$$

B.6 **Integration**

Integration is the converse of differentiation. In situations where we only have an expression for the rate of change of something, e.g. the number of susceptible individuals, we would want to integrate that expression to obtain the actual number of susceptible individuals over time.

The integral of a given expression corresponds to the area under the curve representing that expression when it is plotted graphically. If we have some expression y which depends on t (using mathematical notation, we would refer to it as $y(t)$), then the integral of this expression between points $t = a$ and $t = b$ would be written as:

$\int_a^b y(t)dt$ and it would be represented by the shaded area in the Figure B4.

Technically, when we are calculating the shaded area under the curve in Figure B4, we are subdividing this area under the line into small vertical bars which are of a very small width δt and of height $y(t)$, and summing up the areas of these bars, with t ranging between $t = a$ and $t = b$, as shown in Figure B5.

If we are only interested in the expression for the integral of $y(t)$ (i.e. we are not interested in the integral of the $y(t)$ between the points (a) and (b)), then we would use

the following notation: $\int y(t)dt$.

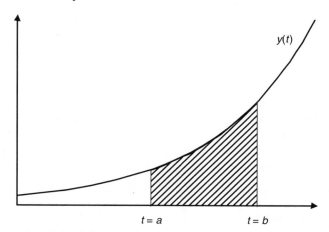

Fig. B4 Illustration of the definition of the integral of a given expression $y(t)$ between points $t = a$ and $t = b$.

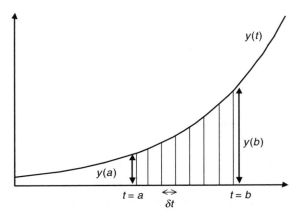

Fig. B5 Illustration of the definition of the integral of a given expression $y(t)$ between points $t = a$ and $t = b$. The area of any given bar is given by width of that bar (γt), multiplied by the height of that bar. The height of each bar differs—that for the first bar is $y(a + \delta t/2)$; that for the last bar is $y(b- \delta t/2)$.

The rules for integrating an expression are closely related to those for differentiating an expression. The simplest rules which can be obtained from any standard text on calculus include:

1) The sum of the integral of several expressions is equal to the integral of the sum of all the expressions.

2) The integral of an expression (e.g. $y(t)$) multiplied by a constant (e.g. c) is just the constant multiplied by the integral of that expression, i.e. $\int cy(t)dt = c\int y(t)dt$

3) The integral of t^n is $\dfrac{t^{n+1}}{n+1}$. However, if we are not specifying the values for t between which the expression is being integrated (see below), we would write the following for the integral of t^n:

$$\int t^n dt = \frac{t^{n+1}}{n+1} + c$$

where c is some constant, which we can identify once we know more about the values of the expression that we are integrating at different points. The addition of a constant term results from the fact that the derivative of any number (e.g. 5, 6 etc) is zero, which means that the integral of zero must be some constant term.

4) The integral of $1/t$ is $ln(t)$, i.e. the natural logarithm of t.

5) If $h(t)$ is the integral of $y(t)$, i.e. $h(t) = \int y(t)dt$, then the integral of $y(t)$ between the points $t=a$ and $t=b$ (written as $\int_a^b y(t)dt$) is given by the following:

$$\int_a^b y(t)dt = h(a) - h(b)$$

i.e. the difference between $h(t)$ (evaluated at $t=b$) and $h(t)$ (evaluated at $t=a$). The right-hand side of this equation is sometimes written as $[h(t)]_a^b$.

6) The integral with respect to t of e^{rt}, where r is some constant, is $\frac{e^{rt}}{r}$. We can obtain this result by using the expression for e^{kt} (see section B.3) and integrating it using rules 1–3 for integration described above.

7) The integral of the product of two expressions $p(t)$ and $q(t)$, i.e. $p(t)q(t)$ is given by the following expression:

$$\int p(t)q(t)dt = f(t)q(t) - \int f(t)\frac{dq(t)}{dt}dt$$

B9

where $f(t) = \int p(t)dt$. Note that $q(t)$ and $p(t)$ are selected so that the second term on the right-hand side of this equation, is as simple to integrate as possible. The derivation is included after the example below.

Example: Calculating $\int te^{kt}dt$

Here, we set $q(t)=t$ (so that $\frac{dq(t)}{dt}=1$) and $p(t)=e^{kt}$. We can set $f(t)=\int p(t)dt$.

Using the result from rule 6, we obtain the result $f(t)=\int e^{kt}dt = \frac{e^{kt}}{k}$. Substituting

for $q(t)$, $\frac{dq(t)}{dt}$ and $f(t)$ into equation B9 leads to the following equation:

$$\int te^{kt}dt = \frac{te^{kt}}{k} - \int\frac{e^{kt}}{k}$$

The second term on the right-hand side of this equation equals $\frac{e^{kt}}{k^2}$, and so $\int te^{kt}dt$ equals the following:

$$\int te^{kt}dt = \frac{te^{kt}}{k} - \frac{e^{kt}}{k^2}$$

Derivation of Equation B9

We reproduce this derivation for convenience for interested readers; however, it can be found in any standard text on calculus. Equation B9 stems the result that the derivative of the product of two expressions $f(t)g(t)$ is given by the expression:

$\frac{d}{dt}[f(t)g(t)] = \frac{df(t)}{dt}g(t) + f(t)\frac{dg(t)}{dt}$ (see section B.5). If we integrate both sides of this equation, we obtain the following result:

$$\int\frac{d}{dt}[f(t)g(t)]dt = \int\frac{df(t)}{dt}g(t)dt + \int f(t)\frac{dg(t)}{dt}dt$$

The left-hand side of this expression equals $f(t)g(t)$ (since integration is the opposite of differentiation), which implies that:

$$f(t)g(t) = \int \frac{df(t)}{dt} g(t)dt + \int f(t) \frac{dg(t)}{dt} dt$$

After rearranging this expression, we obtain the following:

$$\int \frac{df(t)}{dt} g(t)dt = f(t)g(t) - \int f(t) \frac{dg(t)}{dt} dt$$

We obtain equation B9 from this equation by setting $g(t)$ equal to $q(t)$ and setting $f(t)$ equal to $\int p(t)dt$, and then replacing $f(t)$ with $\int p(t)dt$, and replacing $\frac{df(t)}{dt}$ with $p(t)$.

In some instances, it is not possible to integrate an equation to obtain an explicit expression for something in terms of something else. In these situations, we would need to apply alternative techniques or use specialist software (see section 3.5) to estimate how the various quantities change over time.

Exercise B3

Evaluate the following:

(a) $\int t^2 dt$ (b) $\int 4t^3 dt$ (c) $\int \frac{1}{t^5} dt$ (d) $\int_0^{20} e^{-rt} dt$ (e) $\int 70 dt$

B.7 **Matrices**

B.7.1 **Writing equations using matrix notation**

Matrices provide a convenient means of summarizing sets of equations which need to be satisfied simultaneously. For example, if the following two equations have to be satisfied simultaneously:

$$5x + 3y = 6$$

$$3x + 4y = 3$$

they could be summarized using the following notation:

$$\begin{pmatrix} 5 & 3 \\ 3 & 4 \end{pmatrix} \begin{pmatrix} x \\ y \end{pmatrix} = \begin{pmatrix} 6 \\ 3 \end{pmatrix} \qquad \text{B10}$$

Notice that the matrix $\begin{pmatrix} 5 & 3 \\ 3 & 4 \end{pmatrix}$ just consists of the numbers in front of the variables x and y (i.e. their 'coefficients') in the simultaneous equations. The right-hand side of Equation B10, $\begin{pmatrix} 6 \\ 3 \end{pmatrix}$ contains the constant terms of these equations.

Similarly, the equations:

$$4x + 8y + 3z = 18$$

$$2x + y + 5z = 12$$

$$x + 3y + 8z = 4$$

can be written using matrix notation as follows:

$$\begin{pmatrix} 4 & 8 & 3 \\ 2 & 1 & 5 \\ 1 & 3 & 8 \end{pmatrix} \begin{pmatrix} x \\ y \\ z \end{pmatrix} = \begin{pmatrix} 18 \\ 12 \\ 4 \end{pmatrix}$$

Note that a matrix consisting of n rows and m columns, would be referred to as an $n \times m$ matrix, e.g. a matrix with 2 rows and 2 columns would be referred to as a 2×2 matrix. In general, an $n \times n$ matrix would be referred to as a 'n dimensional' matrix. A matrix consisting of just one column, e.g. $\begin{pmatrix} 6 \\ 3 \end{pmatrix}$, would often be referred to as a 'vector'.

Exercise B4

(a) Write down the following simultaneous equations using matrix notation:

(i) $8x + 2y = 7$ (ii) $2x + 6y = 5$
$ 2x + 13y = 3$ $ 3x + 4y = 3$

(b) Write down the simultaneous equations corresponding to the following matrix equations:

(i) $\begin{pmatrix} 9 & 1 \\ 3 & 2 \end{pmatrix} \begin{pmatrix} x \\ y \end{pmatrix} = \begin{pmatrix} 1 \\ 4 \end{pmatrix}$ (ii) $\begin{pmatrix} 13 & 9 \\ 4 & 4 \end{pmatrix} \begin{pmatrix} x \\ y \end{pmatrix} = \begin{pmatrix} 6 \\ 2 \end{pmatrix}$

B.7.2 What is the determinant of a matrix?

It is relatively straightforward to solve two equations wth two unknown parameters simply by manipulating the equations, as illustrated in Exercise B4. However, this approach can be tedious for solving large numbers of equations, e.g. 20 or 100+ equations with equally large numbers of unknowns, as is the case for some problems in the physical or biological sciences.

With the development of sophisticated mathematical theories in the field of linear algebra, the process of finding solutions to such equations has been simplified considerably. These theories often rely on calculating something which is known as the 'determinant' of a matrix. For a two-dimensional matrix, such as $\begin{pmatrix} a & b \\ c & d \end{pmatrix}$, the determinant is defined as the expression $ad-bc$ and is often written as follows: $\begin{vmatrix} a & b \\ c & d \end{vmatrix}$.

For example, the determinant of the matrix $\begin{pmatrix} 9 & 1 \\ 3 & 2 \end{pmatrix}$ equals $9 \times 2 - 1 \times 3 = 18 - 3 = 15$.

Amongst other things, the determinant provides insight into whether it is possible to find a solution to the equations, and sometimes can be used to solve the equations, as described below.

For example, according to matrix theory if the determinant of the matrix is zero, then it is not possible to find a solution to the system of equations making up the matrix equations.

For example, it can be shown, after some manipulation, that the solution of the matrix equation (i.e. the values for x and y):

$$\begin{pmatrix} a & b \\ c & d \end{pmatrix} \begin{pmatrix} x \\ y \end{pmatrix} = \begin{pmatrix} s \\ t \end{pmatrix}$$

is given by the following equation:

$$\begin{pmatrix} x \\ y \end{pmatrix} = \frac{1}{ad - bc} \begin{pmatrix} d & -b \\ -c & a \end{pmatrix} \begin{pmatrix} s \\ t \end{pmatrix}$$

If the determinant of the matrix $\begin{pmatrix} a & b \\ c & d \end{pmatrix}$ is zero (i.e. $ad - bc = 0$), it becomes impossible to find values for x and y.

For a 3×3 matrix $\begin{pmatrix} a & b & c \\ d & e & f \\ g & h & i \end{pmatrix}$, the determinant is given by the expression:

$$a\begin{vmatrix} e & f \\ h & i \end{vmatrix} + b\begin{vmatrix} f & d \\ i & g \end{vmatrix} + c\begin{vmatrix} d & e \\ g & h \end{vmatrix}$$
$$= a(ei - fh) + b(fg - id) + c(dh - eg)$$

Similarly, for a 4×4 matrix $\begin{pmatrix} a & b & c & d \\ e & f & g & h \\ i & j & k & l \\ m & n & o & p \end{pmatrix}$, the determinant is given by the expression:

$$a\begin{vmatrix} f & g & h \\ j & k & l \\ n & o & p \end{vmatrix} + b\begin{vmatrix} g & h & e \\ k & l & i \\ o & p & m \end{vmatrix} + c\begin{vmatrix} h & e & f \\ l & i & j \\ p & m & n \end{vmatrix} + d\begin{vmatrix} e & f & g \\ i & j & k \\ m & n & o \end{vmatrix}$$

The same logic applies generally for all $n \times n$ matrices. A matrix whose determinant is zero is usually called a 'singular' matrix.

Exercise B5

a) Calculate the determinant of the matrices:

$$\text{(a)} \begin{pmatrix} 5 & 2 \\ 10 & 13 \end{pmatrix} \quad \text{(b)} \begin{pmatrix} 3 & 1 & 0 \\ 0 & 4 & 0 \\ 0 & 2 & 1 \end{pmatrix}$$

b) Show that if the equation $\begin{pmatrix} a & b \\ c & d \end{pmatrix} \begin{pmatrix} x \\ y \end{pmatrix} = \begin{pmatrix} 0 \\ 0 \end{pmatrix}$ holds for some non-zero

values of x and y, then the determinant of the matrix $\begin{pmatrix} a & b \\ c & d \end{pmatrix}$ is zero.

B.7.3 **What is an eigenvalue and an eigenvector?**

Many problems in the physical and biological sciences can be solved by calculating the eigenvalue of the system. For example, the eigenvalues of the equations describing a road bridge provide insight into the frequency at which the bridge will vibrate.

In mathematical terms, an eigenvector of a matrix $\mathbf{M}$ is some vector, denoted by $\mathbf{x}$, which, when it is multiplied by the matrix $\mathbf{M}$, results in the same vector multiplied by some factor. This factor is known as the 'eigenvalue', often denoted using the Greek letter ρ (pronounced rho)). Using mathematical notation, $\mathbf{M}$, $\mathbf{x}$ and ρ satisfy the following equation

$$\mathbf{M}\,\mathbf{x} = \rho\,\mathbf{x}$$

Examples

The matrix $\begin{pmatrix} 2 & 0 \\ 0 & 2 \end{pmatrix}$ has $\begin{pmatrix} 1 \\ 0 \end{pmatrix}$ as an eigenvector and 2 is an eigenvalue since

$\begin{pmatrix} 2 & 0 \\ 0 & 2 \end{pmatrix} \begin{pmatrix} 1 \\ 0 \end{pmatrix} = 2 \begin{pmatrix} 1 \\ 0 \end{pmatrix}$.

The matrix $\begin{pmatrix} 2 & 1 \\ 4 & 2 \end{pmatrix}$ has an eigenvector $\begin{pmatrix} 1 \\ 2 \end{pmatrix}$ since $\begin{pmatrix} 2 & 1 \\ 4 & 2 \end{pmatrix} \begin{pmatrix} 1 \\ 2 \end{pmatrix} = 4 \begin{pmatrix} 1 \\ 2 \end{pmatrix}$; 4 is the

eigenvalue of the matrix $\begin{pmatrix} 2 & 1 \\ 4 & 2 \end{pmatrix}$.

Commonly, the eigenvalue ρ of a matrix $\begin{pmatrix} a & b \\ c & d \end{pmatrix}$ is identified by finding values of ρ which satisfy the equation $(a - \rho)(d - \rho) - bc = 0$, or, equivalently $\rho^2 - (a + d)\rho + ad - bc = 0$.

This equation can be derived by first using the fact if ρ is an eigenvalue of the matrix $\begin{pmatrix} a & b \\ c & d \end{pmatrix}$, then the following equation holds:

$$\begin{pmatrix} a & b \\ c & d \end{pmatrix}\begin{pmatrix} x \\ y \end{pmatrix} = \rho \begin{pmatrix} x \\ y \end{pmatrix}$$

B11

This equation is equivalent to the following equation:

$$\begin{pmatrix} a & b \\ c & d \end{pmatrix}\begin{pmatrix} x \\ y \end{pmatrix} = \begin{pmatrix} \rho & 0 \\ 0 & \rho \end{pmatrix}\begin{pmatrix} x \\ y \end{pmatrix}$$

B12

After subtracting the right-hand side of equation B12 from its left-hand side of Equation B12, we obtain the following equation:

$$\begin{pmatrix} a-\rho & b \\ c & d-\rho \end{pmatrix}\begin{pmatrix} x \\ y \end{pmatrix} = \begin{pmatrix} 0 \\ 0 \end{pmatrix}$$

B13

As shown in Exercise B5.a, if Equation B13 holds, the determinant of the matrix $\begin{pmatrix} a-\rho & b \\ c & d-\rho \end{pmatrix}$ is also zero, i.e. $(a-\rho)(d-\rho) - bc = 0$.

Consequently, the eigenvalue ρ of a matrix $\begin{pmatrix} a & b \\ c & d \end{pmatrix}$ can also be identified by finding values of ρ which satisfy the equation $(a - \rho)(d - \rho) - bc = 0$ or, equivalently $\rho^2 - (a + d)\rho + ad - bc = 0$. Readers may recognize this equation as being that of a quadratic, which means that there may be two possible values of ρ which satisfy this equation. Similarly, in the same way, $n \times n$ matrices may have n possible eigenvalues.

Exercise B6

Find the eigenvalues of the following matrices:

(a) $\begin{pmatrix} 5 & 2 \\ 10 & 13 \end{pmatrix}$ (b) $\begin{pmatrix} 3 & 1 & 0 \\ 0 & 4 & 0 \\ 0 & 2 & 1 \end{pmatrix}$

B.7.4 What happens when we repeatedly multiply a matrix by itself?

According to theory (which is normally taught on Linear algebra courses), a matrix $\mathbf{M}$ can often be written down in terms of a matrix $\mathbf{D}$ and some other matrix $\mathbf{P}$ (see the definitions of $\mathbf{D}$ and $\mathbf{P}$, $\mathbf{P}^{-1}$ below) as follows:

$$\mathbf{M} = \mathbf{P}^{-1}\mathbf{DP}$$

B14

Also, the theory goes on to show that when we repeatedly multiply matrix **M** by itself, which is what we do when we calculate R_0 using the simulation approach (see below and section 7.5.3), we obtain the following equation:

$$\mathbf{M}^k = \mathbf{P}^{-1}\mathbf{D}^k\mathbf{P} \qquad \text{B15}$$

Before describing the relevance of this result for calculating R_0, we provide some key definitions.

Definitions

If **M** is a $n \times n$ matrix, then **D** is defined as $\begin{pmatrix} \rho_1 & 0 & \dots & 0 \\ 0 & \rho_2 & \dots & 0 \\ \dots & \dots & \dots & \dots \\ 0 & 0 & \dots & \rho_n \end{pmatrix}$, where $\rho_1, \rho_2,., \rho_n$, are the

eigenvalues of matrix **M**. $\mathbf{P}^{-1}$ is known as the "inverse" of **P**. It is calculated so that

when $\mathbf{P}^{-1}$ is multiplied by **P**, it gives the so-called "identity" matrix, i.e. $\begin{pmatrix} 1 & 0 & \dots & 0 \\ 0 & 1 & \dots & 0 \\ \dots & \dots & \dots & \dots \\ 0 & 0 & \dots & 1 \end{pmatrix}$.

This identity matrix consists of zeros, but has a 1 down the diagonal from the top left corner down to the bottom right corner. Note that when any matrix **Z** is multiplied by

the identity matrix, it just gives **Z**. For example, $\begin{pmatrix} 1 & 2 \\ 4 & 3 \end{pmatrix}$ multiplied by $\begin{pmatrix} 1 & 0 \\ 0 & 1 \end{pmatrix}$

equals $\begin{pmatrix} 1 & 2 \\ 4 & 3 \end{pmatrix}$. For a 2×2 matrix $\begin{pmatrix} a & b \\ c & d \end{pmatrix}$, the inverse is given by the following matrix

(which readers may recognize from section B.7.3):

$$\frac{1}{ad-bc}\begin{pmatrix} d & -b \\ -c & a \end{pmatrix} \qquad \text{B16}$$

Consequently, when we multiply matrix **M** repeatedly by itself, e.g. k times, we obtain Equation B15, as follows:

$$\mathbf{M}^k = \mathbf{P}^{-1}\,\mathbf{DP}\,\mathbf{P}^{-1}\,\mathbf{DP}\,\mathbf{P}^{-1}\,\mathbf{DP}\,\mathbf{P}^{-1}\,\mathbf{DP}\,\mathbf{P}^{-1}\,\mathbf{DP}\,\mathbf{P}^{-1}\,\mathbf{DP}\dots\mathbf{P}^{-1}\,\mathbf{DP}$$
$$= \mathbf{P}^{-1}\,\mathbf{D}^k\mathbf{P}$$

$$= \mathbf{P}^{-1}\begin{pmatrix} \rho_1^k & 0 & \dots & 0 \\ 0 & \rho_2^k & \dots & 0 \\ \dots & \dots & \dots & \dots \\ 0 & 0 & \dots & \rho_n^k \end{pmatrix}\mathbf{P}$$

Relevance of Equation B15

Equation B15 can be used to explain why the ratio between the total numbers of infectious persons in successive generations always converges to the largest eigenvalue of the Next Generation Matrix (i.e. R_0) when we use the simulation approach (sections 7.5.2 and 7.5.3) to calculate R_0.

For example, suppose we simulate the introduction of infectious persons into a totally susceptible population in which individuals are stratified into children and adults (denoted using the subscripts y and o respectively) who contact each other according to some Next Generation Matrix, **M**. If there is an unlimited supply of susceptible individuals, we can show (see below) that the numbers of infectious children and adults in the kth generation (denoted by $I_{y,k}$ and $I_{o,k}$ respectively) are given by the following equation:

$$\begin{pmatrix} I_{y,k} \\ I_{o,k} \end{pmatrix} = \mathbf{M}^k \begin{pmatrix} I_{y,0} \\ I_{o,0} \end{pmatrix}$$

B17

If ρ_1 and ρ_2 are the eigenvalues of matrix **M**, then, using the result that $\mathbf{M}^k = \mathbf{P}^{-1} \mathbf{D}^k \mathbf{P}$, we see that the number of infectious children and adults in the kth generation is given by the following equation:

$$\begin{pmatrix} I_{y,k} \\ I_{o,k} \end{pmatrix} = \mathbf{P}^{-1} \mathbf{D}^k \mathbf{P} \begin{pmatrix} I_{y,0} \\ I_{o,0} \end{pmatrix} = \mathbf{P}^{-1} \begin{pmatrix} \rho_1^k & 0 \\ 0 & \rho_2^k \end{pmatrix} \mathbf{P} \begin{pmatrix} I_{y,0} \\ I_{o,0} \end{pmatrix}$$

B18

As illustrated below using the matrix $\mathbf{M} = \begin{pmatrix} 5 & 2 \\ 10 & 13 \end{pmatrix}$, the total number of infectious

persons (denoted by $G_k = I_{y,k} + I_{o,k}$) in the kth generation is approximately equal to $q\rho_i^k$, where ρ_i is the largest eigenvalue of matrix **M**, and q is some constant value. Taking the ratio between the total numbers of infectious persons in the $k+1^{th}$ and k^{th} generation (G_{k+1}/G_k) leads to the result that:

$$\frac{G_{k+1}}{G_k} \approx \frac{q\rho_i^{k+1}}{q\rho_i^k} = \rho_i$$

i.e. when infectious persons are introduced into a totally susceptible population mixing according to some Next Generation Matrix, **M**, the ratio between the total numbers of infectious persons in successive generations converges to the largest eigenvalue of that matrix, which is defined to be R_0. The proof of this result is too elaborate for this text, and we therefore merely provide an illustrative example of this result.

Example: Illustration of the result $\dfrac{G_{k+1}}{G_k} \approx \rho_i$ for $M = \begin{pmatrix} 5 & 2 \\ 10 & 13 \end{pmatrix}$

This matrix has eigenvalues 3 and 15 (see Exercise B16). Taking P to equal $\begin{pmatrix} 5 & -1 \\ 0.5 & 0.5 \end{pmatrix}$, and therefore $P^{-1} = \dfrac{1}{3}\begin{pmatrix} 0.5 & 1 \\ -0.5 & 5 \end{pmatrix}$ (which is obtained by applying equation B16), we can rewrite M as follows:

$$M = P^{-1}\begin{pmatrix} 3 & 0 \\ 0 & 15 \end{pmatrix}P$$

Incorporating this expression for M in equation B17 and using the result $M^k = P^{-1}D^kP$ (equation B15), we see that the number of infectious children and adults in the kth generation is given by the following equation:

$$\begin{pmatrix} I_{y,k} \\ I_{o,k} \end{pmatrix} = \frac{1}{3}\begin{pmatrix} 0.5 & 1 \\ -0.5 & 5 \end{pmatrix}\begin{pmatrix} 3^k & 0 \\ 0 & 15^k \end{pmatrix}\begin{pmatrix} 5 & -1 \\ 0.5 & 0.5 \end{pmatrix}\begin{pmatrix} I_{y,0} \\ I_{o,0} \end{pmatrix}$$

which simplifies to the following:

$$\begin{pmatrix} I_{y,k} \\ I_{o,k} \end{pmatrix} = \frac{1}{3}\begin{pmatrix} 2.5\times 3^k + 0.5\times 15^k & -0.5\times 3^k + 0.5\times 15^k \\ -2.5\times 3^k + 2.5\times 15^k & 0.5\times 3^k + 2.5\times 15^k \end{pmatrix}\begin{pmatrix} I_{y,0} \\ I_{o,0} \end{pmatrix}$$

After manipulating this equation, we obtain the following equation for the number of infectious persons in the kth generation ($G_k = I_{y,k} + I_{o,k}$):

$$G_k = 15^k(I_{y,0} + I_{o,0})$$

Dividing G_{k+1} by G_k, we obtain the following:

$$\frac{G_{k+1}}{G_k} = \frac{15^{k+1}(I_{y,0} + I_{o,0})}{15^k(I_{y,0} + I_{o,0})} = 15$$

i.e. the ratio between the numbers of infectious persons in successive generations equals largest eigenvalue of the Next Generation Matrix, M.

Derivation of the result $\begin{pmatrix} I_{y,k} \\ I_{o,k} \end{pmatrix} = M^k\begin{pmatrix} I_{y,0} \\ I_{o,0} \end{pmatrix}$

As discussed in Panel 7.8, if we have a Next Generation Matrix $M = \begin{pmatrix} R_{yy} & R_{yo} \\ R_{oy} & R_{oo} \end{pmatrix}$, the number of infectious children and adults in the first generation is given by the following equation:

$$\begin{pmatrix} I_{y,1} \\ I_{o,1} \end{pmatrix} = M\begin{pmatrix} I_{y,0} \\ I_{o,0} \end{pmatrix}$$

B19

The number of infectious children and adults in the second generation is given by the following equation:

$$\begin{pmatrix} I_{y,2} \\ I_{o,2} \end{pmatrix} = \mathbf{M} \begin{pmatrix} I_{y,1} \\ I_{o,1} \end{pmatrix}$$

B20

Substituting the expression for $\begin{pmatrix} I_{y,1} \\ I_{o,1} \end{pmatrix}$ from equation B19 into equation B20, we obtain the following:

$$\begin{pmatrix} I_{y,2} \\ I_{o,2} \end{pmatrix} = \mathbf{M}\mathbf{M} \begin{pmatrix} I_{y,0} \\ I_{o,0} \end{pmatrix} = \mathbf{M}^2 \begin{pmatrix} I_{y,0} \\ I_{o,0} \end{pmatrix}$$

Repeating the same process until the kth generation, we obtain our intended result for the numbers of infectious persons in the kth generation:

$$\begin{pmatrix} I_{y,k} \\ I_{o,k} \end{pmatrix} = \mathbf{M} \begin{pmatrix} I_{y,k-1} \\ I_{o,k-1} \end{pmatrix} = \mathbf{M}\mathbf{M} \begin{pmatrix} I_{y,k-2} \\ I_{o,k-2} \end{pmatrix} = \ldots = \mathbf{M}^k \begin{pmatrix} I_{y,0} \\ I_{o,0} \end{pmatrix}$$

Summary of the key equations used in the text

Unless otherwise stated, the definitions of the parameters or variables used in the equations are provided in Table 2 (symbols and notation) on page xxvii.

Variable or parameter	Mathematical equation	Assumptions/comments	Chapter/section where first used
Transition rates			
Average rate at which individuals become infectious (f), recover (r), die (m) etc.	$f = 1/D'$ $r = 1/D$ $m = 1/L$	Individuals become infectious, recover, die etc. at a constant rate, irrespective of age or any other factor. The distribution of the time interval until the outcome in question occurs (individuals becoming infectious, recovering, dying etc.) is given by the exponential distribution.	Section 2.7.2
Contact parameters:			
The rate at which two specific individuals come into effective contact per unit time (β)	$\beta = R_0/ND$ or $\beta = c_e/N$	Individuals mix randomly. The number contacted does not change with time since infection or any other factor.	Section 2.7.1
The average number of individuals effectively contacted per unit time (c_e)	$c_e = R_0/D$ or βN	Individuals mix randomly. The number contacted does not change with time since infection or other factor.	Section 2.7.1
Summary measure of mixing between population subgroups	$Q = \dfrac{\left(\sum\limits_{j=k} g_{jk}\right) - 1}{b - 1}$	Q only measures mixing within identical groups, ignoring mixing between similar groups. Q also equally weights mixing within different population groups regardless of the size of these groups.	Section 8.5.2
The basic reproduction number (R_0)			
	$R_0 = \dfrac{\beta N}{r} = \beta ND$ or $R_0 = \dfrac{\beta N}{r + m}$	Individuals mix randomly. The two expressions are approximately equal, when the mortality rate (m) is small, relative to the duration of infectiousness.	Sections 2.4.1 and 2.7.1
	$R_0 = 1/s$	Individuals mix randomly. s is the proportion of the population that is susceptible at equilibrium, or equivalently, the average proportion of the population that is susceptible.	Sections 4.2.2.2 and 4.3.1

$R_0 = 1 + \Lambda D$	The pre-infectious period is very short in comparison with the infectious period, or individuals are infectious immediately after they are infected. The infectious period is assumed to follow the exponential distribution. The growth rate in the prevalence of infectious persons is approximately constant during the early stages of an epidemic	Section 4.2.3. See Table 4.1 for further variants.
$R_0 = -\dfrac{\ln(1-z_f)}{z_f}$	z_f is the proportion of individuals that have been infected by the end of an epidemic, following the introduction of an infection into a totally susceptible population.	Section 4.2.4. See Table 4.2 for further variants.
$R_0 \approx L\lambda \approx L/A$	Individuals mix randomly. The age distribution of the population is rectangular (a 'type I' pattern), i.e. all individuals can be assumed to live until age L and then die. A is the average age at infection.	Section 5.2.3.3
$R_0 = 1 + \lambda L \approx 1 + L/A$	Individuals mix randomly. The age distribution is exponential ('type II'), i.e. the mortality rate can be assumed to be constant for all ages. L is the *average life expectancy*; A is the average age at infection.	Section 5.2.3.3
$R_0 = \dfrac{\lambda' L}{1 - ve^{-\lambda a_v} - (1-v)e^{-\lambda L}}$	Individuals mix randomly; rectangular age distribution; v is the effective vaccination coverage (proportion immunized) among individuals of age a_v; λ' is the average force of infection in the long-term following the introduction of vaccination.	Panel 5.6
$R_0 = \dfrac{1 + \lambda' L}{1 - ve^{-(\lambda'+m)a_v}}$	Individuals mix randomly; exponential age distribution; v is the effective vaccination coverage (proportion immunized) among individuals of age a_v; λ' is the average force of infection in the long-term following the introduction of vaccination.	Panel 5.6

(continued)

Variable or parameter	Mathematical equation	Assumptions/comments	Chapter/section where first used
Number of secondary infectious persons among old individuals resulting from one young infectious person (R_{oy}) in a totally susceptible population	$R_{oy} = \beta_{oy} N_o D$	β_{oy} is the rate at which a specific susceptible old person comes into effective contact with a specific infectious young person; N_o is the total number of old persons.	Section 7.5.1
The basic reproduction number (sexually transmitted infection)	$R_0 = c\beta_p D$	People selected randomly (random mixing). No population heterogeneities.	Section 8.3 and Panel 8.2
The basic reproduction number for a sexually transmitted infection in a population with two activity groups.	$R_0 = g_H R_H + g_L R_L$	Partnerships selected randomly. Two activity groups.	Panel 8.5 and Section 8.4.2
The basic reproduction number for a sexually transmitted infection in a heterosexual population (or a vector-borne infection).	$R_0 = \sqrt{R_{WM} R_{MW}}$	—	Section 8.6
The basic reproduction number for a sexually transmitted infection heterogeneity in sexual activity and any mixing pattern	$R_0 = \dfrac{R_{HH} + R_{LL} + \sqrt{\sqrt{(-R_{HH} - R_{LL})^2 - 4 \times (R_{LL} R_{HH} - R_{HL} R_{LH})}}}{2}$	Two activity groups	Panel 8.8

Net reproduction number (R_n)	$R_n = R_0 s$	Individuals mix randomly. s is the average proportion of the population that is susceptible.	Sections 1.3 and 4.2.2.2
Herd immunity threshold (HIT)	$HIT = 1 - 1/R_0$	–	Sections 1.3 and 4.2.2.2
Force of infection			
Force of infection at time t ($\lambda(t)$)	$\lambda(t) = \beta I(t) = c_e \dfrac{I(t)}{N(t)}$	Individuals mix randomly.	Section 2.7.1 and Panel 2.5
Force of infection at time t ($\lambda(t)$) for a sexually transmitted infection	$\lambda(t) = c\beta_p \dfrac{I(t)}{N}$	Individuals mix randomly.	Section 8.3
Reed–Frost equation for the risk of infection between time t and $t+1$ (λ_t)	$\lambda_t = 1 - (1 - p)^{I_t}$	p is the probability of an effective contact between two specific individuals per time step.	Section 6.3.2
Per partnership transmission probability (sexually-transmitted infection)	$\beta_p = 1 - (1 - \beta_a)^n$	The per-act transmission probability does not vary over time. n is the number of sex acts per partnership.	Panel 8.1
Number of infectious persons			
Number of infectious persons at time t during the early stages of an epidemic ($I(t)$)	$I(t) \approx I(0)e^{\Lambda t}$	Λ is the growth rate in the number of infectious persons.	Section 4.2.3.1

(continued)

Variable or parameter	Mathematical equation	Assumptions/comments	Chapter/section where first used
Inter-epidemic period			
Inter-epidemic period (T)	$T = 2\pi\sqrt{\dfrac{L(D+D')}{R_0 - 1}}$	Immunizing infection; no intervention; individuals mix randomly.	Section 4.3.2.2
	$T = 2\pi\sqrt{A(D+D')}$	Immunizing infection; individuals mix randomly. This equation is applicable irrespective of whether an intervention has been introduced.	Section 4.3.2.2
Proportion susceptible/ever infected			
Proportion of individuals that have ever been infected by age a ($z(a)$)	$z(a) = 1 - e^{-\lambda a}$	The average force of infection (λ) is identical for all age groups; this expression does not account for the presence of maternally derived immunity.	Section 5.2.2. See section 5.2.3.5.1, Panel 5.2 and Table 5.4 for other variants.
Proportion of individuals are susceptible at age a ($s(a)$)	$s(a) = e^{-\lambda a}$	The average force of infection (λ) is identical for all age groups; this expression does not account for the presence of maternally derived immunity.	Section 5.2.2. See section 5.2.3.5.1, Panel 5.2 and Table 5.4 for other variants.
Proportion of the population that is susceptible	$s = \dfrac{1}{\lambda L + 1} \approx \dfrac{A}{A+L}$	Exponential age distribution; individuals mix randomly.	Section 5.2.3.2
	$s \approx \dfrac{1}{\lambda L} \approx \dfrac{A}{L}$	Rectangular age distribution; individuals mix randomly.	Section 5.2.3.2
	$s = \sum_a p_a \dfrac{S_a}{N_a}$	p_a is the proportion of individuals in the population that are in age group a; S_a and N_a are the number of individuals that are negative to the biological test for infection and the number tested respectively.	Section 5.2.3.2

Average age at infection

Average age at infection (A) among individuals who ever experience infection in their lifetime	$A \approx \dfrac{1}{\lambda}$	Individuals mix randomly; the average force of infection is identical for all age groups.	Section 5.2.3.1
	$A = \dfrac{\int_0^\infty a\lambda(a)S(a)da}{\int_0^\infty \lambda(a)S(a)da}$	General equation; $\lambda(a)$ is the average force of infection among individuals of age a.	Section 5.2.3.1
	$A = \dfrac{1}{\lambda}\left(\dfrac{1-(1+\lambda L)e^{-\lambda L}}{1-e^{-\lambda L}}\right)$	Rectangular age distribution; the average force of infection is identical for all age groups.	Section 5.2.3.1
	$A = \dfrac{1}{\lambda + 1/L} = \dfrac{1}{\lambda + m}$	Exponential age distribution; the average force of infection is identical for all age groups.	Section 5.2.3.1
Average age at infection (A') in the long-term following the introduction of vaccination among newborns	$A' = \dfrac{A}{(1-v)}$	Exponential age distribution; the average force of infection is identical for all age groups; v is the effective vaccination coverage (the proportion immunized) at birth.	Section 5.3.3

Average number of new infections

Age-specific number of new infections among individuals of age a at time t	$\lambda(a,t)S(a,t)$	General equation; $\lambda(a,t)$ is the force of infection of age a at time t; $S(a,t)$ is the number of susceptible individuals of age a at time t.	Sections 2.6.1.1 and 5.2.3.4

(continued)

Variable or parameter	Mathematical equation	Assumptions/comments	Chapter/section where first used
Age-specific average number of new infections per person unit time	$\lambda s(a) = \lambda e^{-\lambda a}$	The average force of infection (λ) is identical for all age groups; $s(a)$ is the proportion of individuals of age a that is susceptible.	Section 5.2.3.4
Average number of new infections per person among individuals of age a in the long-term	$\lambda'(1-v)e^{-\lambda' a}$	v is the effective vaccination coverage (proportion immunized) among newborns. The average force of infection following the introduction of vaccination among newborns (λ') is identical for all age groups.	Section 5.3.3
Growth rate and doubling time			
Average growth rate in an epidemic	$\Lambda = \dfrac{\ln(2)}{T_d}$	T_d is the time until the number of cases in the population doubles	Panel 4.1 and Panel 8.10
Doubling time for sexually transmitted infection that kills (eg HIV) in a population with other-cause mortality.	$T_d \approx \dfrac{\ln(2)}{c\,\beta_p - \gamma - m}$	Random mixing.	Panel 8.10

Index

age-dependent contact 95, 143, 177–79, 203
age-dependent force of infection 120
age-dependent mixing 95, 116, 177, 181–203
age patterns 105–43, 179, 181, 328–33
age-specific infection incidence, vaccination
    effects 137–41
age-specific risk of infection 110
AIDS 259–63, 298–300, 303–304, 307–308;
    see also human immunodeficiency virus
    animal models 9
antigenic drift 17, 99
antiretroviral therapy 295–6
arthropods 2
assortative (with-like) mixing patterns xxi, 192,
    200, 202
asymptomatic individual xxi, 82, 259
average age at infection 93, 96–7, 106, 111–13,
    116–137–45
average annual risk of infection 111
average force of infection 105–8, 111–25, 187,
    216, 328–329, 359, 362–4
average life expectancy 33–4, 57–8, 84, 93–4,
    101, 107, 112–4, 116–7, 143, 260, 321,
    328–9, 359
average mortality rate 33–4, 329, 332–3
average number of new infections 117,
    138, 363–4

bacteria 1–2, 226, 259–60
basic reproduction number (*R0*), xxi,
    171–172, 327
    calculated using epidemic doubling time, 74
    calculated using epidemic growth rate 72, 74
    calculating using epidemic size 79
    common diseases 8
    cycles of incidence of immunizing
        infections 93–4
    definition 6, 28, 353
    effect of mixing 247, 249–52
    equations 72–4, 358–9
    estimating 115–16
    fitting models to data 79–82
    gonorrhoea model 230
    HIV, 260, 262–4, 306
    incidence trends 65
    influenza 8, 14, 30–31, 73–4, 79, 82
    matrix determinant approach 213, 215,
        336–7
    mumps 8, 116
    Next Generation Matrix 206–11
    non-random mixing patterns 203–17

rubella 8, 116
sexually transmitted infections 230, 234–9,
    249–50, 256–8, 260, 262–3, 265,
    337–8, 360
simulation approach 211
simultaneous equations approach 212–213,
    236, 250, 257, 335–336
tuberculosis 8, 293
threshold properties 203
basic reproduction ratio 211
Bayesian approach 193
beta (β) xxi, 25–32, 42–5, 65, 85, 106, 152–53,
    168, 181, 184–96, 226–7, 322, 324–5,
    334, 358
bipartite graph 274
birth rate 37, 83–5, 87–9, 94, 100, 107, 128,
    173, 327–8
breakthrough varicella 200, 284

carrier xxi, 135–6, 285–6
case xxi, 353
catalytic models xxi, 109, 119–20, 124–5, 216
catch-up campaigns 96, 134–6, 215
chancroid 224, 272, 304–5
chickenpox (varicella) vaccination 83, 200–2,
    283–5
chlamydia 224, 228, 272
circumcision 272, 308
climatic factors 92
closed population model xxi, 42, 45, 52
clustering 269, 274
cofactor STIs 224, 265, 296
coinfection models, HIV/STIs, 296–306
compartmental models xxi, 19
    continuous time (stochastic) 157, 167–9
    discrete-time (stochastic) 150, 160–6
component of a graph 274
concurrency xxi, 223, 265–8, 272–3, 275
condom use, impact on STIs 228
connected graph 274
contact 2
contact network 269
contact parameters 143, 187–97, 358
contact patterns 17, 37, 92, 96, 123, 125, 160,
    177–219, 242, 335–7
contact rate (*k*) 9, 227
contact surveys 180–1
contact tracing 244–5, 272
continuous time stochastic compartmental
    models 157, 167–9
convergence 45

core group xxi, 16, 37, 271
cross-sectional data 105–26

damp out xxii, 89–90, 328
degree distribution 274
degree of a vertex 274
degree of mixing 243
delta (δ) 35
density dependence assumption xxii, 31
derivative 47, 320, 342–7
determinant of a matrix 213, 349–51
deterministic models xxii, 18–23, 169, 172, 174
diameter of graph 274
diaries of contact 180–1
difference equations 13–37
    compared to differential equation 48–9
    number of immune (recovered)
        individuals 23
    number of infectious individuals 22–23
    number of pre-infectious individuals 21–2
    number of susceptible individuals 21
    reliability 24–5, 41–4
differential equations 41–59, 319–21
    checking 51–4
    compared to difference equation 48–9
    interpretation 46–7
    partial 58–59
    prediction 54–8
    rate of change in number of infectious and
        immune individuals 51
    rate of change in number of pre-infectious
        individuals 50–1
    rate of change in number of susceptible
        individuals 50
    writing down 49–54
differentiation 320, 342–5
diphtheria 8, 125–6
directions of arrows 24, 52–4
disassortative (with-unlike) mixing
    patterns xxvi, 242
discrete-time compartmental models 150
distance 274
dominant eigenvalue 209, 212, 236, 338
doubling time xxii, 74, 263, 298, 364
dynamic model xxii, 217
dynamic transmission model 20, 105, 141–2
dynamics of infections 59, 63–100, 126–43,
    283–285, 321–7
    acute non-immunizing infections 97–9
    long-term, acute infections 82–97
    short-term 63–82
    vaccination effects 126–43

'e' 15, 340
edges 269–70, 274–5
effective contact 25–9, 31, 37, 42, 50, 65, 85,
    106, 152–3, 168, 183–6, 191–3, 195–7, 199,
    201, 204, 219, 227, 238, 240, 242, 325, 334,
    358, 360–1

effective reproduction number xxiv, 6, 10;
    see also net reproduction number
effectiveness of vaccines 354
efficacy of vaccines xxii, 284, 306
eigenvalue xxii, 209–10, 212–3, 236, 338, 351–5
eigenvector 210, 351–2
elimination xxii, 354
Elveback model 173
endemic fade out 173
endemic infection xxii, 187–197
    WAIFW matrix 184, 187, 191, 198–203, 335
epidemic threshold (1/R0) xxii, 67
epidemics
    definition 354
    early stages 69–77
    growth rate (Λ) 70–2, 266–9, 326,
    size prediction 77–9
    theory 63–5
epidemiology xxiii, 1, 10, 12, 14, 55, 70, 271,
    275, 289, 294, 296
equilibrium xxiii, 202, 223, 239, 241, 247–9,
    251–5, 259, 263, 286, 299–300, 328, 358
eradication xxiii, 355
exponential decline or growth 55–8
exposed class 15

fitting models to data 79–82
foot and mouth disease 193
force of infection xxiii
    age-dependency 120–5
    calculating 26–32
    definition 355
    estimating average 106–11
    key equations 357–64
    sexually transmitted infections 337–8
frequency dependence assumption, xxiii, 227
frequency of infection 5

generation time xxiii, 99
genital ulcer disease (GUD) 297
giant component 268, 274–5
gonorrhoea
    dynamics of infection 97–99
    natural history 15–6
    screening 254–5
    transmission model 226–31
gradient of a line 46
graph 46, 179, 269, 274–5
growth rate of the epidemic (Λ) xxiii, 70,
    266, 326

Hamer model 90–1
hazard rate 168, 334
helminths 2
hepatitis A 143
herd immunity xxiii, 1, 6–8, 10, 67–9, 86, 133,
    210, 293, 330, 361
herd immunity threshold (HIT) xxiii, 1, 6–8,
    10, 67–9, 86, 133, 210, 293, 330, 361

herpes simplex virus 2 (HSV-2) xxiii
effect of treatment on HIV incidence 304–5
natural history 224
heterogeneity 4
sexual activity 337–8
heterogeneous mixing xxiii, 177–8
heterosexual mixing model 255–8
Hethcote–Yorke model 223, 226–31
homogeneous mixing xxv, 26
honeymoon period 97
human immunodeficiency virus (HIV) xxiii
antiretroviral therapy 295–6
basic reproduction number 286, 293, 306
cofactor STI impact 296–7, 303
concurrency 265, 267–8
curable STI treatment 302–6
derivation of epidemic doubling time 266–8
epidemic predictions 263–65
evolution of models 306–8
immune outcome 3, 10
influence on tuberculosis
epidemiology 293–6
male circumcision 308
microsimulation models 173–4
models of HIV/STI coinfection 294, 296–306
natural history 15, 224
pattern of infection 4
simple transmission model 259–65

identity matrix 353
immune individuals xxiii, 355
difference equation 22–3, 51
rate of change 51
immune outcomes 3, 10
immune response 3–4, 239
immunization xxiii, 6, 10, 129, 141
immunizing infection xxiv, 321–2
cycle of incidence 82–96
incidence xxiv, 5
cycles 82–96
trends 67–9
incubation period xxiv, 1–3, 10, 283, 285–96
individual-based models 20, 150–60
individual-based simulation network
models 270–1
infected class 15
infections 1–5
definition 1
mild 3
outcome 3–4
patterns 4
transmission 1–2, 5–8
infectious agents 1, 2
infectious individuals
difference equation 22–3, 51
rate of change 51
specific age groups 188–9
infectious period xxiv, 2, 356
infectiousness, rate of onset 25, 33–4

influenza
age-dependent contact 178–79
antigenic drift 17, 99
basic reproduction number 8, 74–5, 79, 82
herd immunity threshold 8, 67–9
pattern of infection 4
serial interval 8
setting up a model 35–36
Spanish pandemic (1918) 15, 74–6, 100
spatial spread 193
instantaneous rate 35
integer xxiv, 56, 95, 172
integration 321, 339, 345–8
inter-epidemic period 63, 93–4, 96, 98, 100, 362

'κ' 9–10, 53, 55, 90

latent period xxiv, 14
Latin hypercube sampling 81
lattice model 269–70
lattice network model xxiv, 356
least squares 80
life expectancy, average 33
links 268–9
log likelihood deviance 81
logarithms 121–2, 326, 341–2
long incubation period 283, 285–94
long-term transmission 17

M. tuberculosis, see tuberculosis
macroparasites 1–2
malaria 2–3, 6–8, 37, 125, 256
male circumcision 308
Markov chain Monte Carlo (MCMC)
methods 81
mass action principle 10, 26
maternally derived immunity 108, 113, 117–9, 362
mathematical models 9, 296
mathematical symbols xxvii–xxviii
matrices 348–51
characteristic value 209, 211, 215
determinant of a matrix 349–51
identity matrix 353
mixing matrices 242–3
singular matrix 350
writing equations using matrix
notation 348–9
maximum likelihood 80–1
measles
average age at infection 106–8
basic reproduction number 115–6
cycles of immunizing infection 82–9
estimating potential for an epidemic 117–20
herd immunity threshold 8, 67–9
immune outcome 3, 10
inter-epidemic period 93–4, 96
pattern of infection 4
serial interval 8
vaccination 96–97

mechanical models 9
median age at infection 108
meningococcal meningitis, age-dependent
    contact 179
meningococcal vaccination 135–6
microparasites 1–2
microsimulation models xxiv, 173, 175
mild infections 3
mixing
    age-dependent 181–203
    assortative (with-like) 95, 192, 200, 202, 242,
    disassortative (with-unlike) 242
    on gender 255–8
    heterogeneous 177–8
    heterosexual mixing model 255–8
    homogeneous 26
    non-random 177–8
    patterns 177–8
    proportionate 232–6, 238, 242–50, 252
    random 18, 26, 77, 105, 226–7, 242, 269,
        271–2, 360, 364
    by sexual activity 241–55
    summary measure (Q) 243–4, 358
mixing matrices xxvi, 242–3
MMR vaccination 96, 129–30, 135, 143, 215
model diagrams 51–2
models 8–10
    accuracy of prediction 16–17
    age-structure incorporation 131–2
    classification 18–19, 20
    complexity 17–18
    fitting to data 79–82
    input parameters 23–35
    optimization 35–7
    prediction 35–7
    setting up 13–14, 35
    specialist packages 54
    steps in development 13–14
    structure 15–18
    time period covered by 16–17
    validation 35–7
mortality rate 33, 55, 57–8, 85, 107, 112, 287,
    321, 358
mumps
    average age at infection 106–8
    basic reproduction number 8, 115–6
    beta (β) calculation 184–7
    estimating risk of infection 117–20
    herd immunity threshold 8, 67–9
    immune outcome 3, 10
    proportion of population susceptible 105–10
    serial interval 8

natural history of infection 224
neighbourhood size 275
net reproduction number (Rn) xxiv, 1, 7–8, 10,
    67–9, 133, 171–2, 177, 215–8, 239, 293, 361
    methods for calculating 215–8
    real-time estimates 76–7
network modelling xxiv, 223, 268–75

new infections
    contact parameters 187–97
    WAIFW matrix
newborns 88–9
Next Generation Matrix xxiv, 203–15, 217, 219,
    236, 257, 336–8, 354–5
nodes 269
non-immunizing infections
    age patterns 105–26
    dynamics of infection 97–9
non-random mixing patterns 177–8
notation 25, 30, 35, 46–8, 185
number of immune individuals
    difference equation 23
    rate of change 51
number of infectious individuals
    difference equation 22–3
    rate of change 51
    specific age groups 188–9
number of pre-infectious individuals
    difference equation 21–2
    rate of change 50–1
number of susceptible individuals
    difference equation 21
    rate of change 50

ONCHOSIM 18, 174
optimizing models 35–7
order of graph 275
outcome of infections 3

pair-wise approximation model xxiv, 271–2
pandemic xxiv
partial differential equations 59–60, 132
partnership concurrency 223, 265–7,
    272–4
path 269–70, 273–5
path-length 269–70, 273–5
patterns of infection 4
per-act transmission 228, 296, 361
per-partnership transmission 228–9
persistence of infection 172–3, 271
pertussis 2, 7–8, 16, 59, 93, 96, 127, 143
pneumococcal conjugate vaccine 285
polio 3, 7–8, 11, 79, 117, 143, 173
population density 271
population size 24, 30, 52, 54–8, 149, 173,
    188–89, 204, 215, 226–27, 246, 254, 261,
    322, 324–25, 327–29, 331, 342
post-exposure prophylaxis 357
prediction
    accuracy 16
    differential equations 54–7
    HIV epidemic 263, 265
    model development 36
    reproduction numbers 169–71
    size of epidemics 75–9
pre-emptive saturation xxv, 238–40, 259
pre-exposure prophylaxis 357
preferential attachment 271, 275

pre-infectious individuals
  difference equation 21–2
  rate of change 50–1
pre-infectious period xxiv, 2–3, 10, 14, 33, 37, 68, 72–3, 85, 93, 132, 188, 359
prevalence xxiv, 4–5, 188
prophylaxis xxv
proportion immune 6, 35, 69, 79, 86, 119
proportion susceptible/ever infected 362
proportionate mixing xxv, 232–6, 238, 242–50, 252
protozoa 2
pseudo mass action assumption 31, 227

Q xxv, 223, 243–4, 358

random mixing xxv, 18, 26, 77, 105, 226–7, 242, 269, 271–2, 360, 364
random networks xxv, 269–70, 274
random number sampling 162
rate of change 46–7, 319–20
  number of infectious and immune individuals 51
  number of pre-infectious individuals 50–1
  number of susceptible individuals 48, 50
rate of onset of infection 25, 33–4
rates 24, 57
realistic age structured population 131
recently introduced infections, contact parameters 198
recovered individuals, difference equation 23
recovery rate (r) 25, 33, 170, 226,232, 256, 300, 334
Reed–Frost equation 151–7, 228, 362
re-emergent infections, WAIFW matrix 219
removed class 16
reproduction number 6, 169–71
research question 13, 15–7, 37, 260, 269, 275–6
respiratory infection
  age-dependent contact 178–81
  beta (β) calculation 194–5
  transmission models 32
respiratory syncytial virus (RSV) 53
reversible model 124–25
risk of infection 9, 26–32, 267, 283, 287, 290–93
  age-specific 110–11
  average annual 111
  small population 151–4, 361
risks 6, 24–25, 47–48, 56–57, 111, 272, 288–90, 292, 294
rubella2, 5, 79, 83, 106, 108–9, 117, 119, 129–30
  age-dependent contact 120, 123, 138, 180
  basic reproduction number 8, 116
  force of infection 187, 190–95
  herd immunity threshold 8
  immune outcome 3
  inter-epidemic period 93
  serial interval 8

vaccination effects on age-specific infection 137–42
WAIFW matrices 198–99

SARS 2, 63, 69–72, 74–6
saturated model 81
scale-free networks xxv, 271, 275
SCHISTOSIM 174
school holidays 89, 91
screening, STIs 254–5
seasonal contact 89–92
secondary attack rate 6, 10, 154
sensitivity analysis 274
serial interval xxv, 1–3, 6–9, 65, 67, 72–74, 76, 90, 99, 151, 154, 157, 160, 166, 170, 206
serological data 36, 105, 143, 194, 216
serotype replacement 283, 285, 308
sexually transmitted infections (STIs) xxvi, 223–76
  basic reproduction number 236, 249–50, 255–8, 267,
  characteristics 223–6
  cofactors 228, 259, 263
  concurrency 265–8
  condom use 225, 228, 272
  control 254–5
  doubling time 263, 266
  equilibrium prevalence 249–52
  force of infection 226–7
  heterogeneity in sexual activity 231–41
  heterosexual mixing model 255–8
  HIV/STI coinfection models 294, 296–305
  mixing by sexual activity 241–55
  mixing on gender 255–8
  natural history 252–5
  network modelling 268–75
  population at risk 223
  screening 254–5
  spread 224, 229–31
  see also specific infections
shingles 200, 283–4
simple catalytic model 107–8, 10, 118–20, 125
SIMULAIDS 174
singular matrix 350
six degrees of separation 270
size of graph 275
slope of a line 46
small populations
  modelling transmission 172–3
  risk of infection 151–6
small world networks xxv, 270
smallpox 2, 8, 79–80, 83, 93
social contact surveys 180–1
solidly immune 3
solution to an equation xxv, 214
solve an equation 357
spatial kernel 270
spatial network model xxv, 270
spatial spread of infection 193
stable population model xxv

static models xxv–xxvi, 20, 141
STDSIM 174, 270, 272–3, 305
stochastic effects, cycles of incidence of
    immunizing infections 95–6
stochastic models xxvi, 169–74
  interpreting findings from 169–72
  numbers of runs 157
straight line equation 70, 120–22, 326, 339
superinfected 3
susceptible individuals xxvi, 13, 17, 24, 29,
    34–5, 42–6, 68, 86–90, 106, 109, 117, 132,
    149–52, 156–57, 161–68, 170, 181, 186,
    188–89, 211, 215–16, 218–20, 254, 272,
    319–20, 323, 325, 327–28, 330, 334–35, 342,
    345, 354, 363
  difference equation 21
  rate of change 49, 50–1, 53–4
susceptible–infectious (SI) model 15
susceptible–infectious–recovered (SIR)
    model xxv, 15–16, 65–6, 124–25, 321, 323
susceptible–infectious–recovered–susceptible
    (SIRS) model 15–16, 98
susceptible–infectious–susceptible (SIS)
    model xxv, 15, 124–25, 241,
susceptible–pre-infectious–infectious–
    recovered (SEIR) model 15–16
susceptible–pre-infectious–infectious–
    recovered–susceptible (SEIRS)
    model xxv, 16
symbols xxvii–xxviii
syphilis
  dynamics of infection 97–8
  natural history 224

taking the exponent/anti-logarithms 341
time step size 34, 42, 152
time to next event compartmental models 150,
    167–9
toxoplasmosis 4, 117
transition rates 358
transmission dynamic model 17, 20
transmission dynamics xxvi, 25, 41, 45, 53–4,
    58–9, 80, 84–5, 174, 177, 225–26, 231

transmission of infection 2, 5–8, 16, 30, 32, 89,
    91, 191, 272
true mass action assumption 31, 227
tuberculosis xxvi, 7, 20, 285–94
  age-dependent contact 178
  effect of HIV epidemic, 295–6
  effective contact 27–28
  immune outcome 3
  pattern of infection 4
  research question 17–18
  serial interval 8
two-stage model 15–16, 65–6, 124–25, 321, 323
typical infectee 236, 247, 250, 257
typical infectious person xxvi, 6, 10, 28, 65,
    211–12, 214

vaccination
  age-specific infection incidence 137–41
  catch-up campaigns 96, 134–6, 215
  cycles of incidence of immunizing
    infections 82–3, 89, 96–7
  dynamics of infections 1265–43, 283–5
  impact of vaccinating at different ages 140
  vaccine efficacy and effectiveness 354
  see also specific vaccinations
validating models 35–37
valued network 275
variable asymptote model 124–25
varicella vaccination 200–2, 283–5
varicella zoster 200, 283–285
vertex 269, 274–75
virus 2

wasted contacts 240
who acquires infection from whom (WAIFW)
    matrix xxvi, 184, 191–3, 195, 198–203,
whooping cough 2–3, 125
with-like (assortative) mixing patterns xxvi,
    95, 192, 199–200, 202, 242–45, 247, 249,
    252, 254–55
with-unlike (disassortative) mixing patterns xxvi,
    192, 242–44, 247–49, 252–53, 255
worms 2